Shapers of
American Health
Care Policy

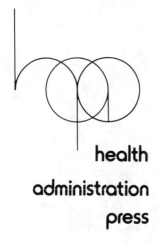

health
administration
press

Lewis E. Weeks • Howard J. Berman

Shapers of American Health Care Policy

An Oral History

Health Administration Press
Ann Arbor, Michigan
1985

Library of Congress Cataloging in Publication Data

Weeks, Lewis E.
  Shapers of American health care policy.

  Bibliography: p.
  Includes index.
  *1. Medical policy—United States—History. 2. Medical
care—United States—History. 3. Health services
administrators—United States—Interviews. I. Berman,
Howard J. II. Title. [DNLM: 1. Delivery of Health Care—
history—United States. 2. Health Policy—history—
United States. 3. Public Health Administration—history—
United States. WA 11 AA1 W3s]*
  RA395.A3W44 1985   362.1'0973   85-17687
  ISBN 0-910701-09-1

*Health Administration Press
School of Public Health
The University of Michigan
1021 East Huron
Ann Arbor, Michigan 48109
(313) 764-1380*

To our wives,
Frances Weeks and Marilyn Berman,
for their patience and understanding
during the writing of this book.

Contents

PART II

Blue Cross: An Evolving Social Movement

PART III

The Emergence of a Profession

PART IV

A Look Backward

Appendix A

Appendix B

Appendix C

Appendix D

Appendix E

Appendix F

Appendix G

Appendix H

Foreword

Some five or six years ago, Lew Weeks, with the encouragement of Howard Berman, began the monumental task of interviewing "movers and shakers" in the hospital and health care fields about their recollections of now-historic developments in which they had played prominent roles. More than 40 such oral histories have been completed so far, and a number of them are now available in the Bacon Library of the American Hospital Association. At some point in the compilation of the histories it occurred to Lew and Howard that many of them were concerned with the same important developments, although from different perspectives and with sometimes significantly varying interpretations or insights. This conclusion happily led to an effort to weave these threads into a whole fabric, of which the result is a fascinating and personalized history, *Shapers of American Health Care Policy*. The book covers a span of more than 50 years and illuminates both the events and the people who helped make them happen.

Here is a sampling:

—I.S. Falk and C. Rufus Rorem discuss in depth the Committee on the Costs of Medical Care, still considered the most far-reaching and compelling study of its kind in American health policy development. Both were staff members.

—John Mannix, Maurice Norby, and Rorem talk about the turbulent and often difficult early days of Blue Cross.

—The struggles to turn the American Hospital Association around from a weak and ineffectual entity to a viable and influential national organization are detailed by Mannix, George Bugbee, and Jim Hamilton.

—Bugbee and Norby review the Commission on Hospital Care and its significance at that time, followed by their account as to how the Hill-Burton legislation "really came about."

—Certainly one of the most intriguing chapters concerns the enactment of Medicare and Medicaid, as described by several key people, including Wilbur Cohen, Wilbur Mills, Nelson Cruikshank, Kenneth Williamson, and Walter McNerney.

—Also covered by various individuals who were influential in such developments are the founding of the American College of Hospital Administrators, the evolution of education in health administration, and the evolution of the Association of University Programs in Health Administration.

Certainly this book provides an unusual and useful examination of the development of American health policy and practice, as candidly related by many of those people who were not only there but made it all possible. The field is indebted to Weeks and Berman for their efforts to gather, collate, and preserve these memoirs, which otherwise might not have seen the light of day.

Andrew Pattullo
Battle Creek, Michigan
October 10, 1984

Preface

When we began the hospital oral history project we were not certain what would eventually result. We did know that the hospital field was relatively young, that its history was for the most part poorly documented, and that many of the people who had made that history were still available to tell their stories. Our goal was to capture those stories while the opportunity still existed and to share them.

The results of this simply stated objective have exceeded our most optimistic hopes. Out of the oral history project have come over 40 published reminiscences, a historical collection in the library of the American Hospital Association, Asa S. Bacon Memorial, and this book. More oral history publications are in progress, and the historical collection is growing into a major national resource.

We have been special beneficiaries of this project. Through collecting the oral histories we have not only learned a great deal, but have also become friends with many people about whom we had only read before. Both as individuals and as a group the people whose stories are told in this book are outstanding achievers. They were able to turn their dreams of what could be into reality. Their contribution to American society has been invaluable. We hope this book meets the standards they have set.

In preparing this volume we have remained true to the spirit of the comments made by all the persons interviewed. From time to time we have edited their remarks to make them "read" as smooth as they sound. If in this process there have been errors of either omission or commission, the responsibility for them lies with us. The credit for any contribution which this work might make, however, lies with the persons interviewed.

This book is the result of the critical appraisal of many individuals besides us. Most of the persons whose oral histories we have quoted, plus other persons with knowledge of the era covered by the book, read all or significant segments of the manuscript. Among those to whom we owe a great expression of thanks are Faye G. Abdellah, George Bugbee, Wilbur Cohen, Nelson Cruikshank, Robert M. Cunningham, Jr., Leon Davis, the late I.S. Falk, Gary L. Filerman, Joan S. Guy, James Hague, James Hamilton, John R. Mannix, Walter J. McNerney, Wilbur Mills, John S. Millis, Maurice Norby, Andrew Pattullo, Daniel Pettengill, C. Rufus Rorem, William Rothman, Robert Sigmond, Kenneth Williamson, and Lynn Wimmer.

We particularly thank Maureen Grazer for her preparation of the manuscript and Eloise Foster, Connie Poole, Patricia Wakeley, and the staff of the Hospital Research and Educational Trust for their advice and background research. Without their help this volume would never have been possible.

Lewis E. Weeks
Howard J. Berman

List of
Abbreviations

AALL	American Association for Labor Legislation
AAMC	Association of American Medical Colleges
ACHA	American College of Hospital Administrators
ACS	American College of Surgeons
AFL	American Federation of Labor
AHA	American Hospital Association
AMA	American Medical Association
AMPAC	American Medical Political Action Committee
AUPHA	Association of University Programs in Health Administration
BCA	Blue Cross Association
CCMC	Committee on the Costs of Medical Care
CIO	Congress of Industrial Organizations
EMIC	Emergency Maternal and Infant Care Act
EPIC	End Poverty in California
FEP	Federal Employees' Health Benefits Program
FERA	Federal Emergency Relief Administration
HEW	Department of Health, Education, and Welfare
HIBAC	Health Insurance Benefits Advisory Council
HIF	Health Information Foundation
HIP	Health Insurance Plan
HMO	health maintenance organization
JAMA	Journal of the American Medical Association

MRI	Magnetic Resonance Imaging
MAC	Medical Administrative Corps
NPC	National Physicians' Committee for the Extension of Medical Service
OASI	Old Age and Survivors Insurance
PHS	Public Health Service
PWA	Public Works Administration
RAB	regional advisory board (of the AHA)
UAW	United Auto Workers
UNESCO	United Nations Economic, Social, and Cultural Organization
WPA	Works Progress Administration

Time Stream
Flexner to Medicare

1899

• *Association of Hospital Superintendents (later the American Hospital Association, AHA) founded in Cleveland.*

1906

• *American Association for Labor Legislation (AALL) founded under the leadership of John B. Andrews.*

1910

• *Abraham Flexner reported a study of medical education which he had done with the assistance of the American Medical Association (AMA). The study had been commissioned by the Carnegie Foundation for the Advancement of Teaching and proved to be a turning point in American medicine.*

• *The AALL advocated compulsory state health insurance paralleling state workmen's compensation. A model, or standard, law was drafted.*

• *The AMA reacted favorably to compulsory state health insurance.*

1912

• *Theodore Roosevelt, former president of the United States, campaigned for the presidency as the candidate of the Progressive, or "Bull Moose," party against Democrat Woodrow Wilson, president of Princeton University, and William*

Howard Taft, the Republican incumbent. Roosevelt advocated many social reforms, including "health insurance for industry," the first time any major presidential candidate had endorsed health insurance.

1916

- *The AMA social insurance committee recommended compulsory state health insurance.*

1918

- *California voters voted down a state health insurance plan.*

1919

- *Uniform accounting was mandated for Ohio hospitals in order to obtain audited cost data for payments to hospitals under workmen's compensation.*
- *The New York legislature defeated a health insurance bill.*

1920

- *The AMA opposed government health insurance.*
- *In the 1920s, industrial productivity was up, but wages were not up in proportion; medical education was improved; medical costs were up substantially; there was growth in specialization among physicians; and prepaid hospitalization plans were developing.*

1921

- *The Sheppard-Towner Act provided federal subsidy for maternal and child health programs.*

1922

- *Insulin as a treatment for diabetes was discovered by two Canadian scientists, Frederick Banting and William Best.*

1923

- *John R. Mannix at Mount Sinai Hospital, Cleveland, moved toward an inclusive daily rate by including laboratory charges in the room rate for an additional 50¢ a day.*

1924

• *Dr. Morris Fishbein became editor of the* Journal of the American Medical Association *(JAMA).*

1926

• *Inclusive rates for maternity and tonsillectomy cases were established at Elyria (Ohio) Hospital by John R. Mannix.*

1927

• *The Committee on the Costs of Medical Care (CCMC) began a five-year study of medical and hospital care in the United States.*

1928

• *Penicillin was discovered by Sir Alexander Fleming in England, thus opening the way for antibiotic therapy.*

1929

• *A prepaid hospital care insurance plan was established at Baylor University Hospital in Dallas. The plan has often been referred to as a forerunner of Blue Cross, even though it was restricted to one hospital.*
• *The Sheppard-Towner Act was allowed to expire.*
• *I.S. Falk took over as research director of the CCMC.*
• *The stock market crashed on October 29, marking the end of the prosperity of the 1920s and, in a sense, the beginning of the Great Depression.*

1930

• *Prepayment rates for hospital care (25¢ a week, $13.00 a year) were recommended by John R. Mannix.*

1932

• *University Hospitals, Cleveland, set an all-inclusive rate.*
• *Prontosil, the first sulfonamide drug to be used against bacterial infections, was introduced in Germany.*
• *The American Federation of Labor endorsed social insurance.*

1933

- *The AHA council on community relations looked at regions developing prepaid hospitalization plans.*
- *Dr. Sidney R. Garfield furnished prepaid per capita medical and hospital care to employees of firms constructing an aqueduct and canal project across the California desert (1933–1938). This was the forerunner of the Kaiser-Permanente Medical Care Program.*
- *The CCMC in its final report recommended that: medical service be furnished by organized groups of physicians and other health personnel; basic public health services be extended; medical services be studied, evaluated, and coordinated; professional education be enhanced; and group payment be instituted for the costs of medical care. A minority report recommended that government activities in medicine be restricted to the care of the indigent, to the care of those with diseases that require institutional care, to the promotion of public health, to the care of military personnel and certain other government employees, and to the care of veterans. The minority wanted the general practitioner in a central position, and it opposed the corporate practice of medicine.*
- *The AHA approved the concept of voluntary hospital insurance.*
- *The Federal Emergency Relief Administration (FERA) indirectly provided money for limited medical care for the needy.*
- *The American College of Hospital Administrators was formed with 108 charter members, one-third of them physicians.*

1934

- *Harry Hopkins, administrator of FERA, announced April 13 that there were 4.3 million families on relief.*
- *A master's degree program in hospital administration was started at the University of Chicago by Michael M. Davis after he convinced Robert Maynard Hutchins that the program was more than a vocational course.*
- *Father Charles Coughlin of Royal Oak, Michigan, "the radio priest," organized the National Union for Social Justice.*
- *Upton Sinclair, writer and candidate for governor of California, promoted EPIC, a plan to "end poverty in California."*
- *Huey P. Long (D–La.) presented the U.S. Senate with his "Share the Wealth" program—"Every Man a King."*
- *Dr. Francis E. Townsend of California proposed the Old Age Revolving Pension Plan to solve the economic problems of the country.*
- *The Committee on Economic Security was appointed by President Franklin Roosevelt from members of his cabinet to address problems of economic security and to make recommendations for a program of legislation.*

1935

• *The Committee on Economic Security reported to Congress on January 17, recommending federal old age insurance, federal-state public assistance, unemployment compensation, extension of public health services, maternal and child welfare services, and vocational rehabilitation services. There were no health insurance benefits.*

• *The Social Security Act was passed on August 14.*

• *To expedite the organization of the Social Security program, President Roosevelt appointed on August 15 an Interdepartmental Committee to Coordinate Health and Welfare Activities. One activity the committee studied was the need for health care and health insurance.*

• *The first National Health Survey was begun.*

1936

• *The Technical Committee on Medical Care, a research arm of the Interdepartmental Committee to Coordinate Health and Welfare Activities, was formed to study health care in the United States.*

1937

• *C. Rufus Rorem went to the AHA with a grant from the Julius Rosenwald Fund to study group hospitalization insurance. This resulted in the setting of standards for these groups.*

1938

• *A report of the Technical Committee on Medical Care was published in February under the title,* A National Health Program.

• *A National Health Conference was called in Washington, D.C., by the interdepartmental committee in July.*

• *The AMA, the District of Columbia Medical Society, the District of Columbia Academy of Surgery, the Harris County (Texas) Medical Society, and 21 individuals (including Morris Fishbein, editor of JAMA, and Olin West, secretary–general manager of the AMA) were indicted on the charge that organized medicine had denied hospital privileges to physicians associated with the Group Health Association of Washington by not allowing them to become members of local medical societies. The AMA won the case in lower court, but the case was appealed to the U.S. Supreme Court, which in 1943 fined the AMA and the District of Columbia Medical Society and found the individuals and the other medical societies not guilty.*

• *The AHA decided on a seal of approval for hospital insurance prepayment plans: the AHA seal was superimposed on a blue cross. The term "Blue Cross" was in general use by 1942.*

> • *Dr. Sidney R. Garfield set up a per capita prepaid medical and hospital plan for employees at the Kaiser Grand Coulee dam construction project (1938–1941).*

> • *The California Physicians' Service was started. This was an insurance forerunner of Blue Shield.*

1939

> • *John R. Mannix founded the Michigan Blue Cross Plan. The plan was faced with the problem of providing national coverage for employees of such corporations as Ford Motor Company and General Motors. There was also a need for physician's services to be covered by insurance. California was the only state trying to start such a plan. The Michigan State Medical Society was encouraged to start such a medical plan, and it did.*

> • *Senator Robert F. Wagner (D–N.Y.) introduced a national health bill that incorporated the recommendations of the National Health Conference. The bill died in committee, after hearings.*

> • *The National Physicians' Committee for the Extension of Medical Service was formed to oppose Wagner's national health bill. Ninety percent of the committee's funding came from the pharmaceutical industry, the remaining 10 percent from individual physicians. The committee's campaign literature was generally quite coarse and inaccurate in its facts. In 1948 the committee broadcast by mail a letter that could be construed as anti-Semitic. The effect was bad for the committee, and consequently it disbanded in 1951.*

> • *The Federal Security Agency was set up to integrate the Social Security Board, the U.S. Public Health Service, the Civilian Conservation Corps, the National Youth Administration, and the U.S. Office of Education.*

1941

> • *The Japanese attacked Pearl Harbor on December 7, causing the United States to enter World War II.*

1942

> • *The Kaiser-Permanente Medical Care Program was established in California, based on the experience of Dr. Sidney Garfield in the California desert and at Grand Coulee dam.*

> • *Rhode Island enacted the first cash sickness law, which provided temporary disability benefits to persons covered under state unemployment insurance law.*

• *The Beveridge report in Great Britain advocated a comprehensive social welfare system there.*

1943

• *George Bugbee became the executive secretary of the AHA.*

• *The Bishop resolution, calling for voluntary health insurance, was passed at the AHA convention.*

• *The Emergency Maternal and Infant Care Act was adopted by Congress to protect the dependents of the four lowest ranks of servicemen. It was administered by the Children's Bureau.*

• *President Roosevelt in a State of the Union speech called for social insurance from the cradle to the grave.*

• *The Wagner-Murray-Dingell bill was introduced in Congress. It called for comprehensive health insurance under Social Security. No action was taken on it.*

1944

• *New York City Mayor Fiorello La Guardia supported the Health Insurance Plan (HIP) by having the city pay part of the premiums for municipal workers.*

• *Michigan Blue Cross raised its family rate from $2.00 a month to $2.25.*

• *Franklin Roosevelt in his State of the Union address called for an economic bill of rights, including the right to adequate medical care.*

• *A Commission on Hospital Care, set up to study the state of hospitals and the care they provided, was established through the efforts of the AHA and the financial support of some foundations. Much of the data collected were useful in the writing of the Hospital Survey and Construction (Hill-Burton) Act.*

• *The Social Security Board in its annual report recommended compulsory national health insurance.*

1945

• *President Roosevelt in his State of the Union address called for good medical care.*

• *Calfornia Governor Earl Warren proposed compulsory state health insurance. The proposed bill was defeated in the legislature after the California Medical Society hired Whittaker & Baxter, a public relations firm, to campaign against it.*

• *President Roosevelt died in Warm Springs, Georgia, on April 12.*

• *President Harry S. Truman called for national health insurance in a message to Congress in November. A revised Wagner-Murray-Dingell bill, asking for national health insurance, was introduced.*

1946

- *The Committee for the Nation's Health was organized to promote the Wagner-Murray-Dingell bill.*
- *The Hospital Survey and Construction (Hill-Burton) Act was passed.*
- *John R. Mannix, president of the John Marshall Insurance Company, attempted to set up a group hospitalization plan offering coverage and service to employees of national corporations. The timing was unfortunate, because medical costs were rising faster than premiums could be increased. After two or three years the company was sold.*
- *The Taft-Smith-Ball bill to provide grants to states for medical aid to the poor was introduced in Congress. No action was taken.*
- *In a reorganization plan, the Social Security Board was abolished and its functions transferred to the federal security administrator, who established the Social Security Administration to carry on the programs of Social Security and the Children's Bureau (except for its child labor functions).*

1947

- *This year marked the centennial of the AMA.*
- *The Wagner-Murray-Dingell bill was reintroduced.*
- *President Truman urged Congress to enact a national health program.*

1948

- *Federal Security Administrator Oscar Ewing called a National Health Assembly in Washington, D.C., May 1–4. Its report endorsed contributory health insurance.*
- *Whittaker & Baxter, the California public relations firm, was hired by the AMA to work against Truman's and Ewing's plans for national health insurance.*
- *The Prall report on the state of education for hospital administration, with recommendations for the future, was published. The study was supported by a grant from the W.K. Kellogg Foundation.*
- *The Association of University Programs in Hospital Administration held its first meeting in Atlantic City.*

1949

- *Robert F. Wagner (D–N.Y.) resigned from the Senate because of ill health.*
- *President Truman again sent a message to Congress calling for national health insurance.*
- *The Republicans introduced a bill in Congress, the Flanders-Ives bill, or the Flanders-Ives-Nixon bill, calling for a federal subsidy to make it possible for low-income persons to buy adequate hospital insurance. The federal government's proportion of the premium would depend on the individual's income. The states would operate the plan and would be required to share in the cost of the subsidy, depending on the average income in the state. The federal government's share would range from one-third to three-quarters. Hearings were held, but nothing else happened.*

1950

- *A National Conference on Aging was called by the Federal Security Agency.*
- *The Social Security Act was amended to provide direct payment to doctors, hospitals, and other providers of care by the states, with matching federal aid.*

1952

- *Federal Security Administrator Oscar Ewing recommended national health insurance for Social Security beneficiaries.*
- *Murray-Humphrey-Dingell-Celler bills were introduced in the House and Senate calling for health insurance for Social Security beneficiaries.*
- *The President's Commission on Health Needs of the Nation reported in favor of health insurance for Social Security beneficiaries.*
- *The Joint Commission on Accreditation of Hospitals began its program.*
- *The Commission on Financing of Hospital Care was established, with the encouragement of the AHA and the financial support of foundations, to study an aspect of health care that the Commission on Hospital Care had been unable to study.*

1953

- *The Federal Security Agency was supplanted by the Department of Health, Education, and Welfare, with Oveta Culp Hobby as secretary.*

1954

- *The Eisenhower administration supported a reinsurance bill under which the federal government would subsidize partial payment of premiums for low-income individuals.*
- *An AHA committee under the chairmanship of E.A. van Steen-wyk studied problems of the elderly and recommended federal help. The AMA was against the use of federal funds. The AFL-CIO said the AHA recommendations were too conservative.*
- *Jonas Salk developed an injectable vaccine against polio.*
- *The Olsen report on education in hospital administration was published.*
- *Dr. Edwin L. Crosby became the executive secretary of the AHA, succeeding George Bugbee.*

1956

- *The Commission on Professional and Hospital Activities was incorporated.*
- *The "Military Medicare" program was enacted, giving health care service to military dependents.*
- *The Social Security Act was amended to give monthly benefits to permanently and totally disabled workers between the ages of 50 and 64.*
- *The executive council of the AFL-CIO took a position favoring government health insurance.*

1957

- *The Forand bill, providing for health insurance for Social Security beneficiaries, was introduced into Congress with the support of the AFL-CIO.*
- *The AMA house of delegates moved against the Forand bill.*
- *Wilbur D. Mills (D–Ark.) became chairman of the House Ways and Means Committee.*

1959

- *The Forand bill was reintroduced in Congress. The House Ways and Means Committee in executive session voted 17 to 8 against it. A stripped-down bill (less surgery benefits) was also defeated 16 to 9 in committee.*
- *A Senate subcommittee held hearings on the problems of the aged (primarily their health problems).*

1960

- *The annual conference of governors recommended medical insurance for the elderly under Social Security.*
- *The presidential Task Force on Health and Social Security for the American People was appointed by President-elect John F. Kennedy.*
- *A Kennedy-Anderson bill was introduced, calling for wider benefits than the Forand bill. It was unable to pass.*
- *The Kerr-Mills bill was passed. It provided federal-state aid for the medically indigent.*

1961

- *A White House Conference on Aging was called by the Department of Health, Education, and Welfare of the outgoing Eisenhower administration.*
- *The presidential Task Force on Health and Social Security for the American People recommended health insurance for the elderly under Social Security.*
- *Newly inaugurated President John F. Kennedy sent a special message to Congress on health.*
- *The King-Anderson bill, an early version of Medicare, was introduced in Congress. It did not progress beyond hearings in the Ways and Means Committee.*
- *The House approved Speaker Sam Rayburn's plan to increase the membership of the House Rules Committee, which had been bottling up liberal bills (including health bills) and preventing them from coming to a vote.*
- *The National Council of Senior Citizens for Health Care Through Social Security was formed in support of the King-Anderson bill.*
- *AMA members formed the American Medical Political Action Committee as a political arm to work against legislation it opposed.*

1962

- *President Kennedy made a televised speech in favor of what later was called Medicare before a crowd of senior citizens in Madison Square Garden. It was probably the worst speech of his career.*
- *Dr. Edward Annis replied for the AMA two days later in an incisive, televised speech to an empty (by design) Madison Square Garden.*
- *An attempt was made to attach a health insurance amendment (the Anderson-Javits amendment) to a welfare bill in the Senate. The amendment was tabled.*

1963

• *Kennedy sent a special message to Congress on the problems of the aged.*

• *A Citizens' Commission on Graduate Medical Education was established under the chairmanship of John S. Millis by the AMA; the commission was to do an external and objective examination of medicine.*

• *The King-Anderson bill (Medicare) was again introduced in Congress.*

• *John F. Kennedy was assassinated on November 22 in Dallas. On that day the House Ways and Means Committee was holding hearings on the King-Anderson bill.*

1964

• *Hearings on the King-Anderson bill were completed in January.*

• *President Lyndon B. Johnson sent a special message to Congress on the health of the nation; in it he advocated Medicare.*

• *The Ways and Means Committee postponed action on the King-Anderson bill.*

• *An amendment (H.R. 11865) to the Social Security Act was reported out by the Ways and Means Committee in July. The proposed amendment included an increase in cash benefits but no health care items. The House passed the amendment in July. Senate hearings were held in August. The bill was reported out without health provisions late in the month. A Medicare measure as a floor amendment to H.R. 11865 passed the Senate in September. Conference committee members were unable to reconcile differences between House and Senate versions in October.*

1965

• *The King-Anderson bill was reintroduced in Congress.*

• *Mills' Medicare proposal (H.R. 6675) was substituted for King-Anderson by the Ways and Means Committee in March. The Mills bill passed the House by a wide margin in April. The Senate held hearings and executive sessions from late April to late June and passed the bill by a wide margin in July. The House-Senate conference committee reconciled the differences between the House and Senate versions of the Mills bill.*

• *The House and Senate passed the conference committee report. Medicare and Medicaid became part of the Social Security Amendments of 1965 after President Lyndon B. Johnson flew to Independence, Missouri, on July 30 to sign the bill into law in the presence of former President Harry S. Truman, thus ending a stage in the process that had begun several decades before.*

PART I

Cornerstones

1

Introduction

In the following chapters we try to capture the beliefs, hopes, and perceptions of some of the people who had a direct hand in the events that helped shape the environment in which hospitals now operate. This book is neither a simple chronology of events nor an analytical political science or public policy text. Rather, it is an oral history, a scrapbook that tells a story of change and of progress.

The story is seen through the eyes and told in the style and language of the people who were part of it. Like all stories, it has some omissions, as well as some exaggerations: memories and perceptions are inevitably imperfect. Reminiscences like these, however, provide a depth of character and understanding that goes beyond either simple recitation of facts or academic analysis. We hope not only that this book will provide an interesting and entertaining experience, but also that it will serve as a steppingstone for the future.

In preparing this book, we have drawn primarily on the Oral History Collection of the American Hospital Association (AHA). The Oral History Collection is a joint project of the Hospital Research and Educational Trust and the AHA. The transcripts are deposited in, and are available through, the AHA's library, the Asa S. Bacon Memorial. Some editing has been done to avoid overt errors of fact and to make the dialogue suitable for reading; it has not, however, changed either the spirit or the point of the speaker's comments. The primary purpose of the editing has been simply to enhance the telling of the story.

Oral History

Oral histories are as old as language itself. In their earliest form they represent our first literature, stories that were told and passed down around tribal campfires from one generation to the next. Oral histories, along with the art of storytelling, were largely supplanted by the written word. Recently, however, they have again captured the public's interest. The work of professional historians and popular writers has enhanced the credibility of oral histories and increased the public's awareness of them. Further, the inexpensive tape recorder has made them do–it–yourself family projects.

In published form, oral histories are typically presented as straightforward recitations of the reminiscences of various interviewees. They are often loosely organized around either periods or general subject areas, with the speakers' comments presented serially and, for the most part, independent of one another. This approach works well for some topics, but a different format was needed for this story. Instead of presenting one speaker's reminiscences and then going on to another's, therefore, we have intertwined the reminiscences of the various speakers. When appropriate, several oral histories have in effect been stitched together to present a whole or at least a wider cloth.

The reader should imagine himself or herself as listening to a conversation. One person begins to speak. As he continues, others who were part of the same event or times interject their comments, adding their perspective to what is being discussed. Occasionally we interject our own comments in order to enhance the flow of the conversation and to ensure clarity. The speakers' different vantage points and roles meld into a single recollection, and the story unfolds.

The events discussed reflect our judgment as to the major forces that have shaped today's hospital environment. In making these judgments, we sought the advice of a number of people. Each was asked the same question: What were the key historical developments whose outcome has significantly influenced the management or operation of today's hospitals? The answers, as might be expected, were varied, exceeding the capacity of a single book. From the variety, however, emerged some common themes. It is around these common themes that we have organized this volume.

Overview

Part I, Cornerstones, focuses on the three major events that many persons have suggested provide the foundation for much of today's hospital operating environment. The first of these (chapter 2) is the work of the

Committee on the Costs of Medical Care (CCMC). The CCMC, organized in 1927, provided the nation with not only an assessment of what its current health care system was, but also a vision of what it could become. It is from the imagination and insight of the CCMC that many of the developments which we now take for granted, for example health planning, health maintenance organizations (HMOs), and Blue Cross, first came.

The story of the CCMC—its aspirations, problems, successes, and ultimate confrontation with the American Medical Association (AMA)—is told primarily by two of its staff members, I.S. Falk and C. Rufus Rorem. In reading chapter 2, it is important for the reader to remember that the ideas of the CCMC, though initially quashed by organized medicine, were powerful enough to survive and to go on to shape both the events of today and events still to come.

The second cornerstone is the Hospital Survey and Construction Act (the Hill-Burton Act). The Hill-Burton Act provided the conceptual plan and the funds for constructing much of the nation's hospital system, a system whose goal was to assure geographic access to care.

The story of Hill-Burton is told in chapter 3. It is presented through the reminiscences of persons (Maurice Norby, George Bugbee, and I.S. Falk) who were able to recognize what problems the post–World War II hospital would face. Those individuals discussed workable answers to the country's needs. Here the strength of an idea—geographic access to care—again dominates the story.

The third cornerstone is Medicare (and Medicaid), which is discussed in chapters 4 and 5. Chapter 4 concentrates on the roots of Medicare. It traces, beginning in the mid-1930s, the development of the political consensus which set the stage for the passage of Medicare. Chapter 4 is essentially a story of legislative failure. From each failed attempt to pass legislation, however, came some progress toward its eventual success. The reminiscences presented in chapter 4 highlight the depth of commitment to that eventual success. The story of the roots of Medicare is told primarily by Wilbur Cohen, Nelson Cruikshank, Robert Sigmond, and I.S. Falk.

In contrast, chapter 5 is a story of legislative success. It looks at the swift movement, after the 1964 general election, toward enactment of the Medicare and Medicaid programs. It focuses on the pre-enactment shaping and later implementation of the legislation. It also tells the story of the pragmatic negotiations and compromises that were necessary to create a workable program for providing the poor and the old with financial access to care. The reminiscences in this chapter are those of some of the people who helped to make Medicare a reality—Wilbur Cohen, Wilbur Mills, Nelson Cruikshank, Walter McNerney, Daniel Pettengill, and Kenneth Williamson.

Part II, An Evolving Social Movement, looks at Blue Cross. It follows the evolution of Blue Cross from a seemingly radical idea to widespread acceptance as a national movement affecting tens of millions of people. It is because of its importance to so many people and its effect on the operations of hospitals that an entire section is devoted to Blue Cross.

The story begins in chapter 6, where hospital prepayment is discussed first as a concept and then as an idea whose time had come. The notion of group prepayment for hospital care had been recommended by the CCMC. The Great Depression was the catalyst in the transformation of the general idea of prepayment into a practical reality. Prepayment met the financial needs of both hospitals and people fearful of the cost of hospitalization. The story of prepayment is told in the main through Rufus Rorem's reminiscences.

Chapter 7 tells the story of how Blue Cross plans developed throughout the country. Although prepayment might have been an idea whose time had come, there was still a huge job to be done in terms of promoting the idea and establishing and managing the administrative mechanisms needed to operate a Blue Cross plan. The story of these problems, successes, and frustrations, as well as the role of hospitals in creating prepayment plans, is told primarily by two of the people who actually created and managed early Blue Cross plans, John Mannix and Maurice Norby.

Chapter 8 looks at the maturation of Blue Cross as a social movement. The story of how the various Blue Cross plans came together into a national confederation is told. The reminiscences of Walter McNerney are the principal narrative. An interesting counterpoint, however, is provided by the comments of Daniel Pettengill, who viewed the national Blue Cross movement from the vantage point of the commercial insurance industry.

Part III, Emergence of a Profession, has taken a somewhat different tack. Instead of focusing on specific major events, as part I does, or a single issue, as part II does, it looks at two phenomena. One is the emergence of the AHA as a national force, and the other is the development of hospital management as a profession and as a recognized academic discipline.

Chapter 9 concentrates on the American Hospital Association. It tells the story of the growth of the AHA as a national organization of institutions, one representing the viewpoint of hospitals while at the same time striving to help hospitals—through technical support, management programs, and continuing education—to better meet the needs of their communities. The story is told through the reminiscences of some of the people who played leadership roles in transforming the AHA—James Hamilton, George Bugbee, John Mannix, James Hague, Kenneth Williamson, and Maurice Norby.

Chapter 10 focuses on the education of hospital administrators. In this chapter Andrew Pattullo talks about the W.K. Kellogg Foundation's leadership in this area, sponsoring commissions to set out the basic design of hospital administration education and funding early graduate programs in hospital administration. James Hamilton and Walter McNerney talk about the philosophy and structure of two of the pace-setting graduate programs. Finally, Edward Connors and Gary Filerman comment on hospital administration education from the perspective of students.

In chapter 11 we attempt to pull together the threads of the previous chapters, providing a context and a perspective for looking backward as well as looking ahead.

Common Belief

Taken as whole, these chapters portray the aspirations of a group of individuals who wanted to make access to hospital care—both financial and geographic—available to everyone. As a group they shared, perhaps unknowingly, many beliefs and values. These formed the basis of today's hospital system, with the administrative personnel and supporting staff needed to manage it and to make it work.

No one would suggest that what they have done cannot be improved. In all likelihood, they would themselves like to see the performance of the health care system improved, to make it better serve the needs of people requiring health care. At the same time, no one would suggest that what they have accomplished has not been of great importance.

The stories told in this book should be seen as part of a larger picture. Recognizing that there are both more stories to be told and more persons who can tell them, we hope that this book will inspire other writers to provide the field with a broader and deeper sense of its history. Ideally, other writers will further "mine" the source material for this book, as well as future oral histories, to tell other stories, enrich other research, and remind us all of our hard-won lessons and accomplishments. Future generations should not be made to stumble along blindly simply because this generation was not thoughtful enough to explain what it believed and what it valued. We hope our work will become part of a series of handholds for the future.

2

The Committee on the Costs of Medical Care

The Flexner report and the work of the Committee on the Costs of Medical Care were major forces shaping today's health care delivery mechanisms.

The Flexner report described the results of a study of medical education early in the century and was published in 1910 under the title, *Medical Education in the United States and Canada, a Report to the Carnegie Foundation for the Advancement of Teaching*. Apparently it came about fortuitously. The Carnegie Foundation was considering supporting a study of the quality and characteristics of the education of members of a learned profession. The first professions proposed for study were law and the ministry, but there were objections or lack of interest on the part of both. Medicine became the third choice.[1]

The timing was fortunate. The AMA had been gathering data on medical education for the purpose of raising the standards of education and licensure, however it did not seem politic for the association to publish a study under its own name. With the foundation financing the study and publishing the findings, the AMA could be helpful in supplying information, and in otherwise assisting in the writing of the report.

Abraham Flexner, a younger brother of Simon Flexner, director of the laboratories of the Rockefeller Institute of Medical Research, was chosen to head the study. In 1886 Abraham Flexner had received his A.B. from the

Johns Hopkins University, which was even then notable for its academic discipline. After his graduation from Johns Hopkins, he returned to his home town of Louisville, Kentucky, and set up a boys' preparatory school which drew favorable attention.

It was in 1909 that Abraham Flexner was chosen to study the medical schools of the United States and make recommendations for their future development. Flexner found the situation deplorable. There were only two university medical schools that required a baccalaureate degree for admission (Johns Hopkins and Harvard), and they sometimes relaxed that requirement. Only 16 out of 155 schools required two years of college, which Flexner believed was the bare minimum.[2]

Many of the medical schools were little more than diploma mills, private schools run for profit. Even the better schools were often little more than lecture sessions, with the lecturers, who were paid a fee, selected from among local medical practitioners. Too often there was little, if any, work done in laboratories and little, if any, instruction in clinical settings. Many of the students were unable to recognize the symptoms of the diseases described in the lectures. The study of basic sciences was generally badly neglected.

One indication of the state of medical education was the failure rate of newly graduated physicians seeking medical positions in the armed forces. Just a few years before Flexner's study, the U.S. Navy had a rejection rate for newly graduated physicians of 46 percent. The Marine Corps' rejection rate was 86 percent.[3]

The Flexner report had widespread repercussions. Higher standards were set for admission to medical schools. The curriculums of medical schools were also changed: in most cases, they began to offer a more thorough grounding in the basic sciences, as well as requiring more laboratory work and clinical training. Many medical schools closed.

What the Flexner report wrought was a revolution in medical education and consequently in medical care.

Eli Ginzberg summed up the effect of the Flexner report:

> In the entire history of this country it is hard to find a more influential social tract than the Flexner Report on American medical education. Released in 1910, this report carefully documented the sorry state of many schools and pointed out the directions for remedial action. These reforms resulted in all future physicians receiving a sound grounding in the biological underpinnings of medicine, in carefully graded educational experiences, and in well-supervised internships.[4]

The genesis of the CCMC can probably be found in the Flexner report. As a result of the report's impact on medical education and the scientific advances that had been taking place in Europe, American medicine made great strides in the early part of the twentieth century. A by-product of American medicine's rapidly increasing ability to improve the quality of life was specialization, which resulted in fragmentation of the provision of medical care, increasing costs, and a rapid change in the role of the hospital. By the mid-1920s, a number of responsible people began asking questions: What was really the state of health care in the United States? Were Americans receiving the care they needed? How was care being paid for? Were there better ways to provide health care? Would health insurance be practicable on a wide scale?

Out of these and other questions, as well as numerous discussions, came a conference in Washington, D.C., on April 1, 1926. About 15 leaders in medicine, public health, and the social sciences attended. The various problems in the health field were discussed, and it was agreed that a committee should be organized. There was some hesitation, however, about immediately instituting a research program. It was decided that further investigation should be made into the feasibility of a research study. A Committee of Five was appointed to investigate the need. About 75 persons, professionals and laymen, were consulted by mail. The response highly favored research into the economic aspects of medical care.

A second conference was held on May 17, 1927, in Washington, D.C., concurrently with the annual meeting of the AMA. About 60 persons attended the conference, and from them came a nucleus for what was initially called the Committee on the Cost of Medical Care. Aided by universities and professional associations, the committee began in 1927 a five-year study of the state of medical care in the United States: an assessment of where we were, where we were going, and how our movement might be directed. Financing for the study ($1 million) was provided by a group of foundations: the Carnegie Corporation, the Josiah Macy, Jr. Foundation, the Julius Rosenwald Fund, the Russell Sage Foundation, and the Twentieth Century Fund. Grants for special studies were given by the Social Science Research Council and the Vermont Commission on Country Life. (See Appendix A for more background on the CCMC.)

It is interesting to note that two important foundations declined to participate in the funding of the CCMC. One was the Filene Foundation of Boston; the other was the Commonwealth Fund of New York City. These two foundations felt that the answers to the questions which the committee planned to investigate were already known. They offered to support an organization to promote some of the necessary changes, but not to study and rediscover what was going on.

Once the CCMC was organized, Dr. Ray Lyman Wilbur, president of Stanford University, former president of the AMA, and later (1929) secretary of the interior under President Herbert Hoover, was chosen as chairman. The vice chairman was Charles-Edward Amory Winslow of the School of Public Health at Yale University. Winthrop W. Aldrich of the Chase National Bank became treasurer. The study director was Harry H. Moore, a health economist from the U.S. Public Health Service. Moore had recently completed his doctorate at American University, with a dissertation entitled "Medical Care for Tomorrow."

Winslow was also chairman of the CCMC executive committee, which had eight members, three of them named by the AMA from its top leadership. In addition to Winslow, the executive committee consisted of Haven Emerson, professor of public health at Columbia University; George Follansbee, chairman of the judicial council of the AMA; Walton Hamilton, professor of economics on the law faculty at Yale; Walter Bower and Walter Steiner, distinguished physicians from Massachusetts and Connecticut, respectively; Michael M. Davis, a medical sociologist and economist; and Mrs. William K. Draper, a member of the public.

Total CCMC membership consisted of 50 persons. Members were drawn from private medical practice, public health, institutions, special interests, economics, sociology, and the public. The entire committee met twice a year; the executive committee met twice a month, except in the summer.

Two of the staff people who were active in the CCMC's efforts were I.S. Falk and C. Rufus Rorem. Both men came to the CCMC from the University of Chicago.

Falk had gone to the University of Chicago in 1923 as an assistant professor of bacteriology. He had attained a full professorship by the age of 30. In 1929 he joined the CCMC staff as associate director. From this position, he became the driving force behind much of the committee's work.

Rorem had been on the faculty of the School of Commerce and Administration at Chicago. He joined the committee's staff on a full-time basis in 1930. Rorem focused much of his effort on what were to become landmark studies of hospital capital investment and clinical group practices.

The reminiscences of Falk and Rorem provide not only a history of the CCMC, but also a feeling for the times; not only the committee's contribution to the development of such forces as Blue Cross, Hill-Burton, and HMOs, but also a sense of its ambitions.

Research and Study Program

FALK:[5]

The committee, as you know, had a five-year study program which was to run until 1932. They had planned a whole series of studies to find out how medicine was being practiced, whom it was reaching and serving, whom it was not reaching and not serving, the costs involved, the sources of the funds, et cetera. Some of the planned studies were library studies. Many, however, were field studies, including extensive surveys of practices by providers of health and medical services, and utilization and financing by consumers. In addition, collaborating studies were planned to be undertaken by such other agencies as: the Public Health Service, the AMA, the American Dental Association, the Milbank Memorial Fund, the Julius Rosenwald Fund, and the National Bureau of Economic Research.

By late 1928 or early 1929, they were, however, encountering difficulties. They had used two or two-and-a-half years of their five-year prospective lifetime and were not well along on what was a very elaborate program of studies. They therefore cast about for some way of strengthening their research undertakings and performance.

Because of some statistical studies I had published in the 1920s and some writings I had done for various journals, I was approached as to whether I might take a leave of absence from the University of Chicago and take charge of the committee's research program. A number of people who were active in the committee knew of my writings and work. Some of them also knew me personally.

At any rate, I was approached. Fortunately or unfortunately, the overture came at just about the time that I was in my most pessimistic mood about the outlook for a school of public health at the University of Chicago. As a result, I was interested.

I went to some meetings of the executive committee and talked with them and they with me about the problems of the committee and its study program. They knew I had something of a reputation of being effective as a director of studies and that I had a fluent pen.

I asked the University of Chicago if I could have a leave of absence. It appeared, however, that I would be gone for two to two-and-one-half years, and they [the university administration] felt they could not approve a leave of that length. So I resigned and became the associate director of the committee, in charge of research.

In passing I should add that this point in time was a troubled period for the University of Chicago. The previous president of the university had retired. A new president had been brought in. However, he had been compelled to resign because of some personal difficulties, and the university was in the process of choosing a new president. About the time I had to make a decision about whether to stay or to leave, the new president came in. However, he wasn't interested in my problem. The vice president was interested in my staying but he was locked into a difficult position by virtue of the financial commitments that had already been made to go ahead with the full development of the Billings Hospital.

The objective of developing a school of public health at the University of Chicago was essentially scratched. As a result, I found that I was spending a good deal of my time and energy working towards a goal that was not going to be achieved.

So I left.

In leaving, my thought was that I would find it interesting to be extensively involved in the work of the committee. The committee could be a landmark in studying the economic aspects of health and disease and lay out a program for the future. Then, after a couple of years of that, if I found I had other interests, I would turn to them.

═══════════

Rorem also came to the CCMC from the University of Chicago, where he and Falk had known each other.

═══════════

ROREM:[6]

In December 1928, while I was teaching as an assistant professor of accounting [at the University of Chicago], I had a conversation with Michael M. Davis, Ph.D. As I'm sure you know, Michael was a medical economist who had just become director of medical services of the Julius Rosenwald Fund in Chicago. He was also a member of the executive committee of the Committee on the Costs of Medical Care.

As part of its work, the committee had been gathering statistical data and general facts about the organization, administration, and resources for health care in this country. They were also beginning to explore some of the financial aspects of hospitals and wanted to add to their staff a person familiar with both accounting and capital investment.

Michael asked me if I could recommend anyone. After some discussion he offered me a temporary, part-time appointment with the committee.

At the outset, I was not a regular member of the committee staff. Instead, I was to work with Michael on a specific study, which was being funded by the Rockefeller Foundation. The study was to examine the amount and nature of the capital investment in the hospitals. No study of this kind had ever been done before in the United States.

The opportunity appealed to me.

I agreed to take the job at the end of the academic year, meanwhile working on a part-time basis through the summer of 1929. Ultimately, I went on the full-time payroll of the committee and moved to Washington, D.C., in January 1930.

═══════════

Falk, as discussed above, was interested in the CCMC and the challenge of attempting to finish the research on schedule. An extraordinary effort would be required; however, as described by Falk, he and the rest of the committee's staff succeeded.

FALK:[7]

As I said, when I joined the staff, two-and-a-half years of the five years were gone. One or two or three publications had been issued. Five or six other studies that were more or less complete were in the doldrums. A half-a-dozen others were either in an early stage of gestation or had not even been started.

Through 1930 and 1931 we made a great deal of progress. We got the study program on a clearer and better track. We completed a number of the studies that had been bogged down for need of additional or updated information and began to publish our reports on a regular schedule. The executive committee, which met nearly monthly throughout the year, and the full committee, which met twice a year, both gave very intense attention to the reports, which were circulated to them in draft form. It was a very carefully patterned program. The committee was not just a showpiece or window dressing. It was a very extensively and actively involved organization. The executive committee gave an endless amount of time to the reports and meetings.

By early 1932, the study program was sufficiently well enough along so that the committee could see that it was going to complete its study program substantially on time. Twenty-six major reports had been published, or were in press, or being readied for publication, and the staff summary report (to be released as Publication Number 27) was well along toward completion. The magnitude of the nation's health costs had been established—their characteristics, impacts, causes, financing, etc.—and their significance for prevention of disease, diagnosis, treatment, the providers involved, etc. A veritable library of information had been built—a basis for planning had been established.

Falk was responsible for the committee's overall research effort, including the landmark longitudinal household survey. Rorem, while an author of the final staff report (along with Falk and Martha D. Ring), focused his research primarily on financial and organizational issues. His efforts were also quickly productive.

ROREM:[8]

As you can appreciate from the number of publications, the committee's total investigation was divided into several separate subdivisions or study areas. Within this overall structure, my own studies were focused on business operations, on the fiscal and administrative side of medical care production.

My first study, *The Public's Investment in Hospitals,* was issued in November 1930 by the University of Chicago Press, which was the official publisher for the committee. It's interesting to recall that we selected the study title because our findings showed that 90 percent of hospital capital had come from public sources, about half from philanthropy and half from taxation, and that these sources expected neither repayment of the original capital nor a return in the form of interest.

My second study, *Private Group Clinics,* was published in February 1931. This study, as its name implies, was an examination of group practice among private physicians. It looked at the trend which had been developing for at least 40 years, having its roots in the Mayo Clinic of Rochester, Minnesota.

I was also the author of a volume titled *The Municipal Doctor System in Saskatchewan.* Additionally, I co-authored, with Robert P. Fischelis, *The Costs of Medicine,* a study dealing with the pharmaceutical industry and the use of the prescription drugs and over-the-counter products.

An interesting part of the capital investment study was that many facts and data were obtained by personal visits to institutions. I would ask each hospital for a copy of its financial statement. During the winter of 1928–1929, the first hospital I visited was the Huggins Memorial Hospital in Wolfeboro, New Hampshire, which had 24 *beds,* and the second was the Massachusetts General Hospital in Boston, which had 24 *operating rooms.* At neither place was there any record of capital investment. For purposes of insurance, some records were maintained, but neither hospital kept a plant ledger, and management was surprised that anyone should ask for such information.

After a few weeks, and after visiting a dozen more institutions, I found that instead of asking questions I was answering questions. This was a field in which I knew very little, but in which the hospital representatives knew nothing. Within a month I became an expert on capital investment in hospitals and began writing on the subject. There was no literature. If I wanted to read something about capital investment, I had to write it myself.

An example of how little I knew about hospitals was that I did not know that attending physicians at hospitals were private practitioners using the institutions to carry on their practice. I did not know that very few deans of medical schools in the country received cash salaries for their work. They donated their services, for the most part, and made their living from serving private patients in their spare time.

For example, a statement from the Presbyterian Hospital in Chicago, the teaching institution for Rush Medical College, showed that the medical school paid $500 for the services of the dean of the medical school, Dr. E.E. Irons, who later became president of the American Medical Association.

One day I was speaking with Dr. Irons and said to him, "I find everything in the statement but your salary."

"That's it," he said.

"That $500? You can't live on that."

"Of course I can't, Rufus. That's just for office expenses."

"Well," I asked, "how do you make your living?"

"I have a private practice on the side."

In 1931 I had moved back to Chicago to work on a full-time basis with the Julius Rosenwald Fund, acting as associate director of medical services under Michael Davis. I still, however, continued to serve as a member of the staff of the Committee on the Costs of Medical Care. I was one of the three joint authors of the final staff report of the committee. The others were Isidore S. Falk and Martha D. Ring. Dr. Falk was the primary author; I wrote the section dealing with financial and organizational matters, and Miss Ring served as editor and coordinator of the volume as a whole. [Rorem stayed with the Rosenwald Fund until December 1936, when the fund's trustees liquidated the program in medical economics.]

Final Statement and Recommendations

As the various studies and final staff report approached completion, Falk turned his attention to the preparation of a final statement from the committee itself. There was some question as to how such a statement should be written—whether it should be drafted for the committee or whether the committee should draft it itself.

FALK:[9]

It was decided that the committee was obligated to produce a statement assessing the findings from its studies, providing interpretations, and giving as it thought appropriate recommendations for the future—recommendations which would lay out a program for desirable developments for the future.

As staff, we made some mistakes in our first attempts to draft such a statement or report. That's not of any consequence, because it had no significance for the outcome. Finally the committee undertook to draft the statement on its own. A subcommittee of the executive committee was appointed to act as a drafting committee. It proceeded to draft a report. The draft was then shared with the other members of the executive committee and at a subsequent point with the members of the full committee.

When the report began to take form in the middle of 1932, it was clear that there were five conclusions that had emerged, as the committee saw it, from the studies that had been conducted and which needed to play a role as a foundation for recommendations that they decided they would want to make. The draft report became a summarization and interpretation of the committee's findings and an estimate of the significance of those findings for the current scene, for the prospective scene, and for the formulation of recommendations.

The drafting committee came up with a report which was titled "Medical Care for the American People, the Final Report of the Committee on the Costs of Medical Care." It's interesting to note that about midway through its work the word "cost" in the committee's name was changed to "costs." This was done because some of the physician members of the committee thought that, unfairly, the public was beginning to think this was just a study of physicians and physician practices. As a result, there seemed to be emerging criticisms just focused on the doctor and the costs of his services. In response to this, various proposals were made to change the title of the committee, to make it clear that this was a much broader undertaking than just looking at the private practitioners of medicine. After considering various alternatives, only one change was made: an "s" was added on to the word "cost." So it began as the Committee on the *Cost* of Medical Care and ended as the Committee on the *Costs* of Medical Care.

The committee's statement, as I indicated, laid out five major recommendations and an extensive text surrounding each. [See Appendix B.] Of these five recommendations, two received particularly intensive attention and precipitated serious controversy.

The first and most important of these was that, because of the developing patterns of fragmented medical care, in the future medical care should be furnished through organized groups of physicians, which would involve generalists, specialists, and supporting ancillary services. Moreover, it also recommended that such groups be organized, preferably around a hospital.

The other particularly controversial recommendation was that, for the future, the costs of medical care should be met by groups of people over periods of time—a group payment concept. This recommendation seems like old hat to us today, but it was not old hat in 1932. It was based on the extensive committee studies which showed that the variable and unforeseeable and, for the individual family, the unbudgetable nature of medical care costs were foreseeable and budgetable for large groups of people—group payment.

In many respects the major recommendations, as subsequent consequences were to indicate, were that the future of medical care should be based on group practice for the availability, the delivery, the provision of care and that group payment, whether by insurance, taxation, or a combination of them, should be the main financial support for the future of medical care.

There were three other major recommendations. One was on the strengthening of professional and technical education. Another was for the strengthening of public health in community activities. The fifth was on the coordination of these various developments.

I should also note that it was the sense, though not the unanimous opinion, of the committee that the developments they were recommending should come about primarily on a voluntary basis.

It should be remembered that when the committee began its work, in the late 1920s, we were seemingly in a period of great prosperity. The United States was flying toward the highest level of economic affluence and prosperity that it had ever known. It was a period in which there were very strong commitments in a broad spectrum of the population for reliance on voluntarism; people would do things for themselves. Except for the formal field of public health, it was felt that health care was not primarily the concern of government. Instead it was felt that it was primarily a concern of people in their private lives and in the private sectors of their lives. So it is not surprising that these recommendations, except for where public health was concerned, anticipated voluntary, private sector action.

As I indicated, a few members of the committee disagreed. They felt the committee should have stood neutral on voluntary versus governmental activity. They nevertheless went along with the majority. Their views, however, were noted in procedurally agreed-upon footnotes.

The committee's draft report was circulated and studied and discussed. At a general meeting of the committee it quickly became apparent that a minority disagreed very strongly with the recommendations on group practice as the means of providing medical care and on group payment as the means of financing it.

Group practice they regarded as a threat to the independence and the sovereignty of professional people to make their own decisions as to how they wanted to pursue their careers, how they wanted to practice. Group payment was viewed as a threatening challenge to the existence of fee-for-service as the principal means of paying for medical care.

Nine members (eight of them M.D.'s) elected to dissent on those two recommendations as well as, in limited degrees, on others. They wrote an independent report which was published as Minority Report Number One [Appendix C].

Their dissent was based mainly on the notion that the future of medical practice should be left to the medical profession to plan, guide, and control. They did not want dilution of their opportunities and their prerogatives through the participation of lay people.

They also took strong exception to the group payment recommendation unless group payment remained voluntary, was elected by the profession, and remained under the control of the profession through its medical societies. In general, their position was a reflection of the position of the medical profession at that time. They took a position which aimed at preserving the sovereignty—not merely the independence, but the sovereignty—of the medical profession in the field of personal health care.

There was another minority report written by two dentist members of the committee. I won't spend much time on that, because they weren't of one mind. They weren't sure of where they stood, and they wanted to be on both sides of the issue.

There was another major report, called a "statement," written by Walton Hamilton, which I thought was the best economic statement on medical care that had been written up to that point by anybody. He felt the committee had failed to meet its primary obligation because it had made too many compromises in the development of its major recommendations and in the development of the supports for those recommendations. There was also a personal statement by Edgar Sydenstricker in which he took the same position as Hamilton. Sydenstricker did not, however, spell it out.

The majority report, as the formal report of the committee, had the support of a majority of the physicians who were on the committee. The physicians who signed Minority Report Number One were a minority of the total physicians on the committee. That's a point that has not always been clearly understood.

The majority report and the minority reports were released on October 31, 1932, at an important series of meetings at the New York Academy of Medicine.

When the report was released, at the New York Academy of Medicine, there was consternation, because on the table laid out for the press there was also a preprint of an editorial which was to be published in the *Journal of the American Medical Association,* prepared by the then-editor, Dr. Morris Fishbein. In his editorial, Dr. Fishbein damned the majority report of the committee from here to kingdom come. He referred to it in blistering terms, saying that the report and its recommendations were "Socialism and Communism—inciting to revolution." He consigned the majority report to "innocuous desuetude."

There was consternation, and, in a sense, the ceiling fell in on October 31, 1932.

The plans that had been considered for a follow-up organization to publicize the recommendations, to serve to explain them, to assist groups in society to make use of the committee's work—all that went down the drain. They went down the drain because the AMA called a special meeting of its house of delegates and the house formally endorsed the principal minority report [Minority Report Number One].

As a sort of a footnote, I should tell you that by no stretch of my imagination can I conceive of how the AMA could possibly have taken a less productive and less constructive, and a less intelligent position than they took through the pressures on their representatives on the committee to participate in the development of the Minority Report Number One, or the position they took in their house of delegates in endorsing the minority report. At that time the AMA had a clear choice of a road to follow in the development of the design and the rules under which medical care would develop in the United States.

They had the examples that had been followed by the British Medical Association, by the Medical Association of France, by the medical association in Canada, when confronted with somewhat similar situations. It was as though they were deaf, dumb, and blind—or, their senses apart, they were indifferent to the experience of other medical associations in seeking to provide any constructive or useful guidance. Instead they chose to stand pat and perhaps even be obstructive.

As you can sense, in my view the consequence was disastrous for the whole field of medical care. At that time there was no major group or force in the United States that could play a countervailing role to the AMA and its house of delegates. They were damning the recommendations of a majority of the committee and endorsing the potential monopolistic position of the medical profession, to the exclusion of practically everybody else.

So it came about as ordered from 535 North Dearborn Street in Chicago [AMA headquarters]—except for one important factor. The committee had begun its work in 1927, when the country was rising toward the highest level of economic comfort and affluence that it had known. By October 1932 the country was plunging toward the worst economic depression of recent times. Thus, the committee's work had started in 1927, on the upcurve toward prosperity and great economic resources, but it had ended in late '32, when the country's economy was winding toward a nearly total halt. The "innocuous desuetude" could not be accepted by a nation that was finding itself in very grievous circumstances.

COHEN:[10]

A most significant development occurred when the Committee on the Costs of Medical Care made its report in 1932. At that time Dr. Morris Fishbein was the editor of the *Journal of the American Medical Association* and he wrote a rather significant editorial commenting on the report, indicating that any kind of health insurance proposal was "Socialism and Communism—inciting to revolution." His characterization of health insurance, whether voluntary or public, served to set the dominant ideological and controversial note for some 33 years after that, a third of a century.

During that time, anyone who advocated national health insurance was usually tarred with the epithet of being a socialist or a communist or a radical. It was not until the passage of Medicare in 1965 that those who advocated some kind of a program were able to overcome that kind of criticism. It was extremely unfortunate, because by injecting that kind of emotional element into the discussion, many of the technical, professional, and substantive issues were overlooked in the battle of the ideological terminology.

It's interesting, however, that Morris Fishbein, before he died, told me that he thought Medicare was a very acceptable and reasonable program and that none of what he said in 1932 had come to pass, at least with respect to the Medicare program.

Morris Fishbein was able later to revise his approach, which some others were not able to do. Nevertheless, it was only with the passage of Medicare that the fateful criticism of socialism-communism was erased. Nobody was socialized or communized by the passage of Medicare, despite the fact that such fateful predictions were made.

The Spirit of the CCMC

Another factor, besides the AMA's stance, that robbed the work of the CCMC of its effectiveness was the despair of the times. Within ten days of the issuance of the report, a complete turnover of political philosophy took place. The inability of the Hoover administration to cope with massive unemployment, bank failures, mortgage foreclosures, and hunger and hopelessness led to the election of Franklin D. Roosevelt as president. Roosevelt promised quick and decisive action, but, despite his massive action campaign four months later, the minds of the people were on basic bread-and-butter issues, with the problems of medical care seeming less urgent.

No matter how despondent the leaders of the CCMC were because their recommendations had been rejected by the AMA, their data and recommendations did have lasting effects. For many years, the data developed by the committee provided a basis for most efforts to reform or understand health care in the United States. Some of the health legislation recommended by the cabinet-level Committee on Economic Security (from whose deliberations Social Security developed) was based on CCMC data.[11]

The data developed in the household surveys, in fact, were the basic source of such information until Odin Anderson instituted a similar household survey at the Health Information Foundation some 20 years later.[12] (Anderson's mentor at the University of Michigan had been Nathan Sinai, a principal in the committee's household survey.)

The five principal recommendations of the committee were ultimately effective in influencing the course of health care. From these recommendations came, in whole or in part, the roots, strong or tenuous, of prepaid hospital care (Blue Cross), the Hill-Burton Act, health care planning, Medicare and Medicaid, and HMOs. The thread started in 1927 thus continues to be spun out.

A few years later, when writing his history of the AMA, Morris Fishbein, editor of the *Journal of the American Medical Association* and reputed author of the editorial opposing the CCMC report, softened his remarks a bit. He said the studies published by the CCMC indicated the value of such studies as a basis for conclusions and recommendations. He recommended continued studies, particularly in industrial medical services and in corporate practice. He said the minority report was "particularly resentful" that the majority made recommendations based on inadequate studies.

Fishbein added that the minority felt that the majority presented the situation in a distorted sense—that the "evils of contract practice are widespread and pernicious."

He charged that the CCMC showed only favorable aspects, that they were chosen because they were thought to be favorable examples of this type of practice in the United States. The minority, in turn, added that for each favorable example "a score of the opposite kind can be found."

Fishbein reverted to the position he had taken in his editorial, in which he condemned the CCMC majority report by using the terms "Socialism," "communism," and "inciting to revolution." He summed up the majority and minority reports in his history by saying that the two represented the "difference between incitement to revolution and a desire for gradual evolution based on analysis and study."

Finally, it should be noted that, while the AMA opposed the committee's recommendations, the American Hospital Association firmly agreed with the recommendation for group prepayment of hospital care. John R. Mannix of Cleveland was actively involved in promoting the hospital prepayment idea, as shown by his work with Blue Cross plans in Cleveland, Detroit, and Chicago. From the 1930s on, Mannix played a major role in shaping the policies of both the AHA and the Blue Cross movement.

MANNIX:[13]

One of the resolutions we offered suggested American Hospital Association activity in what was then called group hospitalization, or periodic payment for hospital care. This resolution resulted in action by the AHA trustees in January 1933 to establish approval standards for hospital prepayment plans and recommended the study by hospitals at the local level of periodic payment for hospital care. This came immediately after the issuance of the final report of the Committee on the Costs of Medical Care, which recommended experiments with the financing of hospital care on a periodic payment basis.

During the next two years, 1933 and 1934, there were seven plans established, which later became Blue Cross plans and, in my opinion, were the basis of the whole Blue Cross and Blue Shield development.

Following this action of its trustees, the AHA established a group hospitalization committee of five: Dr. Basil MacLean, Dr. S.S. Goldwater, Monsignor Maurice Griffin, Dr. Robin C. Buerki, and C. Rufus Rorem. They strongly advocated local hospitals' establishing programs of prepayment for health care.

The spirit of the CCMC lives on today in pluralistic approaches toward finding a practicable, affordable method, or methods, of insuring all Americans or of finding more than one option, if need be, to solve the problem.

The CCMC also had a lasting influence on patterns of health care research, as shown by remarks of Odin W. Anderson, who became a researcher nearly two decades after the committee's work.

ANDERSON:[14]

I was appointed the research director of the Health Information Foundation in 1952. I was 38 years old with a Ph.D. in sociology from the University of Michigan. . . . My primary interests were in the application of social science research to public policy problems in the health services. . . . My entry to the health field was through a former staff member of the Committee on the Costs of Medical Care, Nathan Sinai, D.P.H., professor of public health administration, School of Public Health, the University of Michigan, who hired me as a research assistant in 1942, while I was a graduate student at the university. The link between Sinai's connection with the Committee on the Costs of Medical Care and subsequent research conducted in national household surveys by me at the Health Information Foundation is a direct one. It is an interesting example of research continuity. Among the scores of staff members on the CCMC, Sinai was the only one who continued his interest into an academic position. Others, notably Falk, Klem, and Louis Reed, became very active in the Public Health Service. C. Rufus Rorem became active in hospital prepayment and had enormous influence on the development of the Blue Cross system. I, in fact, have always regarded myself as a research descendent—and the only primary one—of the CCMC research base.

Notes

(Transcripts of the oral histories cited here are housed in the Library of the American Hospital Association, Asa S. Bacon Memorial, 840 North Lake Shore Drive, Chicago, Illinois 60611. The Oral History Collection is a joint project of the Hospital Research and Educational Trust and the AHA.)

1. Much of the information about the circumstances that resulted in medical education's becoming the subject of the Carnegie study comes from conversations with George Bugbee and John Millis (see Profiles of Participants, in the center of this book, for biographical information).

2. J.C. Furnas, *Great Times* (New York: Putnam's, 1974), p. 175. See also J.T. Flexner, *An American Saga: The Story of Helen Thomas and Simon Flexner* (Boston: Little, Brown, 1984).

3. Furnas, *Great Times,* p. 174.

4. Eli Ginzberg, *The Limits of Health Reform* (New York: Basic Books, 1977), p. 84.

5. *I.S. Falk, In the First Person: An Oral History.* See Profiles of Participants for biographical information.

6. *C. Rufus Rorem, In the First Person: An Oral History.* See Profiles of Participants for biographical information.

7. *Falk, Oral History.*

8. *Rorem, Oral History.*

9. *Falk, Oral History.*

10. *Wilbur J. Cohen, In the First Person: An Oral History.* See Profiles of Participants for biographical information.

11. The cabinet-level Committee on Economic Security, appointed by President Franklin D. Roosevelt in 1934, was charged with making recommendations on unemployment and old age insurance. Frances Perkins, secretary of the treasury, chaired the committee.

12. For a description of the activities of the Health Information Foundation, see *Odin W. Anderson, In the First Person: An Oral History.* See Profiles of Participants for biographical information.

13. *John R. Mannix, In the First Person: An Oral History.* See Profiles of Participants for biographical information.

14. *Odin W. Anderson, In the First Person: An Oral History.* See Profiles of Participants for biographical information.

3

The Hospital Survey and Construction (Hill-Burton) Act

Hospital construction, renovation, and repair were greatly curtailed during the Great Depression and World War II. The depression years were simply years of want and despair, during which work of all kinds came to a near standstill. Money was scarce, unemployment was widespread, and the future seemed bleak; consequently, planning for the future seemed futile.[1]

After the inauguration of Franklin D. Roosevelt as president in 1933, there was some renewal of hope. Roosevelt was a picture of optimism, saying there was nothing to fear but fear itself. Under his administration, direct relief programs were undertaken with great speed by the federal government. Work programs followed quickly, and public works projects followed with less haste and more planning under the direction of Harold L. Ickes, secretary of the interior and head of the Public Works Administration (PWA).

The PWA constructed public buildings: post offices, municipal and county buildings, state university classrooms and other schools, and so on. In a few cases, hospitals benefited from the PWA programs.

More than bricks and mortar and labor were needed to build hospitals, however, as the following story about Governor Frank Murphy[2] of Michigan illustrates. Murphy, a favorite of Roosevelt's, went to Washington to ask the president for money to build hospitals in rural areas of Michigan, where inpatient care was unavailable. Roosevelt directed Murphy to Ickes. Ickes, in turn, consulted with Josephine Roche, assistant secretary of the treasury, who was in charge of the Public Health Service (then a part of the Department of the Treasury).

Roche was concerned because the program that Murphy was proposing for the construction and equipping of hospitals did not even include start-up money for the operation of the hospitals. There was a meeting between Murphy and Ickes, which was also attended by Josephine Roche; Abe Fortas, under secretary and general counsel of the Department of the Interior; and I.S. Falk from the Bureau of Research and Statistics of the Social Security Administration. Falk remembers that meeting:

FALK:[3]

I remember that meeting in Mr. Ickes' office because I had the unhappy task to say, "This is no go, because the very communities for which the governor wants the help for these small rural hospitals are, in general, communities that don't have hospitals because they can't support them. What will you do with these hospitals if you build them? How will you maintain them? Let's give some thought to where the money is to come from to support them."

We had a long session in which I was the most unpopular person in the room.

Another aspect to the situation was that, not only would assistance be needed for operating expenses, but also the medical and nurse staffing would be a problem in rural areas. It has been the unhappy discovery of many rural areas that new buildings alone will not attract the desired professional staff. During this time, schools of medicine and schools of nursing, along with everything else, were feeling the effects of the Great Depression and were not growing with an eye to future population increase and its needs.

Many of the leaders of the health field realized the inadequacy of existing facilities and the need for national planning for the construction of medical care facilities, for support for educating professional and paraprofessional health care personnel, and for providing access to and financing of health care for all.

George Bugbee became the executive secretary of the AHA in 1943, just when some persons were asking, What will we do when the war is over? (Victory seemed inevitable then.) Within a reasonable time after the end of the war, millions of men and women in the service would be returning home and would expect, rightly, that health care, education, and social programs sufficient to take care of everyone's needs would be in place. Bugbee was conscious of the necessity of planning for the postwar period. The federal government, at least in the person of Dr. Thomas Parran, the surgeon general of the U.S. Public Health Service, was thinking of postwar health care needs also.

As a first, formal step in planning for the future, the AHA passed what became known as the Bishop resolution. This resolution provided the foundation for a series of initiatives that culminated in the Hill-Burton Act.

George Bugbee recalls the role of AHA in establishing the Commission on Hospital Care, and lobbying for Hill-Burton.

BUGBEE:[4]

At the American Hospital Association's 1943 convention, the house of delegates passed a resolution which had taken a great deal of work. It was called the Bishop resolution.

The resolution essentially recommended three things: voluntary health insurance; federal aid for the construction of hospitals where they were needed; and government aid for those who couldn't pay for care. It's interesting that that's always the proposal made contrary to national health insurance. You either have entitlement for everyone, or you only give it to those who need it. The association took the conservative side. You could argue whether it should have or should not have. That's a different story and a philosophical dividing point.

On the last day of the convention, a group of us were in what I suspect was Jim Hamilton's[5] suite. He was president of AHA that year [1943]. I don't recall exactly who was there. Hamilton was and E.A. van Steenwyk[6] [one of the early pioneers in Blue Cross] was and I was. There were about eight or ten people in total.

I remember van Steenwyk saying: "Now that the association has a policy [the Bishop resolution], what are we going to do about it? There isn't any use in it just sitting there, we'd better do something!"

That resolution, in a sense, gave me authority to move. I thought: He's right, I'd better move. I had been in office only two or three months, but action was indicated. You will recall that one of the three items of policy was, build hospitals where they are needed.

Commission on Hospital Care

There was at that time no complete directory of hospitals listing the location, ownership, number of beds, or services offered. The principal source of information about health care in the United States was still the report of the Committee on the Costs of Medical Care.

As a first step, Hamilton and Bugbee and Bugbee's colleagues decided that a study was needed to assess the current situation, evaluate existing facilities and services, make projections, and offer recommendations for action after the war was over. The ultimate result of this decision was the establishment in 1944 of the Commission on Hospital Care.

The commission's charge was to study the nation's need for hospital and medical facilities and to make plans for the postwar period. Many persons believe that it was partly as a result of the commission's work that the Hill-Burton Act was passed in 1946.

Although created by the AHA, the commission was an independent entity. It was financed by outside sources, including the W.K. Kellogg Foundation, and its report was published by the Commonwealth Fund. The commission also operated under its own board of directors. (See Appendixes D and E.)

The commission's report, "Hospital Care in the United States," not only collected information, it visualized a regional hospital system, with primary, secondary, and tertiary care given on the basis of hospital size and available services.

George Bugbee and others, particularly the commission's associate director, Maurice Norby, discuss the forming and operation of the commission.

BUGBEE:[7]

Jim Hamilton and I—I think Hamilton was the primary leader, although Graham Davis[8] was high in the association's councils and he was in charge of the hospital division of the W.K. Kellogg Foundation—were a part of an effort made to create a Commission on Hospital Care. It was hard going to raise the money for the commission. The Kellogg Foundation pledged a certain amount, and we solicited many other people. I can remember going to the Carnegie Foundation. They said that all that we were trying to do was measure leaves in a whirlwind. However, largely due to the help of Morris Fishbein [editor of the *Journal of the American Medical Association*], we were able to get to Basil O'Connor,[9] who was the chairman of the March of Dimes. He gave us some money, and there was, I believe, a little from a third source. It didn't amount to much. Later the Public Health Service supplemented the funds.

We persuaded Dr. Arthur Bachmeyer, then associate dean of biological sciences at the University of Chicago and superintendent of the University of Chicago Hospitals and Clinics to become the commission's director. He said that he would do it, but he couldn't spend more than half time. It was then that we persuaded Maurice Norby,[10] who was working with Rufus Rorem[11] at the Blue Cross Commission, to take the principal staff job. The orderliness of the commission's report and its success were partly due to Art Bachmeyer, but due a great deal more to Maurice Norby.

The commission was chaired by Thomas S. Gates, the president of the

University of Pennsylvania, a very public-spirited man. We spent a lot of time, some with Mr. Gates, who was to do the appointing [of the commission members], trying to figure out who should be on such a commission. I would say there were about 25 members. It became a pattern for foundation-supported commissions, including a few years later the Commission on Financing of Hospital Care.[12]

Maurice J. Norby, who was the staff member that probably did the most work on the Commission on Hospital Care, and I consulted with quite a few people on how you establish such a commission. The ingredients we wanted were representatives from all walks of life. We wanted labor and industry and farmers, who, at that time, were more powerful because their numbers were a great deal greater. We wanted providers, blacks, whites, women, etc. We had really quite a representative commission. It was important, because later the fact that it was representative was very helpful in the passage of the Hill-Burton Act.

Bugbee, Bachmeyer, and Norby were quite successful in putting together a strong commission.[13] In addition to Gates as chairman, the commission included Edward Ryerson, chairman of the board of Inland Steel Corporation, as vice chairman; Sarah Gibson Blanding, president of Vassar College; Willard C. Rappleye, dean of the medical school at Columbia University; Joseph W. Fichter, head of the Ohio State Grange; Albert W. Dent, president of Dillard University in New Orleans; Clinton S. Golden, assistant to the president of the United Steel Workers; and Herbert C. Hoover, former president of the United States.[14]

BUGBEE:[15]

There's always been a question whether the Commission on Hospital Care and its findings and report led to the Hill-Burton Act. Well, having been there, I am inclined to think they are related, but hardly as direct a lead-in as later the Public Health Service said. They were the ones who indicated that it was the source. I don't feel it was.

Maurice Norby was the associate director of the commission. He went there from Blue Cross, partly because he felt that "someone ought to be identified with hospitals who was in Blue Cross." As associate director, Norby carried the day-to-day responsibility for the commission and, as suggested by Bugbee, did most of the commission's work. His observations on the commission, its work, and its accomplishments follow.

NORBY:[16]

The American Hospital Association, with the Bishop resolution, demonstrated an awareness of the need to provide care for people who needed assistance. They also showed that they understood that the demand for hospital-based services would increase and that more hospitals would be needed. The AHA also recognized that a fact base and data were needed to document what existed in the way of hospital physical facilities and to guide the future development of hospitals.

To obtain these data, the AHA, and really I think it was George Bugbee working with a committee of the board, drew up a plan for a study which could be presented to outside agencies in order to obtain financial assistance. The result of this effort, as you know, was the Commission on Hospital Care.

Once financing was obtained and the commission was formed, it operated completely independently of the AHA.

I got involved because, though Arthur Bachmeyer was the commission's director, he could only spend half time on the project. As a result, he wanted an assistant. Later he changed the title to associate director. Whether he asked for me or whether George Bugbee suggested me to him, I don't know. I do know that the two of them approached me together and asked if I would be willing to work full-time on the commission.

I studied the commission's prospectus and decided to do it. At the time, I was the director of research at the Blue Cross Commission with Rufus Rorem. In fact, part of my reason for taking the job was that I thought that someone ought to be identified with hospitals who was in Blue Cross. At that time no Blue Cross administrator had been a hospital administrator [except John R. Mannix]. None of them had been identified as people knowledgeable about hospitals. All they were supposed to be worrying about was dollars. Let the hospital administrators run hospitals.

It was my feeling that trouble was brewing between Blue Cross plan directors and hospital administrators, basically because hospitals knew Blue Cross directors did not fully understand the problems of hospital administrators. Plan directors were just asked to provide the dollars to run hospitals.

I thought that, if I could work for this national study, I might be identified as someone in Blue Cross who knew the hospital problem. I would be looking at what hospitals are. The Commission on Hospital Care was created to find out what the hospital is and to identify what it should be doing in the future.

So I took a leave of absence from the Blue Cross Commission. I thought I would spend two years on the Commission on Hospital Care.

The commission's first task was to determine what the present hospital was. To, in effect, define the creatures we were dealing with and determine where they were located.

The American Medical Association had a list of hospitals, however their list had no detailed information and only included about a fourth of the nation's hospitals.

I went to the Census Bureau and, after some cajoling with the director, developed a good working relationship. He assigned me one of his assistants. Together, we built a list of all the places where people had died in the United States. We went through that list and eliminated lots of things just by the name of the place. Finally he let us go deeper into the records and see the characteristics of the places on the list, by the replies that they had made on income tax records. Actually, we shouldn't have had that data. It was a tedious job.

We also asked the state hospital associations for the names of all their hospitals. We asked the nursing home association for all of theirs, and we asked the state health departments for all the health facilities they licensed. We sifted all these names until we finally got some 14,000 places that we thought might be hospitals. Then we developed a questionnaire that we then mailed to all these places. We asked them questions which would help us to identify whether or not they were hospitals.

At the same time that we were doing this, we also were thinking about the questions we were going to ask hospitals to find out the kinds of services they rendered, what their financial condition was, what it was costing them to run the place, what their plans were for the future, and so on.

Paralleling the interest of the Commission on Hospital Care was that of the Public Health Service (PHS), particularly Surgeon General Thomas Parran.[17] Parran was concerned with what would be expected of his department with respect to meeting postwar health care needs. What he wanted was definitive data, updated data.

Parran had taken several steps to prepare for a potential federal program of planning and building hospitals. One was to have Dr. Vane Hoge, of the Public Health Service, enroll at the University of Chicago in the graduate course in hospital administration in order to prepare himself for administration of any program that might be enacted. (Hoge in fact did become the first Hill-Burton administrator.) Another was to have a PHS physician assigned to the staff of the Commission on Hospital Care to participate in the work of the commission. The first person assigned was Dr. Robert Morey, who resigned from the PHS shortly afterward to enter private practice. He was succeeded by Dr. David Wilson, who later went on to become president of the AHA.

The relationship of the PHS to the commission, however, was more than just assigning a liaison person to the commission staff. The PHS was involved in writing legislation. To do this, it needed data—information such as the commission was collecting. The commission, on the other hand, did not have the capacity to process its data.

Norby saw an impossible situation unless he got help, so he went to Parran.

_____

NORBY:[18]

We recognized, however, that we were also going to need even more technical help. So I went to see Dr. Parran, who at the time was surgeon general of the Public Health Service.

I initiated the meeting with Dr. Parran. However, before I went I knew, from other sources, that he needed information and that he had a couple of hundred thousand dollars of postwar planning money available. Parran needed the data in order to administer properly the hospital construction program which was anticipated to begin after the war.[19]

We reached an agreement with the Public Health Service. They eventually provided us with help in first devising the questionnaire we needed and then in tabulating the data.

Parran loaned me a fellow named Rollo Britten, a statistician on the Public Health Service staff. He worked for me on a half-time basis, about every other week. Rollo was devising a questionnaire we needed. Bachmeyer was very good at anticipating the kind of information we should have. He knew hospital operations, so he could get the ideas for questions to Rollo and Rollo would word them and put them in sequence.

_____

At the time the questionnaires were being prepared for mailing, the W.K. Kellogg Foundation asked the Commission on Hospital Care to do a study of Michigan hospitals; the foundation needed data on which to base their considerations of requests for grants and other support.

The timing was propitious, because it enabled the commission to conduct a pilot study in 200 or 300 hospitals.

_____

NORBY:[20]

We got the questionnaire all ready, then Kellogg said they would give us some money if we would do a pilot study in Michigan, thus testing our questionnaire for the national study.

We actually ran this small study, a pilot study for the state of Michigan. There was a special report—it was all bound in a special book—reporting findings. In the process, we identified errors in our questionnaire and in methods and procedures.

We finally devised a 41-page questionnaire. Then we thought, when we get all these answers coming in, what are we going to do with the volume of information?

Dr. Parran said, "You send out the questionnaire because I need the information." He liked the big questionnaire. This information was available nowhere else. He said, "I'll help you tabulate it and handle the data."

He employed me as a dollar-a-year man to supervise a staff of about 20 people, whom he paid and who worked in our building in Chicago. They were to code the data from the questionnaires. Rollo had set it up so that the data could be transferred to punch cards for tabulation on IBM machines. I think we had 12 cards for each questionnaire.

I should say that Parran agreed to give us this assistance with the understanding that the data was to be considered as having been collected by his staff and that it would all be available to him—so he could say when he came up before Congress, "This is the information I have collected."

The commission considered it a necessary function of the staff to keep the public and the health field informed as to the progress of the study. This reporting was done principally by means of a newsletter. Norby talks about the newsletter and its distribution.

NORBY:[21]

I had assembled a list of some 15,000 names. I had obtained the names and addresses of presidents of school boards, for example, the presidents of farm bureaus, presidents of trade associations, professional associations, and so forth—all kinds of groups. They became the mailing list for our newsletter. After we got a chapter approved by the commission's board, I would have a staff editor summarize it into a four-page printed report, a newsletter, setting out the thoughts of the Commission on Hospital Care on whatever the particular subject was. These short reports in effect became a preview of our final report.

The Hill-Burton Legislation

Besides establishing the Commission on Hospital Care, the AHA did other things to obtain legislation aiding hospital construction.

BUGBEE:[22]

The establishment of the Commission on Hospital Care was only one expression of the intent of the association to drive for legislation to aid in the construction of hospitals.

One of the major issues in any legislation was whether nonprofit hospitals should be eligible for grants. There had been major work relief programs for years prior to the war, and only one of those programs allowed grants to be made to nonprofit hospitals. Since nonprofit or voluntary hospitals were providing most of the nation's short-term hospital care, it did not seem right that they be excluded from being eligible for assistance. Certainly, the nonprofit group didn't like it.

In addressing this issue, a planning committee—Postwar Planning Committee was its title—was set up under the AHA's council on government relations. It met in Washington. It began trying to figure out what might be done to see that the nongovernment hospitals were considered in any postwar building program.

On the Postwar Planning Committee was Dr. Vane Hoge. I think the action of the committee was due to Vane and his boss, Surgeon General Dr. Thomas Parran.

Parran thought, "Things are coming together. Let's draft legislation for aid to hospitals." He brought the draft to the Postwar Planning Committee. The committee said that the draft was just what they had been looking for.

The essential points were that each state have a plan, pick the neediest areas, and federal aid was to be varied between the states according to need. The aid was to go within the state to government and nonprofit hospitals by priority of need. This in a way is what Hill-Burton turned out to be, with considerable embroidery, one way or another.

The bill, as first drafted by the Public Health Service, seemed good. Then the question was how to get it introduced. I won't go through all of it, but about that time I became registered as a lobbyist. I intended that we pass that bill. Its passage was one of the successes of my life. However, even with that success I certainly was an amateur lobbyist. In fact, I never liked lobbying. I think some of the most disagreeable jobs I was confronted with were hanging around outside the House or Senate waiting to catch some person who didn't want to see me to ask how he was planning to vote. Or going to his office and trying to get in.

In any event, we had a bill. The question was, who were we going to get to introduce it? When I went to Cleveland to succeed Jim Hamilton at the Cleveland City Hospital, I was appointed by the then-mayor, Harold Burton. Harold Burton later became a United States Senator, and after that a justice of the Supreme Court. At the time I am talking about, he was in the Senate. So I went to see Harold Burton. He agreed to introduce the bill, with one reservation—and that was that Senator Robert Taft, the senior senator from Ohio, had to agree.

I went to see Taft and he did agree. He was getting ready to run for the presidency. He said, "I have a labor bill and I have this and that—education bill—and I need a health bill." He later rewrote the bill, because he said he was going to make it a model for federal grants-in-aid programs.

He believed (and, I believe, too) that states in such a program should have some independence of action. His interest was fueled by the fact that the state of Ohio about that time had done something that caused the federal government to hold up millions in Social Security benefits. This included the pay of those in state government administering the program. The federal government said that the state was not administering the Social Security program the way it should be. Taft was furious about the federal government's action. He was going to fix the Hill–Burton bill so it wouldn't happen with that.

The bill was introduced January 10, 1945 [and signed into law on August 13, 1946].

CRUIKSHANK:[23]

I know a little about what that was.

It was an incident involving Social Security and unemployment compensation, which was administered by the state. The funds, however, came out of the federal government. The federal government could declare a state out of compliance.

Arthur Altmeyer was then the chief administrator of the Social Security Act (unemployment insurance was then a part of Social Security). Davey, who was at that time Governor of Ohio, had introduced politics into the checks that went out to the unemployed. Altmeyer declared them out of compliance and shut off the funds to the state of Ohio, which was a risky thing to do, but it was a thing which established the authority of the federal government in that whole area. Of course Taft didn't like that: Davey was one of his buddies.

John Mannix was an important part of the Cleveland scene when George Bugbee was administrator of the Cleveland City Hospital during the time that Harold Burton was mayor of the city. Mannix spoke of Bugbee's and Burton's interest and efforts in hospital planning several years before the Hill–Burton Act.

MANNIX:[24]

The major development in hospital planning came about 1941, when George Bugbee, who was administrator of Cleveland City Hospital, which later became Metropolitan General Hospital, became interested in facility planning. For all practical purposes, there had been no hospitals built during the 1930s. No one had money to build facilities during the depression years.[25] At that time, Harold Burton was mayor of Cleveland, and George Bugbee's boss. Concern on the part of both Bugbee and Burton regarding hospital facilities resulted in the establishment of a joint hospital committee. This was a committee of 30 people, 10 appointed by the mayor, 10 by the hospital association, and 10 by the Council of Social Agencies (Cleveland Welfare Association).

The interest of Bugbee and Burton during this period affected the national situation, because Burton became a United States senator.

While in the Senate, Burton became interested in the whole problem of hospital facilities. It should be remembered, we had a period of about 15 years during the 1930s and World War II years when there was a large increase in population, with little building of hospitals in the country. There was a tremendous shortage of hospital beds nationwide in 1945. The interest of Senator Burton resulted in the Hill-Burton Act and the federal financing of hospital facilities.

Introduction of the legislation was only one step. Bugbee's next task was to help develop support for its passage.

BUGBEE:[26]

We asked members of the Commission on Hospital Care for support on the Hill-Burton legislation. The representative of the farm bureaus [the grange] was terribly key in getting support in the House for the bill. With the labor man [Golden], we immediately went to Nelson Cruikshank, who was on the staff of the health and welfare committee of the AF of L. He was very supportive.

When I went to the American Medical Association they had been so against everything that they essentially said they needed something to be for. So they agreed to support it, and they did testify in support of it, but reluctantly as far as their inner circle was concerned.

It was almost two years before the Hill-Burton Act was passed—with great authority to the states. Taft was thinking that what the states did wrong would be less bad than what would happen if it were a national program. That was his philosophy.

James Hague, who came on the AHA scene later (1953–1977), underscored Bugbee's point, both with respect to Taft's role and the operation of the Hill-Burton program.

HAGUE:[27]

As I am sure you know, Burton is just a name on Hill-Burton. It's Taft's name which probably belongs there, because it was Taft who did the work, who came up with the grants-in-aid program.

Hill-Burton was really intended to provide seed money for hospital construction, and it surely did. I have seen charts of the money that went into hospital construction during the Hill-Burton years. Hill-Burton was a substantial fraction, but it was a minority of the funds that were spent.

Taft insisted on local control. That's why there has been no scandal. I know of no Hill-Burton scandal. That's because individual hospital boards had to raise local community money. Their reputations were on the line.

[On reviewing the manuscript, Hague asked that this narrative carry an explicit statement that his comments are based on extensive interviews he had with Bugbee and Norby, who, unlike himself, were at the scene of the action. He believes his remarks are accurate but thinks the reader should know that they are based on hearsay—reliable hearsay, to be sure, but hearsay nonetheless.]

The Hill-Burton Formula

Senator Taft wanted to make Hill-Burton a model for federal grants-in-aid programs. As finally devised, the act provided a higher percentage of aid to poorer states. Bugbee commented on the question of whether it set a pattern for later federal programs.

BUGBEE:[28]

I think certainly it set a pattern, and I'll tell you why.

How much a previous pattern there was, I don't really know. I sat in on the executive sessions of the Senate committee which rewrote the bill. On that committee were Senator Murray, who seldom came and deputized Lister Hill to chair the committee; Robert Taft; Robert LaFollette, Jr., from Wisconsin; a senator from Missouri; and another from Louisiana.

The consequential ones were Taft and Hill. Hill tended to give Taft anything he wanted, within reason. I think Lister Hill felt that help in passage from the Republicans and the priority he would get for aid to the South were what he needed. They probably were.

Later, when Oveta Culp Hobby became secretary of the Department of Health, Education, and Welfare under Dwight Eisenhower, she somehow was able to persuade the administration and Congress to make the Hill-Burton formula apply for all Department of Health, Education, and Welfare grants. The cities certainly got a blow when that happened.

The Senate committee, with the Hill-Burton program and its grants-in-aid formula, was creating not only new law, but also the basis for new public policy. I.S. Falk was involved in the policy discussions. Falk was the director of research and statistics for the Social Security Administration. He and his staff played a key role in developing the Hill–Burton formula.

His recollection of the events, problems, and accomplishments follow.

FALK:[29]

The Hill–Burton bill began as a bill-drafter's rehash of the hospital construction program that had been Title XII in the Wagner National Health Act of 1939, S. 1620. It also drew on S. 3230, of the 76th Congress—the Wagner-George National Health Act of 1940—which provided for both construction and early year maintenance support grants and which was favorably reported by Senator Murray (Committee on Labor and Education) in Report Number 1558, April 30, 1940, but which was not enacted. It was subsequently in the Wagner-Murray-Dingell bill.

The bill was introduced in 1943 and was referred to Senator Murray's committee. A subcommittee of the full Senate committee actually did the work on the bill. Lister Hill was chairman of the subcommittee on that bill for executive committee review in the Senate (not public hearings).

The situation was somewhat complicated because the bill had been introduced in the Senate by Hill and Burton. Before the bill came up for review, Burton had been appointed to the Supreme Court, so that, when the bill was to go through executive hearings and markup, it was all on the Senate side, with Hill handling it alone because Burton was no longer there.

I remember those executive sessions very well, having been heavily involved. Vane Hoge, Louis Reed, and others in the Public Health Service, George Bugbee from the AHA, and others also participated in those sessions.

The bill was in difficulties because the financial proposals in it, the federal distribution of funds to the states, were unacceptable to the states represented in the subcommittee (mainly Senator Allen Ellender of Louisiana). Also, LaFollette from Wisconsin and Robert Taft had problems with the bill—but for different reasons.

Lister Hill was in a quandary about what to do. He and Murray put their heads together. They called me one day and told me the situation behind the scene. They asked me if I would figure out some kind of financing arrangement that would make the bill potentially acceptable. Bob Taft had said that there was no point in giving a lot of federal money to the rich states but that it was OK to give it to the poor states. LaFollette had said, "Which are the rich states? None of us is rich enough to deal with this problem."

Allen Ellender said, "Why should we give money to New York State and Massachusetts in order to build hospitals? They have got all the hospitals they can use and more. We need them down in poor little Louisiana."

I can remember pulling some of my staff together and saying, "I am not altogether happy with some of the provisions that the Public Health

Service and the AHA have put into this bill. I liked it better the way we had it in the 1939 Wagner bill or in the Wagner-George bill of 1940 or in the Wagner-Murray-Dingell bill, but that's past history. Let's see what we can do to straighten this out." So we drafted a whole series of alternative financing provisions.

The main problem was to get a financial formulation that would be applicable to the perspectives of rich states and poor states, big states and small states, and so on, because the needs and issues were diverse. The key problem was that the drafters had been working with specifications that were based on fixed formulas for grants. You couldn't get enough flexibility in the programs with a provision of that kind. So, two or three people of my staff who were very knowledgeable in this field (we had been working extensively on diverse federal grant patterns for public assistance and health programs) really put their heads together with me and said, "We'll have to put together a variable plan formula that is peculiarly adaptable to the hospital field."

Of course, in the hospital field there were two different categories of variables that produced coinciding results: the question of the need of the state or the community for federal aid in general, and the question of the particular community's need for hospital care. The key to that problem is that, if the community, statewide or part of a state, is poor, generally it has fewer hospital beds, and it has a higher need for support. If it is a well-to-do area, or a well-to-do community, it has a more generous supply of hospitals, more generous support for them, and less need for general federal support. So we said, "Let's play with that kind of formula."

We tried various approaches to a variable grant formula. Finally, we came up with a particular variant that was accepted by the subcommittee and enacted.

It is a peculiar formula. I have never really understood why it was accepted. The second or third time at the executive sessions of the subcommittee we had a list of the states on a blackboard and showed how this formula would work; when we got through with a presentation, Lister Hill took a canvass of the committee—the subcommittee was there and some other members of the full committee. He asked, "How many here understand what we have been talking about?"

One hand went up. It was Senator Taft's. He said, "Because I know what he means when he says a square of the allotment percentage derived according to the factors required to be considered."

We had formulas through which the states with per capita income equal to or above the national average would get lesser shares of the federal appropriations. It was a compromise formula. We had to work in that square in order to get big enough grants to the poorest states, granting them the

credit, so to speak, in the formula because (a) they had more financial need
for hospitals than the richer states, and (b) they had more need for hospital
care. So we squared the formula.

Alanson Willcox had been sitting in.[30] He was the assistant general
counsel for the Public Health Service. He drafted the report for the Lister
Hill–Murray committee. If you read that report you will find some very
skillful writing.

The bill went through the full Senate committee, the Senate, and the
House in a breeze.

That is how the Hill-Burton formula came into being, with its famous
(or infamous) square formula. The fellow whose ingenuity made that formula possible was a member of my staff named Daniel Gerig. I never forget
to give him credit for it.

Hill-Burton was quite a step forward in federal support.

FALK:[31]

It [the Hill-Burton Act] was not only the first major health legislation
enacted after the war, but it had another nearly unique quality. It was the
first bill enacted by Congress with a grant formula since the days of 1870 or
1880 or 1890, when a variable grant formula was used in the land grant and
related acts.

Under Hill-Burton, the federal government was to make money available under prescribed conditions; for example, it required a state plan, matching funds from local applicants, and so on. The states certified that they
would observe the various conditions, thereby becoming eligible for their
share of the federal funds.

At the level of the individual institution, the Hill-Burton grant was
only intended to provide partial funding for any approved project. The applicant—as opposed to the community—had to bear the nonfederal share of
the project's cost. The applicant also had to agree to various conditions for
construction and for subsequent operations.

The portion of a project's costs that had to be met by the applicant
could be determined individually, within specified limits, by each state.

FALK:[32]

The states got the federal money. The state could say to the applicant
that was going to build a hospital that it—the applicant—would have to find
the money, not the state agency. A state could say that we get so many
million federal dollars (according to the formula), we have applications for
so much money, any applicant that meets such and such conditions can get
up to (not to exceed, let's say) 50 percent of their expected costs from this

federal grant pool, or 40 percent, or 33 percent. Some states had a 50 percent formula, I don't think there were any higher than that. Connecticut had a 33 percent provision. That was a variable with the state, dependent on how best to spread the federal grant which they got through the federal formula among the applicants whom the state agency could properly approve.

The state didn't have to put any of its own money into the program except for the support of their own administrative expenses.

As good as the bill was, there were two provisions that caused trouble. One caused a potential problem immediately and the other later. The first was President Truman's objection that an advisory council of nongovernment persons could override the surgeon general on some provisions for approval or nonapproval of applicants. The president thought it was at least bad policy and possibly unconstitutional. When he signed the bill into law he said he had first considered a veto, then accepted the bill, but announced he would ask Congress later to amend the act.

The other element in the bill that caused a problem was the provision that allowed federal grants despite "equal but separate" operation of aided institutions. Until the Supreme Court's decision came on that, the bill remained intact except for amendments later.

In general, except for the separate but equal provision, the act was flawless, at least in providing federal grants to the states, with no required matching by the states (the applicant institution had to provide the matching funds) but with a carefully developed set of conditions which the state and the federal agency would be required to see that the applicant met. It was not until the 1970s that we got the beginning of a new battle about the Hill-Burton Act, about the availability of "free" services from Hill-Burton–aided hospitals or other facilities for people who couldn't pay. That issue is still going on. The performance by the federal bureaucracy on this has been outrageous, because they have blatantly amended the contract agreements under which grants were received by applicants, and spent by them, by putting on requirements that go beyond those that were contracted for when the original aid was awarded.

———

Every state that wished to participate in the Hill-Burton program was required to develop a plan for implementing the program. Richard Stull, who later became president of the American College of Hospital Administrators, was a young man with much of his career ahead of him when he was approached to perform this task for the state of California.

———

STULL:[33]

Graham Davis left the Duke Endowment to go to work for the W.K. Kellogg Foundation. There Graham was approached by a Dr. Phillip Gilman, retired chief of surgery at Stanford Medical School, in San Francisco, California. He asked Graham about getting somebody to do the statewide planning for their Hill-Burton program. They couldn't find anybody; they didn't know anybody. Graham told them they should contact me. I got a letter from Gilman. I had never planned a major state program. I didn't know anything about it, but I had the confidence of youth.

So I took the gamble and accepted the job, much to my wife's dismay because she thought there were still Indians west of the Mississippi. Nevertheless, I took on the assignment and went to the California State Department of Public Health. My first responsibility was to develop the survey approach, direct the study, and write the plan to be adopted by the state and subsequently by the Public Health Service for approving Hill-Burton programs in California.

I recruited a staff. A lot of them were ex–military people. We trained them in the use of the survey forms and then initiated the surveys, learning all about the state and all about the health facilities in the state and what had to be done. Then we began the process of developing a state plan. Concurrently with this I worked with the legislature to pass enabling legislation in the state of California so that the state would then match federal and local funds. So the funds were one-third national, one-third state, and one-third local, which was quite important for California.

Hill-Burton's Accomplishments

It is both a flaw and strength of human nature that one tends to forget the circumstances that surrounded the need for and that shaped certain decisions and actions. The recent criticisms of the Hill-Burton Act are an example of this. The following observations of Kenneth Williamson, former head of the AHA's Washington bureau, provide a final perspective within which to consider the importance and contribution of Hill-Burton.

WILLIAMSON:[34]

The Hill-Burton Act was a big thing. Hill-Burton is under the gun now, you know. Hospitals are criticizing it all over the place.

I read a letter in the *New York Times* recently from a man who should have known better but [who] exhibited an enormous lack of information and knowledge of the past, because he criticized the federal government for its participation. He mentioned Hill-Burton. He mentioned Medicare and Medicaid and so on. Without those things there would be no hospital field today. Hospital care would be a government program.

Hill-Burton came at a time when we had just had World War II. There had been little invested in the hospital field for some years before the war. It was a period of great neglect of the hospital plant of America and of neglect of all the areas of the country that had no hospitals.

Also, a new kind of physician came out of the war. In fact, he came out discarding the little black bag. He was a guy who was used to having organized means at his disposal. He was trained differently, too. So, a new kind of doctor had come back, and the American people were hearing about the great advances in "modern medicine." Yet in thousands, I mean thousands, of communities all over America there was absolutely no means for modern medical care. You can imagine the pressure that came out of that.

Really from George Bugbee's leadership the hospital field saw that and realized that something had to be done or it was going to burst the bounds some day. There had to be a means by which the health needs of the American public would be met, and that meant more hospitals.

So the Hill-Burton program came about. It was terribly important to the hospital field. There isn't anybody who can see 25 or 30 years ahead and be sure about how certain words will later be interpreted. There is language in the act which said that the hospitals would have to give, within their ability, some free care. It was a very casual thing. It was put in to give a kind of assurance. Now those words are being interpreted in a hard way by the government. Hospitals are being pinned down; they are damning Hill-Burton, but, if they only knew it, Hill-Burton is one reason we still have voluntary hospitals.

———

After the long preparatory work of the Commission on Hospital Care and the planning and lobbying of George Bugbee and some of his colleagues at AHA, plus the extensive involvement of officials and staff people of the Public Health Service, Congress passed what is commonly called the Hill-Burton Act.

The Hospital Survey and Construction Act was signed into law by President Harry Truman in August 1946, becoming Title VI of the Public Health Service Act.[35] The act was designed to be a federal-state partnership, with the federal government providing grants to assist states in inventorying their existing hospitals; surveying the need for the construction of public and nonprofit hospitals; and constructing public and nonprofit hospitals in accordance with the programs developed by the states.

The act carried an initial annual appropriation of $75 million. By the time the program expired in the late 1970s, it had provided approximately $4 billion in grants to nearly 4,000 hospitals and $1.9 billion in loans and loan guarantees to almost 300 hospitals.

George Bugbee once said that passing Hill-Burton was one thing, but that eternal vigilance was needed to protect the act from the tinkering and tampering of well-meaning and ill-meaning persons and forces. Some amendments were made through the years as they became necessary, but many attempts to drastically change the act were turned aside. To see Bugbee in action defending Hill–Burton, read his testimony before a Senate committee considering a change in the act (Appendix F).

Regardless of how it is viewed today, the Hill–Burton program was a landmark effort, establishing the foundation of much of today's hospital system. Not only did it accomplish its goals of increasing the nation's supply of hospital beds and of improving their distribution through regionalization, but it did so in a manner that established a new template for future federal-state relationships.

Notes

(Transcripts of the oral histories cited here are housed in the library of the American Hospital Association, 840 North Lake Shore Drive, Chicago, Illinois 60611. The Oral History collection is a joint project of the Hospital Research and Educational Trust and the AHA.)

1. There was at least one exception to the stoppage of hospital building during the war: Congress in 1941 passed the Lanham Act, which provided for the building of hospital facilities in burgeoning war industry areas.

2. Murphy was mayor of Detroit from 1930 to 1933, when he resigned to accept an appointment by President Franklin D. Roosevelt as governor general of the Philippines. In 1936 he returned to Michigan and was elected governor. He failed to be reelected in 1938, probably because of his refusal to remove sit-down strikers from the automobile plants in Flint by force. Roosevelt appointed him attorney general in 1939. He remained in that job only a short time, until Roosevelt appointed him an associate justice of the U.S. Supreme Court in 1940. Murphy served on the Court until his death at age 59 in 1949.

3. *I.S. Falk, In the First Person: An Oral History.* See Profiles of Participants, in the center of this book, for biographical information.

4. *George Bugbee, In the First Person: An Oral History.* See Profiles of Participants for biographical information.

5. See Profiles of Participants for biographical information.

6. Van Steenwyk, director of the Blue Cross plan in Minneapolis, was a pioneer in the field and the first person to use a blue cross as the symbol for a group prepayment plan.

7. *Bugbee, Oral History.*

8. Davis was president of the AHA in 1948 and was probably the only non–hospital administrator ever to serve in that post. He was head of the hospital division of the W.K. Kellogg Foundation for a number of years. Before that, he had been with the Duke Endowment in a similar position.

9. O'Connor was a former law partner of President Franklin D. Roosevelt.

10. See Profiles of Participants for biographical information.

11. See Profiles of Participants for biographical information.

12. The Commission on Hospital Care did not study the financing of hospital care, so a few years later the Commission on Financing of Hospital Care was formed to do so.

13. Bachmeyer was a good choice to direct the commission. He was a prodigious worker, and he had first-hand knowledge of the problems of hospitals and of providing health care. His associate director, Maurice J. Norby, had had extensive experience in the Blue Cross Commission, as director of statistics and research under C. Rufus Rorem, as well as experience as the developer and first director of the Blue Cross plan in Pittsburgh. Norby was also knowledgeable about the operation of the AHA, because in his Blue Cross Commission work he had been housed at AHA headquarters and had worked alongside AHA officials.

14. The remaining members of the Commission on Hospital Care were Katharine J. Densford, director, School of Nursing, University of Minnesota; Evarts A. Graham, chairman, department of surgery, Washington University School of Medicine; Wilton L. Halverson, director of public health, State of California; Charles F. Kettering, vice president and director, General Motors Corporation; Ada Belle McCleery, former administrator, Evanston (Illinois) Hospital; James Alexander Miller, professor of clinical medicine, Columbia University; Leroy M. S. Miner, former dean, School of Dentistry, Harvard University; Claude W. Munger, director, St. Luke's Hospital, New York City; Rt. Rev. Msgr. Thomas O'Dwyer, director of Catholic charities and hospitals, Archdiocese of Los Angeles; William F. Ogburn, chairman, department of sociology, University of Chicago; Clarence Poe, editor, *Progressive Farmer*, Raleigh, N.C.; J. Barrye Wall, editor, Farmville (Virginia) *Herald*; Frank J. Walter, administrator, Good Samaritan Hospital (Portland); and Matthew Woll, vice president, American Federation of Labor.

15. *Bugbee, Oral History.*

16. *Maurice J. Norby, In the First Person: An Oral History.*

17. Parran was appointed surgeon general in 1936 by President Franklin D. Roosevelt. He continued to serve as surgeon general under President Harry S. Truman, leaving to become dean of the School of Public Health at the University of Pittsburgh.

18. *Norby, Oral History.*

19. James Hague, director of publications and corporate secretary of the AHA, observed that:

> Dr. Parran had a notion of a big program that finally turned out to be Hill-Burton. He needed data to sell it to the Congress. . . . Dr. Parran had a political, legislative problem on his hands and he wanted those data and he wanted the fact-finding well done. So the PHS was the hidden financier of the whole thing. All the statistical work was done by PHS people. As the reports came out, they went to the PHS, so the PHS was privy to the data before those data were public. That work, of course, made the Hill-Burton legislation possible *[James Hague, In the First Person: An Oral History]*.

20. *Norby, Oral History.*

21. Ibid.

22. *Bugbee, Oral History.*

23. *Nelson Cruikshank, In the First Person: An Oral History.* See Profiles of Participants for biographical information.

24. *John R. Mannix, In the First Person: An Oral History.* See Profiles of Participants for biographical information.

25. Bugbee said of that period, "Every hospital was planning a building fund drive."

26. *Bugbee, Oral History.*

27. *Hague, Oral History.* See Profiles of Participants for biographical information.

28. *Bugbee, Oral History.*

29. *Falk, Oral History.*

30. Years later, Willcox became the chief counsel for Aetna.

31. *Falk, Oral History.*

32. Ibid.

33. *Richard Stull, In the First Person: An Oral History.* See Profiles of Participants for biographical information.

34. *Kenneth Williamson, In the First Person: An Oral History.* See Profiles of Participants for biographical information.

35. Bugbee had held out for giving the federal council more than advisory powers in the Hill-Burton bill. This position was unpopular with President Truman. There was some intimation that the president might veto the bill for this reason and because of its separate but equal clause. When talking about the pens used in the signing of the bill Bugbee said, "I got two of the pens—sort of a consolation prize from friends. I wasn't invited to the signing, which was, I imagine, a calculated insult that I was too naive to care about. I had gone back and forth between Chicago and Washington so much I was delighted not to make another trip."

4

The Roots of Medicare

Medicare, which was passed by Congress in 1965 and became effective in 1966, made the federal government, through the Social Security Administration, directly responsible for the health care of Social Security beneficiaries. This action has been called a watershed, a breakthrough, and a decisive step in federal-state relationships and responsibilities. No longer could it be said that the states were basically responsible for the health care of the aged, either as a prime factor or in partnership or shared responsibility with the federal government.

This historic legislation did not come about through a single action of Congress, however, but through evolution. The Committee on the Costs of Medical Care furnished basic statistical data and recommendations for assessments of health care needs. Its data were updated by the work of the Commission on Hospital Care and the Commission on Financing of Hospital Care.

Some observers trace the direct lineage of Medicare much farther back. They see the first step in federal involvement as the provision of hospitals for American seamen in the early days of the republic and in the emergence of the Public Health Service in 1799 to administer the hospitals and to protect the nation from disease and pestilence.

Probably more to the point is the influence of the Wisconsin group of economists, which led the country in many social advances. Members of the group were proteges of John R. Commons,[1] many of whose ideas were seminal in the social and labor reform movements of the early twentieth century.

The American Association of Labor Legislation (AALL) was formed out of this Wisconsin group in 1906 under the leadership of John B. Andrews. The AALL grew to 3,000 or more members, including economists, political scientists, attorneys, social workers, and other public-spirited persons.

The AALL's first major effort was passage of state workmen's compensation legislation. Its next step, in conjunction with AMA leaders, was the formation in 1912 of a social insurance committee to study health insurance.

Health insurance also became an issue in the 1912 presidential campaign, in which Republican incumbent William Howard Taft, was opposed by Democrat Woodrow Wilson and former President Theodore Roosevelt as the Progressive, or Bull Moose, candidate. In a dramatic appearance at the Bull Moose convention, Theodore Roosevelt made an emotional presentation which he called his "confession of faith."[2] Among other things, he called for social welfare for women and children, women's suffrage, recall of judicial decisions, workmen's compensation, farm relief, and health insurance in industry. This was the first time health insurance had been an issue in an American presidential campaign.

In the meantime, the AALL committee designed a model health insurance bill for state legislatures. This bill was ready by 1915, and it appeared that it would be considered favorably in many states. In 1916 the AMA's social insurance committee recommended government health insurance plans, and several state legislatures began considering the model bill.[3]

Then the United States entered World War I.

One can only speculate as to whether attitudes in this country changed during the war. It is true that the government set up restrictions, asserted the authority necessary to support the war effort, and became a compelling force in the daily lives of the population. Thus, when the war was over, it is likely that people reacted against government restriction and interference and wished to return to the old ways.

In any case, after World War I the tide turned against health insurance. In 1918 California defeated a referendum for state health insurance; in 1919 the New York State Assembly failed to pass a health insurance bill; in 1920 the AMA reversed its position and opposed state government insurance. Doctors returning from the war wanted independence because they feared government interference. Even labor unions were afraid that government health insurance would be a step toward reducing union influence in bargaining. In addition, after a slight economic decline in 1920, the country repudiated Woodrow Wilson's idealistic visions and elected as president Warren G. Harding, who promised a return to "normalcy."

During the near-decade of prosperity that followed, there were agitations for a government health care program. In 1921 Congress passed the Sheppard-Towner Act, which subsidized child and maternal health care.[4]

The Sheppard-Towner Act, however, was the exception to the rule: rarely during this period did the federal government inject itself into a social issue.

Of greater influence on later events was the five-year study by the Committee on the Costs of Medical Care (see chapter 2). The CCMC recommended group health care insurance, group practice for physicians and other health professionals, and statewide planning for health needs. It also suggested improving health education—for physicians, dentists, nurses, nurse midwives, pharmacists, and nurses' aides. This study was done so skillfully that for the first time the United States had a picture of where its health care system was and where it might want to go in the future.

Another factor entered the scene: voluntary hospital insurance. The popular example used to mark the beginning of voluntary hospital insurance is the experiment at Baylor University Hospital in Dallas. In 1929 Justin Ford Kimball, executive vice president of the university, proposed a prepayment plan under which school teachers in Dallas could assure themselves of up to 21 days of hospital care at the Baylor University Hospital for a premium of 50¢ a month.[5]

The rapid growth of hospital service plans modeled on the Baylor plan and others of that period is discussed in later chapters, however it should be noted that the growth of hospital service plans, along with commercial insurance coverage, began to have political significance. Some of the more conservative politicians saw voluntary prepaid hospital insurance as the answer to national health insurance. Some began to talk about voluntary plans supplemented by government subsidies for the poor and near-poor in general, and for the aged poor in particular.

Other events were taking place in health affairs as the nation moved into the Great Depression. The American Federation of Labor (AF of L), the strongest union group in 1932, changed its position and endorsed social insurance. A year later, the AHA approved private and voluntary health insurance.

When Franklin D. Roosevelt took office as president, on March 4, 1933, he faced many problems that had to be dealt with immediately. Fifteen to 17 million persons were unemployed, and many of them were unable to feed their families. Almost overnight the banks of the country were closed. Everything seemed to be at a standstill.

In that first month, the government acted under the president's leadership in what Nathan Miller has called the "Roosevelt whirlwind."[6] Congress voted $500 million in 1933 for immediate relief under an agency called the Federal Emergency Relief Administration (FERA). This agency was headed by Harry Hopkins, who had headed New York's relief organization when Roosevelt was governor. Within hours of the passage of the federal legislation, millions of dollars were shuttled to the states for direct relief—

for food, clothing, fuel, rent, whatever the immediate needs were. Some small part of that money may have helped with medical care, but the majority of it went for food and shelter.

The relief measures, although welcome, were stopgaps at best. The state of the economy was still the major problem. At Roosevelt's urging, Congress created many agencies to correct the system. This "alphabet soup" of agencies—AAA, CCC, FERA, NRA, PWA, WPA, and so on—was fair game for the humorists of the day. All of the agencies, however, were established in an effort to put people back to work, to set fair agricultural prices and fair wages, and to feed the hungry.

No matter how hard Congress and the president worked to find solutions to the problems of the day, there was always the danger that Americans would be misled by persons propounding radical social movements and utopias. Senator Huey Long (D–La.) told his followers that he had a plan for sharing the wealth in which every man would be a king. In California, Dr. Francis E. Townsend said that his Old Age Revolving Pension Plan was the solution to the economic crisis. He would have the federal government pay each unemployed person over 60 years of age a pension of $200 a month. (This amount was far greater than the average industrial or clerical worker earned at that time.) The entire $200 would have to be spent during the month in order to be eligible for a payment the next month. The plan would be financed by a 2 percent sales tax. Hundreds of Townsend clubs were formed among the elderly. Meanwhile, the president was under pressure to do something to counteract the demagoguery of Townsend, Long, and others who were exciting the emotions of the millions of people who were suffering in the depression.[7]

Roosevelt's move was to appoint a cabinet-level Committee on Economic Security to study the situation regarding unemployment insurance, old age assistance and pensions, and health care. It is significant that this was a cabinet-level committee and therefore under the direct control of the president. Roosevelt called for quick action: the committee was named in June 1934 and had instructions to report and recommend action by the end of the year.

Frances Perkins, secretary of labor, was appointed chairman. Other members of the committee were Henry Morgenthau, Jr., secretary of the treasury; Homer Cummings, attorney general; Henry Wallace, secretary of agriculture; and Harry Hopkins, then administrator of FERA.

The Committee on Economic Security used staff members and facilities of the various departments represented. It was financed, partially at least, by funds from the WPA. Edwin E. Witte, chairman of the department of economics at the University of Wisconsin, was chosen as executive director of the committee. Witte was outstanding in the field of labor legislation. Arthur J. Altmeyer, an assistant secretary of labor who was also from Wisconsin, was selected to head the technical committee, whose duties were to assist the executive director and to direct the larger committee's studies and investigations.[8] There was also an advisory council of 23 members: 5 labor leaders, 5 employers, and 13 members of the public interested in social welfare. The function of the council was to:

> . . . convey to the committee the views of interested individuals and groups outside the government, but the council was not expected to make a formal report. . . . The advisory council functioned much more independently than had been originally contemplated. It also made a lengthy report which contained recommendations differing in some respects from the final recommendations of the Committee on Economic Security.[9]

The Committee on Economic Security worked hard and fast, reporting to Congress in January 1935. The committee had been able to design a social security system that was not based on a dole. In a casual conversation with Supreme Court Justice Harlan F. Stone, Frances Perkins expressed fear that any social security program might fail if tested in the Supreme Court. The justice whispered in reply, "The taxing power of the federal government, my dear; the taxing power is sufficient for everything you want and need."[10]

That was the secret: unemployment insurance was based on taxation of employers; old age pensions were based on payroll taxes levied on both employer and employee. There was expected to be no need for general federal funds as long as actuarial figures were correct and Congress was willing to levy sufficient taxes.

The committee wanted to recommend a health insurance measure, but at least two things prevented it. First, no plan had been developed for recommendation. Second, and perhaps just as important, the AMA was adamantly opposed to federal health insurance. Some of the president's advisors feared that, if the administration recommended health insurance, other parts of the Social Security program—old age pensions and unemployment insurance in particular—were likely to be defeated in Congress or delayed in enactment.

Roosevelt needed a positive social security program passed before the election of 1936, and he felt that he could not afford a long-drawn-out battle with the AMA. It seemed best to enact as much of the program as possible. He was urged by secretary Perkins and Arthur Altmeyer to try another time for health insurance.

The Social Security bill without health insurance passed in August 1935, Roosevelt won in 1936, and he continued to refer to health insurance as a subject that needed to be addressed.

Wilbur Cohen, who in 1968 was appointed secretary of health, education, and welfare by President Lyndon Johnson, originally went to Washington, D.C., in 1934, after graduating from the University of Wisconsin with a degree in economics. He went to work for one of his Wisconsin professors, Edwin Witte, the executive director of the Committee on Economic Security. Cohen recalls how and why the committee was formed.

COHEN:[11]

The Social Security program was the very major result of the Great Depression of 1929. That depression really completely demoralized not only the American economy, but by 1932 it had really demoralized America's faith in itself, its institutions, and its people.

The result was that many people felt that they'd lost everything. The fact that they had saved and worked hard didn't result in their being able to sustain themselves. It was the most catastrophic blow that could be imagined. As a result, when Roosevelt became president of the United States in 1933, there were pending in Congress a number of bills on unemployment insurance and/or old age assistance.

Roosevelt's advisors recommended that instead of going forward piecemeal on these ideas, that they be studied in a comprehensive way. Harry Hopkins and Frances Perkins were the leaders in the effort, and it was as a result of their suggestions and others that a cabinet-level committee—the Committee on Economic Security—was established.

I.S. Falk, who had previously contributed so much to the research of the Committee on the Costs of Medical Care (see chapter 2) also joined in the work of the Committee on Economic Security—particularly in the health studies. He describes the makeup and the work of the new committee.

FALK:[12]

By mid-1934 the president had issued an executive order creating the Committee on Economic Security and directed it to explore measures to deal with the risks of economic insecurity, including the risks of loss of income arising out of illness and the costs of medical care. The committee was formed near the end of June, and it went to work to produce a program for the president and the Congress. A comprehensive structure was created using government people and bringing in many nongovernment people who were knowledgeable about the problems that were going to have to be confronted.

With respect to the field of health—public health, personal health care, medical care, disability, and the risks and losses and the economic burdens arising out of illness—two of us were asked to become members of the cabinet committee staff. Edgar Sydenstricker, who was chief of research at the Milbank Memorial Fund, with which I had been working between the end of the Committee on the Costs of Medical Care and this period, was asked to take charge of the committee's health staff. He accepted on condition that I would join him. I did. So he and I were the primary staff members for those studies and programs relating to health and disability problems.

The committee had advisory committees for the overall structure of the program. They also had a technical board of very distinguished people and a series of actuarial consultants. On our suggestion, because of the complexity of the public relations involved and the complexity of the technical problems, the committee set up a medical advisory committee, with representatives from the various aspects of the medical profession; a public health advisory committee; a hospital advisory board; and a dental advisory committee. Collaterally, because of the proposals that were coming up in the areas of maternal and child health and welfare and related subjects, on recommendation from the people in these fields, there was a committee on child welfare, a nursing advisory committee, and so on.

So, as we were developing analyses and proposals, we met with these various advisory committees and tried out our ideas. We had extensive discussions with them and some considerable disputes, particularly with the medical advisory committee, whose members included some who had been selected from the American Medical Association and related organizations.

The idea of having these various advisory committees was smart for public relations, but it was a stupid idea for the purpose of getting the job done because there were utterly irreconcilable elements in the medical advisory committee. The outlook for getting any consensus was nil. Also, some of the committee members didn't play fair with us. Although it had been agreed that we would be working in camera until the time came for approved and agreed releases, the AMA people immediately broke that promise and began releasing the intramural discussions. This meant floods of telegrams and letters pouring in on the White House, on the members of the committee, and on the chairman and members of the congressional committees that were going to have jurisdiction. This led to a complex and very uncomfortable situation.

At any rate, we proceeded with the studies with the help of our ancillary staff, some of whom came directly from the AMA and acted fairly. I wasn't referring to them; it was a few members of the advisory committees who played games.

We developed a program for federal support for a federal-state system of health services availability. I hesitate to say health insurance, because latitudes would be given to the states as to what kinds of programs they might prefer or might want to enact. In addition, we developed proposals for strengthening the public health services and then the programs for disability insurance.

When we came up with the proposal for a federal-state program in the health field, two things happened to us that were very significant. One is that we caught hell from the AMA and various other groups that didn't want any such thing as "government intrusion" in medical care; and we caught hell from the labor union people, who didn't want any such thing, saying, "You are going to come up with a program that will depend on state benefits, state insurance programs, you give them [the states] choices and so on. We, the labor union people, are going to have to fight these battles out in 48 different states. We don't want any of that. We want a straight national system."

On the other hand, there were other national groups that said, "A national system in the health field! You are out of your minds. This is not for money payments, this is for service provisions. Service provisions have to be geared to the local scene, and local control, and local options."

We were on the horns of a dilemma. We had to opt for something, so we developed a program on a federal-state basis, knowing that some of our strongest potential supporters weren't going to like it.

When the economic security (later to be known as Social Security) bill went to Congress, it had in one section authorization for the Social Security Board to continue further studies in this, that, and in health insurance. Those three or four words precipitated so many telegrams and so many telephone calls and so much pressure from the medical world, obviously carefully orchestrated, that the chairman of the House committee and the chairman of the Senate committee really were so plagued by the opposition from the medical world that they said, "Look, take your whole economic security bill away, we want no part of it," or words to that effect.

Secretary of Labor Frances Perkins, as chairman of the cabinet committee, became frightened that the whole economic security program, as it was being called, would go down the drain because of the dispute about health insurance. So the matter was taken up to the president.

Roosevelt decided to take advantage of the fact that our medical advisory committee had asked for more time to study the health program proposals. The president approved that delay. A draft of guidelines was given to Congress in a preliminary report, but our definitive reports on the health insurance proposals never were submitted to Congress; and by agreeing to moderate a few words in the bill bearing on further health insurance studies, matters quieted down.

So the health insurance program was deferred and did not see the light of day until some years later. The excuse was given that the health insurance studies had not been carried to the point that a bill was ready for submittal to Congress, which was partly but not quite true.

The public health recommendations did go to Congress. They were enacted, substantially as we submitted them, as Title VI of the Social Security Act. The maternal and child health and welfare programs went in as Title V of the act. They were enacted practically unchanged.

Wilbur Cohen continues with his description of the committee.

COHEN:[13]

Mr. Altmeyer, who came from Wisconsin, and Mr. Witte, who came from Wisconsin, were two of several of the very important leaders who worked with the Committee on Economic Security. That committee really developed the outline of the major provisions that became the Social Security Act of 1935.

However, Roosevelt, Witte, Altmeyer, Perkins were not people who were merely theoreticians. They had all given a lot of thought to the history of social reform; they had been administering programs; they had had contacts with legislators; and they realized that the Social Security program of 1935 would only be a beginning. Franklin D. Roosevelt, when he signed the act, called it a cornerstone in a developing program, and he recognized that there would have to be other changes coming along later.

The act was passed by Congress in less than eight months. It was certainly a tremendous, successfully developed legislative event. It could only have taken place with the backdrop of the depression and under the leadership of Franklin D. Roosevelt.

Though a health insurance program was not included in the Social Security program of 1935, some positive steps were taken to keep the subject of health insurance alive. The day after the Social Security bill was signed, President Roosevelt established an Interdepartmental Committee to Coordinate Health and Welfare Activities. Following this was the National Health Survey. A further step was taken in 1937, with the establishment of the Technical Committee on Medical Care under the interdepartmental committee. The next year the technical committee published a report titled *A National Health Program*. Careful follow-through came with the sponsorship of the National Health Conference. A year later (1939) Senator Robert Wagner (D–N.Y.) introduced a national health bill comprised basically of the recommendations of the National Health Conference. The bill would make matching funds available to states to assist them in meeting minimal federal standards for public health services, child and maternal health care, health services, temporary disability insurance, construction of hospitals and health

centers, and health insurance programs. Matching funds would vary according to the states' per capita wealth. As might be expected, the state health
insurance proposal generated much opposition.

All of this careful preparation of a legislative path came to nought at
the moment, for the AMA organized an effective campaign to defeat the bill,
which died in committee.

Wilbur Cohen talks about the interdepartmental committee.

_____

COHEN:[14]

Immediately upon the passage of the Social Security Act, Mr. Altmeyer
decided that he had to begin research and studies leading to its improvement.
Just a couple of days after the act was passed, he was able to get President
Roosevelt to establish the interdepartmental committee on health to study
how health insurance and other aspects could be developed. In addition, Mr.
Altmeyer began to set up a research staff, which ultimately was headed by
Dr. I.S. Falk. As a result of these efforts, studies relating to health, disability,
death benefits, unemployment insurance benefits, and changes in the welfare
program became a major part of the research and planning work.

_____

Franklin Roosevelt continued to talk about the need for complete social
security from birth to death. A friendly dispute arose about who had originated the term "from the cradle to the grave." When the Beveridge report,
which suggested birth-to-death national health coverage, was published in
England in 1942, some journalists used "from the cradle to the grave" to
describe it. Roosevelt considered that friendly plagiarism.

Some progress in health coverage was made during World War II. In
1943 Congress passed the Emergency Maternal and Infant Care (EMIC) Act
to cover dependents of military personnel. This was direct federal support
for a health program, probably not greatly opposed because it was supportive
of families of the military during wartime.

In 1943 the first of the noted Wagner-Murray-Dingell bills was introduced in Congress. The bill was sponsored by Senator Robert Wagner
(D–N.Y.), Senator James Murray (D–Mont.), and Representative John Dingell (D–Mich.). The bill was the result of many consultations and much
cooperation among labor leaders, physicians, the Public Health Service, the
Social Security Board, the Children's Bureau, the U.S. Employment Service,
and others. It was an ambitious bill, calling for compulsory national health
insurance, nationalized and extended unemployment insurance, expanded
coverage and benefits for old age insurance, new national systems of temporary and permanent disability payments, paid-up Social Security benefits
for veterans for the time they spent in the service, unemployment benefits
for veterans while getting back into civilian life, a nationalized employment

service, and a restructuring of grants-in-aid to states for public assistance. Huthmacher[15] points out that the bill stressed nationalizing programs that had been state administered even though support may have come from federal grants-in-aid or matching funds. The bill failed in committee.

Roosevelt kept referring to the need for health insurance after the demise of the first Wagner-Murray-Dingell bill. In 1944 he talked about an individual's *right* to adequate medical care. That same year the Social Security Board in its annual report recommended comprehensive national health insurance. In his 1945 State of the Union speech, Roosevelt again referred to the right to good medical care; however, in that same year, the California legislature defeated Governor Earl Warren's proposal for comprehensive state health insurance. Physicians labeled it "socialized medicine."

Franklin Roosevelt died in Warm Springs, Georgia, in April 1945. Harry S. Truman, although largely unprepared for the presidency when he succeeded Roosevelt, was a decisive man. He was willing to take the responsibility for making tough decisions, and he was stubborn once he had made one.

In spite of having an unfinished war on his hands, a difficult ally in the USSR, and a powerful and colorful leader to follow, Truman took a determined position supporting national health insurance.

He was the first president of the United States to do so, and he did it forthrightly, time and again—in messages to Congress and in other public statements, as well as in remarks to the press.

For example, in a letter of September 9, 1949, to Dr. Sam Roberts, who had warned him of the danger of national health insurance, Truman said:

> . . . there is something wrong with the health of this country and I am trying to find a remedy for it. When it comes to a point where a man getting $2,400 a year has to pay $500 for prenatal care and then an additional hospital bill on top, there is something wrong with the system and I am going to try to remedy it. I suggest you doctors had better be hunting for a remedy yourselves unless you want a drastic one.[16]

On July 11, 1952, in a letter to his cousin Ethel Noland, Truman wrote, "I am sorry that Nellie has had to go back to the hospital. What a bunch of robbers they are! Why can anyone be against my health program? We'd be able to meet situations like Nellie's if we had it."[17]

Truman was in New York City in January 1954, after President Eisenhower had delivered his State of the Union address to Congress, and reporters asked him to comment on the address. In his diary Truman wrote:

I told them that Ike's New Deal recommendations merited support, that his political statements had the usual demagogic sound. I was thinking particularly about his statement that he is against "Socialized Medicine." So is everyone. The American Medical Association in 1952 had a mild case of hydrophobia over my suggestion that a health tax be levied by the federal government so the ordinary fellow could pay his doctor and hospital bills when an emergency arose in his family.

Most people can't pay $12.50 to $25.00 a day for a hospital room and $500.00 for a minor operation in addition to nurse hire and incidentals. So I thought, and I still think, that a nest egg held out of the regular pay as is social security might meet the situation. If the propaganda of the AMA is studied, you'd find the doctors don't want guaranteed payments for fees. Why I'll never know.[18]

In his first health message, in 1945, Truman recommended to Congress comprehensive prepaid medical insurance for persons of all ages as a part of Social Security.[19] Truman said everyone should have "ready access" to all necessary medical, hospital, and related services. Coverage was recommended for all employed persons and their dependents. The financing suggested was a 4 percent tax on wages and salaries up to $3,600 a year. Needy persons and other groups he said could be taken care of with funds from the general revenue. Truman wanted the proposed plan to cover doctor, hospital, nursing, laboratory, and dental services. He countered the arguments of "socialized medicine" by saying there should be a free choice of doctors and hospitals.

A second Wagner-Murray-Dingell bill was introduced in Congress in 1945; this one included the provisions recommended by President Truman. (A request for veterans' benefits was not carried over from the 1943 bill, because the GI Bill of Rights had been enacted in the meantime.) A committee for national health insurance was organized to promote the new bill, but to no avail. The bill foundered.

The following year, 1946, was one of substantial activity but little in the way of results in health legislation. The Republicans introduced the Taft-Smith-Ball bill to counter the Wagner-Murray-Dingell bill. The Republican bill called for $200 million in matching funds for states to provide medical care for the poor. This failed to pass. One bright spot, however, was that the Hill-Burton Act was passed in 1946 (see chapter 3).

In 1947 a familiar routine was played. President Truman sent a message to Congress asking for a national health program; the Wagner-Murray-Dingell bill was re-introduced; the Taft-Smith-Ball bill was re-introduced. Neither of the bills passed.

The next year, 1948, was a presidential election year. Truman, running for reelection, again advocated national health insurance. He instructed Oscar

Ewing, the federal security administrator, to call a national assembly to consider the problems of health care. The assembly approved all the previous recommendations of the president except national health insurance as a method of financing medical care.[20] The AMA organized resistance to national health insurance through what it called a "national education campaign." Truman was reelected, and a Democratic Congress was returned. Many party members considered this a mandate for enacting a national health insurance law.

The Republicans brought forth in 1949 their version of a health bill, the Flanders-Ives bill, which many considered merely a rewarming of the Taft-Smith-Ball bill of 1946. It called for support of health care through subsidies to private insurance companies.

The AMA reacted to the reelection of President Truman and the return of a Democratic Congress with great alarm. It quickly assessed each member $25 and hired a public relations firm to organize a campaign against any national health insurance legislation and to educate the public about the dangers of such a system of insurance. Apparently the AMA felt that the rise in the number of Blue Cross and other private insurance subscribers might obviate the need for a federal or state system of insurance, so it supported private insurance.

I.S. Falk and Wilbur Cohen reflect on the events in which they were participants during the period of the Wagner-Murray-Dingell bills and the development of proposals for insurance for Social Security beneficiaries.

———

FALK:[21]

The impasse on the Wagner-Murray-Dingell bills persisted year after year. The impasse led me to begin to think about the possibilities of having a paid-up health insurance plan for the beneficiaries of the Social Security system particularly, but not limited to the aged, recognizing that it might later extend to the disabled when they might become beneficiaries. (They weren't yet under the Social Security program at the time.) But it could extend to survivors of covered and insured persons. I undertook, with members of my Bureau of Research and Statistics staff, a systematic exploration of how such a compromise proposal might be designed, what its specifications could be, what its scope and potential impact and effectiveness might be, what such a proposal might cost, and how it would fit within the framework of financial measures such as payroll taxes, general revenue support, or otherwise. We worked out the specifications systematically and developed the design of the program and the cost estimates rather quietly and with very little about this work known throughout the Social Security Administration.

When we arrived at the point where we had a systematic presentation ready, I showed a copy of it in April 1952 to Wilbur Cohen, who was then technical assistant to the Social Security commissioner. He in turn called this

possible program development to the attention of Mr. Oscar Ewing, who
was the federal security administrator.

Mr. Ewing seized upon it very vigorously. He had been displaying
indications of presidential ambitions and was very much concerned with the
possibilities of broadening the scope of the social insurance program, particularly with reference to what might be done in the health insurance field. He
had been less than enthusiastic about the Wagner–Murray–Dingell bills. He
indicated that he thought that this was potentially a useful, perhaps even a
promising alternative approach to be pursued. He read the draft report and
asked me to confer with him about it. He explored it, had various members
of his immediate staff and the general counsel review it. He also made drafts
of it available to some other people outside of federal government, people
he knew well, whose judgment he respected.

Attention to the proposal became quite extensive, long before I thought
it was ready for general public discussion. However, the development and
spread couldn't be contained, so Mr. Ewing submitted the proposal for review to the various responsible authorities in the federal government: the
Bureau of the Budget, the Treasury Department, and other departments of
the government. He also made copies available to some of the staff in the
White House.

President Truman was a little cool about acting on our proposal, because the Magnuson Commission on the Health Needs of the Nation was
approaching completion of its studies. Mr. Truman, I was told, was reluctant
to inject a new set of proposals into the political scene, since it might intrude
into the issue he had delegated to that commission. But he did authorize the
Bureau of the Budget to, in turn, authorize Mr. Ewing to proceed to make
the proposal public and to make the design of the program available to
possible sponsors of legislation in the Congress.

Accordingly, in the middle of 1952, Mr. Ewing released the content
of the proposed program at a press conference, and a bill was prepared and
was made available to Senators Murray and Hubert Humphrey [D–Minn.],
and to Representatives Dingell and [Emanuel] Celler [D–N.Y.], and through
them in turn to others. The proposal was that beneficiaries, primarily old
age beneficiaries, of the Social Security program should become eligible for
a paid-up program of health benefits, rather broadly designed to extend to
hospital, physician, and some collateral services. The costs of the program
were to be met by a relatively small adjustment of the payroll taxes that were
being paid by employers and employees covered by the Old Age and Survivors Insurance program.

The program, as a whole, was very well received except by the American Medical Association and some related health professional organizations.
It was quite well received by most of the insurance industry, which had long

been plagued by the difficulties of embracing within their programs the aged—the people who had the greatest need for health care and, generally speaking, the least means for obtaining health insurance. Insurance carriers in very broad measure thought that they would be relieved under this program of an obligation to extend their insurance carrier functions to the aged.

The bill Falk mentions was different from the Wagner-Murray-Dingell bills in that it was designed for Social Security beneficiaries. This new bill was generally known as the Murray-Dingell bill or the Murray-Humphrey-Dingell-Celler bill. It was introduced into Congress in April 1952. This was a presidential election year, so Truman took no position on the bill out of deference to the Democratic candidate who would be nominated that summer. (Senator Wagner's name does not appear on the bill because he had resigned from the Senate in 1949 due to poor health.)

Cohen also comments on this period when emphasis was changing from the national coverage of the Wagner-Murray-Dingell bills to coverage for Social Security beneficiaries only.

COHEN:[22]

In about 1950, after it appeared that the Wagner-Murray-Dingell bill and the Truman health proposal were not going to go anywhere, Mr. Oscar Ewing, who was then the federal security administrator, asked Mr. Altmeyer whether he had anybody to help him in developing some kind of alternative or substitute health proposal. Mr. Altmeyer assigned that responsibility to me. I checked around with various staff members, and, after talking with them, I produced a memorandum which included in it what we would now call Medicare. When Mr. Ewing received that memo, he was very enthusiastic about that idea and asked us to draft it up. That major responsibility fell to Dr. I.S. Falk. So in 1950–1951, Dr. Falk and I spent a lot of time designing, with the help of other staff members, what ultimately became Medicare, and it was introduced in Congress.

We were not able to get any of the major members of Congress to introduce it. We had to take whatever we could. A number of other people outside the House Ways and Means Committee, like Representative Emanuel Celler and Senator James Murray, originally introduced the bill, but while it was reintroduced each session, it never got anywhere until 1957. Then [in 1957] Representative Aime Forand, a member of the House Ways and Means Committee from Rhode Island, introduced it and thus gave it major public attention. There were hearings on it, and this resulted in making it a major issue in the 1960 campaign.

General Dwight D. Eisenhower, who opposed national health insurance, was elected president of the United States in 1952. On the face of it, little happened in the health field in the early years of the Eisenhower administration except organizationally. A Department of Health, Education, and Welfare (HEW) was formed; it included the Federal Security Agency, of which Social Security was a part. The new department was headed by Oveta Culp Hobby, of Houston. Hobby had formerly been a Democrat of some influence in Texas. Her acceptance of a post with a Republican administration made her relations with leading Democrats, especially Sam Rayburn of Texas, Democratic leader in the House, a little unpleasant sometimes. This was true when she tried to promote administration alternatives to national health insurance.

The administration favored the extension of unemployment insurance, the extension of old age pensions under Social Security, and "a limited government reinsurance plan that would permit the private and non-profit insurance companies to offer broader protection to more of the many families which want and should have it."[23]

Several things that were significant in the evolution of Medicare legislation did take place during the early Eisenhower years.

—A federal program was established in 1956 to provide health care for dependents of military personnel.

—Medical vendors were paid directly for welfare patients (this required federal subsidies to the states for health care).

—A special subcommittee on aging (which later became a special committee) was appointed, with Senator Pat McNamara (D–Mich.) as chairman.

—Disability cash benefits were allowed to totally and permanently disabled persons age 50 or older under an amendment to the Social Security Act.

—The American Hospital Association called for public hearings on various insurance bills.

—The AFL-CIO joined with others in an effort to secure government-sponsored health insurance.

—The first Forand bill was introduced in the House, late in 1957, calling for 60 days of hospital care, surgical, and nursing home benefits for all Social Security beneficiaries.

—The AMA hired a public relations firm to oppose the passage of the Forand bill.

—A Joint Council to Improve Health Care of the Aged was formed to see whether the health care problems of the aged could be taken care of without government participation. The AMA, the AHA, the

American Nursing Home Association, and the American Dental Association were members of the joint council.

—The AMA urged physicians to cut fees for the aged.

—The Kerr-Mills bill was enacted to provide aid to the poor and the aged poor.

One event not listed above was the establishment of the Commission on Financing of Hospital Care. This took place early in the Eisenhower administration, and the commission worked between 1952 and 1954. It was an outgrowth of the Commission on Hospital Care, which had reported almost a decade earlier. The earlier commission had been unable to study the financing of hospital care within its allotted time, thus it had been suggested that financing be covered later, by a separate research group (see Appendixes G and H).

The Commission on Financing of Hospital Care was formed in 1952 with the support of several foundations.[24] The group was chaired by Gordon Gray, president of the University of North Carolina, and had a distinguished membership. A malignant fate seemed to dog the directors of the study. The first director, Graham Davis of the W.K. Kellogg Foundation, resigned early on because of illness. Davis was followed by Arthur Bachmeyer of the University of Chicago, who had been the director of the Commission on Hospital Care. Bachmeyer died in the Washington airport after attending a meeting of the Commission on Financing of Hospital Care. Bachmeyer was succeeded by John H. Hayes, who had retired as superintendent of Lenox Hill Hospital in New York City. Maurice J. Norby, deputy director of the AHA and chief staff person for the Commission on Hospital Care, acted as a special consultant to help see this project through to a successful conclusion.

Robert M. Sigmond, who served on the staff of the Commission on Financing of Hospital Care, commented recently on the commission and the study.

―――――

SIGMOND:[25]

Sometime in 1952 I was approached by Maurice J. Norby, at that time the deputy director of the American Hospital Association under George Bugbee, to consider a position with the newly established staff of the Commission on Financing of Hospital Care. At that time I remember taking a trip to Chicago and staying overnight with the Norbys at their home and having a long talk with Maurice about the situation. He reported that the commission was formed as a logical outgrowth of the Commission on Hospital Care, which had not dealt with issues of financing operations, as contrasted with the issues of capital financing. George Bugbee had decided that they should try the national commission approach again and had raised over one-half million dollars to fund the new commission.

Norby had wanted to name Harry Becker of the United Auto Workers as the director, but George Bugbee was concerned that he would be viewed as being too radical. George Bugbee convinced Graham Davis to head up the new commission, and Norby was successful in convincing Becker to sign on as the associate director. Graham Davis eventually left the commission for health reasons. At that time, Bugbee and Norby brought Bachmeyer in as director.

Becker's primary interest was in the financing of hospital care, but the commission was committed to devoting a significant part of its energies to the issue of rising costs. Norby wanted me to come on and head up that section of the work, explaining that Bachmeyer was not in a position to give direct leadership to this phase of the work and that Becker did not have the background.

Norby indicated that the major issues would be on the financing side, centering around prepayment plans and government role, but that he wanted a really good job done on issues centering around control of hospital costs and wanted someone in charge of that who knew something about hospitals. He told me that I would find it difficult to work with Bachmeyer because of his virtual total deafness and that I would find Harry Becker to be an extremely stimulating guy, who might be hard to handle. Norby assured me that he would help me with handling either Bachmeyer or Becker if I took the job. Subsequently, I met with Harry Becker and found him to be a fascinating person and learned to respect Art Bachmeyer.

I took a leave of absence from the Albert Einstein Medical Center and came to Chicago and spent two years working with the commission. This was a very stimulating experience for me, as very little work had been done on control of hospital costs. So I was dealing with a relatively new field. Also, being with the staff of the national commission gave me an opportunity to meet a great many key people throughout the country and to become quite close with many of them.

As is well documented in the foreword by the chairman, Gordon Gray [Appendix G], at the beginning of each of the three volumes that were published from the commission studies, Arthur Bachmeyer was very much involved in developing the plans for the study and served not only as the director of the study, but also as a member of both the commission and the commission's executive committee. Unfortunately, Bachmeyer died suddenly, immediately following a meeting of the commission in Washington, D.C., on May 22, 1953. He was succeeded by John H. Hayes, who had just retired as director of Lenox Hill Hospital. Hayes was a very fine gentleman and a respected hospital administrator, however he had no special skills in the field of studies and commissions.

The most helpful person to me in connection with my work on the commission was Morris Fishbein, M.D., who served on my committee and offered to give me editorial advice and consultation. I was scared to death that he would inject his philosophy into the report, but he never did so. He read every page and made detailed editorial suggestions, line by line, all of which were extremely helpful. He really taught me how to write. I would meet with him at his home for lunch about once every two weeks and he couldn't possibly have been more helpful.

I was not directly involved in the other two reports of the commission, namely, the report on prepayment and the report on financing hospital care for nonwage and low-income groups.

The weakest part of the work on the commission, I believe, was in the category of financing hospital care for nonwage and low-income groups. This was under the direction of Carl Schmidt, but Harry Becker insisted on taking over. Harry tried to resolve the fundamental differences between the traditional folks in the health establishment and those associated with organized labor, etc., but failed. As a result, the book essentially centers around the problems of the "needy," and divides those who are needy into the aged, the unemployed, the disabled, the low-income group, and public aid recipients. Of the entire book, about 20 pages are devoted to problems of the aged. The recommendations centered around the "needy" aged.

In fact, those who were promoting national solutions had not yet begun to focus in on insurance for the aged as contrasted with national health insurance generally. The labor members of the commission filed dissents against the commission report because it did not pay special attention to the problems of the aged as such. As I recall, the only person who paid special attention to the commission's recommendations for the aged was the guy from commercial health insurance, who was against any attachment of health benefits to OASI [Old Age and Survivors Insurance], even for the needy. As I recall, the entire report with respect to the aged was focused almost exclusively on "means test" approaches, and the commission generally accepted that approach, except for the labor folks.

In another interview, Sigmond spoke about Hayes again and about his own disappointment at the reception the commission's report received.

SIGMOND:[26]

I concentrated on the cost of hospital service. That's volume one. . . . He (John Hayes) theoretically supervised me in the preparation of volume one, with Harry Becker concentrating on volumes two and three. We spent two years on that, and, in my opinion, we came up with some of the best early studies and best ideas on what to do about rising hospital costs, all of which are in the first volume. That commission report came out at a time when nobody cared. Nobody was interested in the problem.

James Hague,[27] an official of the AHA in the days of the Commission on Financing of Hospital Care, spoke of one of the outcomes of the commission's work: drawing attention to the health care needs of the elderly.

HAGUE:[28]

The Commission on Financing of Hospital Care was an outgrowth of the unwillingness of the Commission on Hospital Care to tackle the subject of health care financing. They just weren't going to get anywhere on that issue, so they decided to put it aside. George Bugbee, then the executive director of the American Hospital Association, recognized this and created in 1951 another commission, the Commission on Financing of Hospital Care.

The Commission on Financing of Hospital Care did do one thing: it focused the attention of the AHA on health care for the aged. A committee was appointed by the AHA board to study the findings of the Commission on Financing of Hospital Care. What should the position of the AHA be with respect to the health care of the aged? E.A. van Steenwyk (president of Philadelphia Blue Cross) made the recommendation and the AHA board adopted it. From that point on, it seems to me that the AHA debate was more methods than anything else.

The AHA quickly accepted the need of the aged for health care help and the need for federal assistance in the solution.

The AHA's approach was to be via a Blue Cross card for everyone, destroying the differential between those who couldn't pay because everyone would have a Blue Cross card. It would base a person's contribution to that premium on some income basis but applied with some humaneness. No hardbench [sic] means test approach.

Such a lack of entitlement was attractive to many of the hospital conservatives. It's an acceptable thing, if done properly, to liberals such as I. I found, despite my liberal beliefs, and I am much more liberal than most people in the hospital field, that I could live in this AHA climate. I couldn't live in the American Medical Association climate. The AMA came up with Kerr-Mills as a way of stopping Medicare. It didn't stop Medicare, of course.

At the time the commission's reports were published, there may not have seemed to be much enthusiasm for their findings and recommendations. Nevertheless, the commission's work was valuable to the writers of the stream of bills introduced into Congress and evolving ultimately into Medicare.

One notable legislative event was the passage of an amendment to the Social Security Act in 1956 making possible disability cash benefits for totally and permanently disabled persons age 55 and over. The amendment came about because of the determination of the newly merged AFL-CIO to take a positive and meaningful step in the health field.

Nelson Cruikshank talks about the efforts of the AFL-CIO to promote the passage of the disability amendment.

CRUIKSHANK:[29]

In the disability thing we in a way made that a test of the first thing we could do in our field following merger. We put on the agenda what would be the first piece of legislation the merged organization would try to enact. We decided that disability insurance would be our test. The disability insurance idea had been around for a long time. It was first reported in 1938 by the advisory committee that made changes in the old age thing and added survivors. They had tried to get disability adopted then. That was in 1938, now this was in 1956. We knew we couldn't get Medicare or national health insurance. We thought that disability was the test. Of course, AMA opposed it with all the vigor and enthusiasm and venom that they had directed toward other policy things. They said, and we agreed, that it was a foot in the door for health insurance.

What is generally unknown about the action that took place in pushing the disability amendment through Congress is the sacrifice that Senator Earle C. Clements (D–Ky.) made and the eloquence of Senator Walter F. George (D–Ga.) in holding the bridge against the opposition while Senator Lyndon Johnson (D–Tex.) mustered enough votes to pass the measure in the Senate. (The bill had narrowly passed in the House.) Nelson Cruikshank gives a first-hand account of the behind-the-scenes action—especially what happened to swing one or two key votes.

CRUIKSHANK:[30]

In 1956 Senator George was up for reelection and he felt that under the unit rule in Georgia he couldn't win against Herman Talmadge because it was badly weighted against him. So he withdrew. He announced he was not going to run again. Then at that time he announced he didn't want to see any people. The disability thing was very tight. It had passed the House by a narrow majority. It had been turned down by the Senate Finance Committee. We knew we needed somebody of great prestige on the floor, particularly with Southern colleagues. There were a number of people, senators from the South, that would be able to say to their constituents, "Look, I went along with Senator George."

There was a congressman by the name of Page whose son was an assistant to Senator George, on his staff. Andy Biemiller (of our legislative staff) said to me, "I think we can see Senator George and get him to make this his kind of swan song. I think I can get to see him."

I said, "He isn't seeing anybody."

Andy said, "We can see him on a Saturday morning, if we are going to be willing to go down there and wait and hang around."

"Well," I said, "I usually go over to the [Chesapeake] Bay on Saturday."

I remember my wife and I packed up the car. I told her we probably would have to wait around a while. So I parked on the Capitol grounds and went into George's outer office. He had somebody in there, somebody from the sugar interests or Coca Cola from Georgia. Anyway we saw them file out.

We heard him say to young Page, "You mean to say these men have stayed here all morning?"

Hour after hour went by; my poor wife was sitting out in the car.

We heard Senator George say, "Tell them I'll see them for five minutes."

So he came out and ushered Andy and me in. We made our pitch. He would lead the battle to override the Senate Finance Committee, of which he was a member. He was in a clear position because he had voted for us but he was not in the majority. So he was not reversing his personal position; but to take on the Senate Finance Committee was a major job. But, he carried on that battle.

Lyndon Johnson also was with us. He was the Senate Majority Leader at the time. We met in his office with Clements of Kentucky, who was the Majority Whip, and we counted noses. We went down every member of the Senate and where we thought they were. We had a bare majority.

Clements then said, "Look, you have counted me with you. I can't be with you. I am up for reelection, and the AMA in Kentucky has vowed to defeat me if I vote for disability." Lyndon Johnson was pretty upset.

He said, "This is a party position. You are the Majority Whip, you can't go against us." He argued with him. Finally Johnson said, "I'll tell you. If we need your vote, if it's that close, can we have your vote?"

Clements said, "Yes. If my vote makes the difference, you can have my vote. Please don't call me. Let me get out of this if I can. I'll not vote one way or the other unless my vote is critical."

It came up on the floor in August. I was in the gallery. The debate was started. Senator George was speaking. I saw Lyndon Johnson searching around the gallery. He caught my eye and pointed down. I knew he wanted me to meet him down in his little private office off the floor. I rushed down.

He said, "How many votes have you got, Cruikshank?"

I said, "We've got a bare majority."

He said, "I can't believe that."

He showed me a list that he had of guys that had gone back on what we had thought was their position. So I went out in the hall and gathered together all the labor and welfare people I could round up. We divided up those names and started working on them.

Johnson said, "I'll pass a note to George to keep talking for an hour. He'll have the floor for an hour. You've got an hour to get those six votes."

One of the peculiar votes that we rounded up was Joe McCarthy. Now Joe McCarthy was a very conservative guy, of course. Joe McCarthy had been taken to task by Nixon. Eisenhower sent Nixon, who was then vice president, to McCarthy to ask him to slow down on his Communist drives. He was sore at Nixon for having done this. Nixon was in the chair as vice president. Very seldom did the vice president actually occupy the chair; however, he had come over that day knowing that it was going to be close and that he might have to cast the deciding vote in case of a tie.

The machinists' representative said, "I know how to get Joe McCarthy. Tell him that he will embarrass Nixon." So we worked on him, and McCarthy voted with us. Then, when he saw his vote wasn't needed, he called up to the clerk and reserved his vote, which made it a tie. You see, it carried the first time, but then, when McCarthy reversed his vote, it made it a tie.

At that point I saw Lyndon Johnson stride up the aisle in six-foot strides and hold up the arm of the reluctant Clements, who cast his vote. It wasn't a tie. We carried it in the end by two votes. At that moment Clements' vote was the vote that was needed to break it.

Incidentally, that was in August, and in November the AMA defeated Clements. It cost him his seat in the Senate to put disability on the rolls. But today there are 7 million people in their wheelchairs in hospitals and so forth that benefit because of that vote. I don't think Clements would regret it.

Another event that occurred during the Eisenhower presidency was the introduction of the Forand bill in the House late in 1957. The Forand bill was the successor of the long series of health insurance bills going back to the Wagner health bill of 1939 (or to earlier events), and it was followed, in turn, by a whole series of Wagner-Murray-Dingell and Murray-Dingell bills. The Forand bill presented a new approach: if health insurance legislation could not be passed for the entire population, why not concentrate on a federal program for Social Security beneficiaries? The bill called for 60 days of hospital care and certain nursing home and surgical benefits.

It became the Forand bill because Aime Forand (D–R.I.) was induced to introduce it. The bill was written by legislative specialists and was supported by, among others, the AFL-CIO. The sponsoring groups looked for someone to introduce the bill in the House. Jere Cooper, then chairman of the House Ways and Means Committee, said, according to Cruikshank, that he didn't want to touch it. Finally the labor group went to Forand, who was third in rank among the Democrats on the committee. Forand had worked closely with the American Public Welfare Association over the years; it is questionable whether he had any direct interest in the subject of health insurance. Cruikshank talked about going to Forand seeking his help.

CRUIKSHANK:[31]

He said, "We'll look it over and see."

We kept going back to him: well, he was busy, he hadn't had a chance to look at it yet. Meanwhile, there was a chap by the name of Greenberg who was kind of a medical expert on the Providence *Journal* and had written a number of articles we thought were pretty good. Most journalists don't know what they are talking about in the health field. He was of a different stripe. He had written a series of articles for the Providence *Journal*. I had met him at a couple of conferences. I called him and said, "Your Congressman is thinking about putting in a bill." I said, "If he gets some support in Rhode Island it will strengthen his hand. There is no reason I can't give you a scoop, if he does this."

He said, "Fine! Great!"

Then Forand, when we went back to him, said to Andy Biemiller and me, "Will you fellows guarantee me that this is a good, sound bill?"

We said, "We have worked it over. It's got the advice of the medical group. It's got the advice of our social security committee. It's endorsed by the AFL-CIO, and now the combined organization. It's gone through several refinement procedures. We can tell you, you don't need to be worried about this bill. Your people in Rhode Island will be happy about it too."

He said, "I haven't had time to look it over. Write me a speech of introduction."

So we went back and wrote him a speech. He introduced the bill. I sent a copy of the speech up to Greenberg with a note on it saying that when Forand made the speech I would give him a call and that if there were any departures from the speech I would let him know.

He made the speech word for word. I called Greenberg, and the next day the Providence *Journal* came out with banner headlines with everything in favor of it. Forand was absolutely delighted. From then on, Aime Forand thought he invented the whole idea. We didn't bother to disillusion him. He was a great friend. That's the way it was done.

The Forand bill received the support of many labor and professional groups, but it was opposed by the AMA, the Chamber of Commerce, insurance groups, and the Farm Bureau, among others. The bill was not reported out by the Ways and Means Committee after hearings were held in June 1958. The Ways and Means Committee stated that it needed more information before it could act and called upon HEW to study the problem of health care for the elderly. The department reported back in April 1959. Its report outlined the problems of the aged but ended equivocally, by questioning whether the government should do something directly to aid the elderly at that time or whether the government should wait to see if the growing enrollment of citizens in private insurance would eventually solve the problem without government intervention.

The Forand bill was on the scene until 1960. The last form of the bill was stripped of surgical benefits, hoping to lessen the animosity of physicians, but to no avail.

Falk, who had been busy with Cohen and others in writing legislative proposals for health insurance since the days of Wagner's original health bill, discusses the latest reincarnation (the Forand bill) and the substitution of the Kerr-Mills program for it in an attempt to care for the aged and indigent.

FALK:[32]

By 1958 there were indications that a health insurance bill might be able to be enacted. This led to very vigorous countermeasures from some who were strongly opposed to expansion of the Social Security system. Finally—skipping a lot of intermediate steps—it resulted in development of an expanded means test program as an alternative to a paid-up insurance program—the Kerr-Mills program.

The Kerr-Mills program was intended to broaden the availability of public assistance medical care so that it would extend to the medically indigent and not be limited to the indigent in need of money payments for support. That program, enacted in 1960, if I remember correctly, was expected to be very effective. This was the expectation, because the financial support to the states from the federal government was increased—to buy the support of the states—so that they could undertake broadened public assistance, medical care programs with very little additional cost to them. The additional costs were borne by increased federal grants-in-aid to the states.

That program was very quickly picked up and developed in six to nine relatively wealthy states that could put up their matching funds. Otherwise it was a general disaster. Most of the states could not afford to take advantage of the program's opportunities, even though the federal grant support had been considerably increased. Within two or three years it was evident that the majority of the federal money was going to a few of the wealthiest states and only a miniscule portion was going to the states in which the needs were greatest.

I mentioned the catastrophies of the Kerr-Mills program because through the early 1960s its failure led to expediting, augmenting, and accelerating the acceptability of the paid-up insurance concept that was going to become Medicare in 1965.

[Shortly before his death in October 1984, Falk read a draft copy of this chapter. He added a note at this point: "The Clements story is particularly moving to me. I had spent more years on the design of disability insurance—since 1936—than on any subject other than health insurance. I was particularly piqued at the insurance industry for their opposition, because, after some early bad experiences with it, they lost money on it and had no intention to take it up. Theirs was a dog in the manger opposition to it. It pained me greatly for years."]

The Kerr-Mills program lasted less than five years and was succeeded by Medicaid in 1966. Kerr-Mills did not solve the problems it set out to correct (unless it was meant to delay the passage of Medicare, which it may have done).

Looking back at the Eisenhower years, we might summarize by saying that, even though not much seemed to be happening in the health field, there was some simmering under the surface that would bubble over in the mid-1960s. Action picked up during the Kennedy and Johnson years and culminated in the passage of Medicare and Medicaid in 1965. That action is described in the next chapter.

Notes

(Transcripts of the oral histories cited here are housed in the library of the American Hospital Association, 840 North Lake Shore Drive, Chicago, Illinois 60611. The Oral History Collection is a joint project of the Hospital Research and Educational Trust and the AHA.)

1. Commons was a professor at the University of Wisconsin from 1904 to 1932.

2. Henry F. Pringle, *Theodore Roosevelt* (New York: Harcourt, Brace, 1956), pp. 396–97.

3. For background reading see Peter A. Corning, *The Evolution of Medicare* (Washington, D.C.: Office of Research and Statistics, Social Security Administration, U.S. Department of Health, Education, and Welfare, 1969).

4. The act was not renewed in 1929.

5. See Odin W. Anderson, *Blue Cross Since 1929* (Cambridge, Mass.: Ballinger, 1975).

6. Nathan Miller, *FDR: An Intimate History* (Garden City, N.Y.: Doubleday, 1983), pp. 306–25.

7. For a description of the utopian movement in the United States in the 1930s, see George Creel, *Rebel at Large* (New York: Putnam's, 1947).

8. Altmeyer later became one of the three members of the first Social Security Board.

9. Quoted from Arthur J. Altmeyer, *The Formative Years of Social Security* (Madison: The University of Wisconsin Press, 1968), pp. 8–9.

10. Frances Perkins, *The Roosevelt I Knew* (New York: Viking Press, 1946), p. 286.

11. *Wilbur Cohen, In the First Person: An Oral History.* See Profiles of Participants, in the center of this book, for biographical information.

12. *I.S. Falk, In the First Person: An Oral History.* See Profiles of Participants for biographical information.

13. *Cohen, Oral History.*

14. Ibid.

15. J. Joseph Huthmacher, *Senator Robert F. Wagner and the Rise of Urban Liberalism* (New York: Atheneum, 1968), p. 292.

16. Robert H. Ferrell, ed., *Off the Record: The Private Papers of Harry S. Truman* (New York: Harper & Row, 1980), pp. 165–66.

17. Ibid., p. 262.

18. Ibid., p. 303.

19. Robert J. Donovan, *Conflict and Crisis: The Presidency of Harry S. Truman, 1945–1948* (New York: Norton, 1977), p. 125.

20. Altmeyer, *Formative Years,* p. 163.

21. *Falk, Oral History.*

22. *Cohen, Oral History.*

23. Altmeyer, *Formative Years,* pp. 237–38.

24. Grants totalling $556,000 for the support of the Commission on Financing of Hospital Care were forthcoming from the Blue Cross Commission, the Health Information Foundation, the John Hancock Mutual Life Insurance Company, the W.K. Kellogg Foundation, Michigan Medical Services, the Milbank Memorial Fund, the National Foundation for Infantile Paralysis, and the Rockefeller Foundation.

25. See Profiles of Participants for biographical information.

26. *Robert Sigmond, In the First Person: An Oral History.*

27. See Profiles of Participants for biographical information.

28. *James Hague, In the First Person: An Oral History.*

29. *Nelson H. Cruikshank, In the First Person: An Oral History.* See Profiles of Participants for biographical information.

30. *Cruikshank, Oral History.*

31. Ibid.

32. *Falk, Oral History.*

5

The Evolution of Medicare Legislation

The lack of health care legislation during the Eisenhower years should not be attributed entirely to Republican control of Congress, because between 1953 and 1954, when the Republicans had a majority, it was very slight and tenuous. When "Mr. Sam" Rayburn was again elected Speaker of the House in 1955, he also had a very slim majority. Even the election of President John F. Kennedy in 1960 was very close. In fact, the Democrats never had a comfortable majority until the 1964 Johnson landslide, which came on a wave of sympathy after the assassination of John F. Kennedy. A substantial majority of Democrats was needed to pass legislation over the opposition of the AMA and other conservative forces in both parties.

During the Eisenhower administration, various studies were done on the needs of the aged, liberal Republicans began to approve of health insurance for the aged, and the first White House Conference on Aging was planned.

The White House Conference on Aging

The White House Conference on Aging, which was to become a traditional meeting every ten years, was first held in 1961. Planning for it took place during 1960, the last year of the Eisenhower administration, and was carried out by Republicans, closely watched by the AMA.

Nelson Cruikshank, director of the department of social security of the AFL-CIO, had great influence in the organizing of the conference and in the orchestration of the proceedings.[1]

Part of his influence was due to an arrangement George Meany, president of the AFL-CIO, had with Nelson Rockefeller, then under secretary of HEW. Rockefeller wanted to be on good terms with labor, particularly with Meany, and labor was eager to have sympathetic persons appointed to federal posts. One sensitive appointment was the commissioner of Social Security. During the early years of Eisenhower's administration, Rockefeller telephoned Cruikshank saying he wanted labor's opinion of Charles Schottland, a Republican from California whom Eisenhower was considering as commissioner. Cruikshank checked with California labor leaders and learned that Schottland, a "Warren Republican," was well thought of by labor. Schottland was appointed. Cruikshank relates how this appointment fit in with the White House Conference on Aging.

=====

CRUIKSHANK:[2]

Schottland, as Social Security commissioner, was on the small steering committee from the administration that set up the machinery of the White House conference. The first thing was to get a chairman. We knew it had to be a Republican, because he was to be appointed by the president. There was a congressman from New Jersey—Kean it was spelled, but he pronounced it "Kane"—he had been very friendly to us on a number of occasions. He was a very broad-gauged fellow. He was on the Ways and Means Committee. He had *not* sponsored Medicare legislation, but he was on the Ways and Means Committee and he had given us several favorable votes on social security issues.

I think it was Arthur Flemming's suggestion that they could get Kean to chair the thing, and I said, "That would be great with us." He would not wield the power of the chair against us.

Then Schottland, on the planning committee, agreed with us that Medicare should be put in the income maintenance section. Medicare was a proposed amendment to the Social Security Act and therefore fit in income maintenance and as opposed to the health section. We also agreed that we would keep this assignment decision quiet.

Meanwhile the AMA was getting all of its constituent bodies to sign up for the health section. We said that was fine, we encouraged that. We knew that Medicare wouldn't be assigned to that section.

By this time we had developed quite a coalition of organizations that were for Medicare. We sent letters to them all asking who were their delegates to the White House conference. We asked them if they would mind checking in with us and telling us what their room was, and where they were, and so forth. We had a card for everyone so that we knew the organizations and what committees they were assigned to, or what subgroups they were assigned to, what their room number was, what their phone number was, and all that.

Any time anyone tried to bring up Medicare in the health section or the education section or anywhere else, one of these delegates would phone our central office, then we would make a bunch of telephone calls, and people would converge on that meeting and object that it was out of order to bring up Medicare. Finally the doctors found out what was going on. They tried to object to the thing at the final plenary session. Kean was in the chair, of course. It was the final windup of the thing. The doctors all got together and were going to make an objection.

I went up to the platform and said to Kean, "These guys are trying. . . ." He said, "Take it easy, Nelson. I know what I am doing. Don't worry!"

They went on and on. I thought he was letting them get away with murder and all. Finally he banged the gavel and said, "I find there isn't a quorum present and therefore the issue is out of order. Next question?"

He knew what he was doing all the time. They never got their objection before the body. Under the rules we had set up, the plenary session could not pass on policy issues. The policy issues were to be determined within the different subsections.

Of course, the White House Conference on Aging could not pass a bill. Cruikshank was asked if the report of the conference was generally favorable to Medicare.

CRUIKSHANK:[3]

Yes, but it was in the section that I can say now was loaded in its favor.

We knew it wouldn't pass a bill. It was just a recommendation of the White House conference. It didn't do an awful lot of good to forwarding the bill. However, had it gone the other way, it would have been an awful lot against the bill.

One of the positive outcomes of the conference was that several of the liberal Republican leaders were able to show their support for Medicare without overtly expressing an opinion counter to that of the Eisenhower administration. Cruikshank commented on this:

CRUIKSHANK:[4]

The interesting thing about that was that we had the administration people with us right under Eisenhower's nose. Charlie Schottland, Arthur

Flemming, and Congressman Kean—they were all Republicans.[5] This is the way they could be for Medicare without openly challenging the administration's position.

One other positive outcome of the White House Conference on Aging was the formation of the National Council of Senior Citizens from the many organizations that had worked hard to get a favorable report on Medicare out of the conference. Some 500 groups had supported Medicare on the floor in the conference.

Aime Forand saw the potential of a united effort among these organizations in publicizing the need for Medicare. He suggested an organization be formed to carry out this effort. Cruikshank explains the situation:

CRUIKSHANK:[6]

The delegates from the White House Conference on Aging met with Aime Forand. He wanted to meet with us. He was the author of our bill.

He said, "You've got a victory here in a way, and you have done a good job, but that isn't going to pass the bill. What you need is an organization that will implement this and carry it through. I think you people ought to form some kind of a permanent organization that will allow groups to work together actively in the legislative process."

The steelworkers put up some money, the autoworkers put up some money. They came to me and I put the arm on Mr. Meany and he put up some money. We got a little nest egg together to start what became the National Council of Senior Citizens.

It was an organization inspired primarily by Forand and primarily directed at the passage of Medicare.

The Kennedy Years

Forand didn't stand for reelection to Congress; he became the first president of the National Council of Senior Citizens and worked actively through the council to promote Medicare.

President-elect Kennedy in 1960 appointed a Task Force on Health and Social Security for the American People, chaired by Wilbur Cohen.[7] The task force reported on January 10, 1961, and recommended health insurance for the aged under Social Security. Doctors' fees were excluded to avoid confrontation with the AMA. Cohen speaks of the task force recommendations:

COHEN:[8]

In 1960 President Kennedy appointed me chairman of his Task Force on Health and Social Security, in which, with a number of other people, I recommended not only Medicare, but federal aid for construction of medical schools and tuition grants for physicians and other health personnel.

Although President Kennedy in his first State of the Union address, in January 1961, mentioned the need for health insurance under Social Security, he was realistic enough to know that there was little chance of such legislation's being passed in the current Congress. The Democrats had a 20-seat majority in the House and barely retained control of the Senate.

Nevertheless, Kennedy persisted. He sent a special health message to Congress on February 10 reiterating his request for action in this area. Three days later, Senator Clinton Anderson (D–N.M.) and Representative Cecil King (D–Calif.) introduced a health insurance bill in Congress. This was a successor to the Forand bill.

Possibly just as important as the national council's efforts in bringing the health insurance issue to public attention was the opposition action of the AMA. The AMA apparently felt the medical profession was threatened by the King-Anderson bill. The AMA assumed the attitude that there could be no compromise; the movement had to be stopped. In fact, a campaign was waged in which radio and television commercials were used extensively. Several million pamphlets were distributed. A speakers' bureau was established to spread the word, and a "letter to your congressman" effort resulted in a cascade of thousands of letters on Washington, D.C.

In the summer of 1961, members of the AMA also established the American Medical Political Action Committee (AMPAC) in anticipation of the 1962 elections.

In the meantime, the implementation of the Kerr-Mills program was going forward. Many of the opponents of Medicare hoped that Kerr-Mills would take care of the medical problems of the aged and poor. If so, they argued, it would obviate the need for Medicare. It was soon evident that Kerr-Mills was not solving the problems of the aged ill and indigent ill, particularly in the poorer states.

All in all, a great deal of publicity, pro and con, was generated about Medicare. On the pro side were labor unions, churches, the American Public Health Association, and others. Several prominent physicians formed the Physicians' Committee for Health Care Through Social Security.

Blue Cross, Blue Shield, and some of the commercial insurance companies began developing low-cost insurance programs for persons 65 and over. It was hoped that private insurance could help relieve the needs of the elderly.

Walter J. McNerney had moved from the University of Michigan to the presidency of the Blue Cross Association (BCA) in 1961. One of the first problems he faced was determining what the Blue Cross plans could do to offer health insurance coverage to the elderly at a cost they could afford.

McNERNEY:[9]

It would take a long time to spell out all that happened.

When the aging issue began to heat up in the early 1960s, there was a lot of tension and a lot of politicking.

I convinced Ed Crosby [executive director of the AHA] that the American Hospital Association and the Blue Cross Association should do a study on the aged and that its initial focus should be on what the problem was; that is, number of aged, age distribution, sex distribution, the amount they spent on health, their length of stay versus the same for the under-65 population, and so forth. We were trying to get a grasp of what the problem was. My thought, at the time, was that if we were able to define the problem better we would be serving a good public purpose. It would also make it clear we were not afraid of the problem.

In general terms, I think the AHA and BCA took some very responsible steps. We made some mistakes but, by and large, we took responsible steps.

We also took the initiative. We were the ones who came out during the debates and said, "There is absolutely no question that the aged are in a unique position. At a time in their lives when they can afford it the least, they have the most health care expenses." We documented that this was true and that there was an obverse relation between income and incidence of illness and that the private sector was incapable of producing, through subsidization from the insured working population, enough money to make health insurance premium rates generally affordable to the aged. Something had to be done about it.

Clearly there were quarrels about the best way to go about it. But AHA and BCA were on the line saying we have a problem here and also saying that the low-income group, whether they were aged or not, had a similar problem that had to be dealt with as well.

I said we made some mistakes. When the debate dragged out and it wasn't clear what was going to happen, I, particularly, took the point of view that, since we don't know when this is going to be resolved, how about Blue Cross making a special effort? So we talked about a national program that would improve our offerings to the aged. By that time we were doing better than any of our competitors. If everyone had the same percentage of aged enrolled as we did, there would have been a lesser problem. There would have still been a problem, but a far smaller problem.

I encouraged the Blue Cross plans to have some special open enrollments to make it possible for the aged who hadn't been enrolled to come on board, and to do a better job for those who were on board. This was interpreted by some as an effort on my part to try to solve the problem naively, through just the private sector, undercutting, if you will, the legislative process. I don't think I was dumb enough to think our effort could or would fully solve the problem. On the other hand, I was a bit naive in regard to the timing and how our encouragement of this effort would be interpreted. I didn't anticipate that it would be used against us later the way it was, but that passed.

John R. Mannix was actively involved in the Blue Cross movement.[10] He was asked what he remembered about the Blue Cross attitude toward the elderly, particularly in the years before Medicare.

MANNIX:[11]

I was very much interested in Blue Cross and Blue Shield offering a program for the care of the elderly and advocated a program which I called the Golden Age Program.

I tried to develop such a program in the Cleveland area, in which the individual would pay a somewhat higher premium during his working years which would be adequate to cover the cost of his care after he retired. I did some work on a plan which would pay 75 percent at that time. The premium was on a graduated scale depending on his years of membership as a worker.

One of the interesting things about this was that labor opposed it. In the early 1960s, labor was very much in favor of a federal health insurance program. When I presented this program to the Ohio Insurance Department for approval, labor opposed it.

Medicare came a couple years later, and I think it leaves a lot to be desired. Medicare is paying only approximately 40 percent of the cost of health services of the elderly. Blue Cross and Blue Shield and private insurance companies supplement this with what is generally referred to as fill-in programs where they cover the benefits Medicare does not cover. This is a problem for the elderly.

Daniel W. Pettengill[12] was with the Aetna Life Insurance Company from 1937 to 1978. From 1964 to 1978 he served as a vice president of the company. During his career, Pettengill was a major force within the commercial insurance industry on matters of national health policy. He discusses how the commercial insurance companies approached the problem of how to provide health insurance protection for the elderly.

PETTENGILL:[13]

The hard fact remained that, for any employer, health care coverage for a retiree was about three times as expensive as for an active employee and hence was not a coverage to be purchased voluntarily. Furthermore, many unions were wary about using their bargaining power in this area. So insurance companies were left with the problem of how to provide coverage for the aged who needed it the most but who could afford it the least.

No one insurer could handle this problem alone. A joint effort was needed in order to obtain the large volumes of insureds needed to cover the extra risk and the expense. Unfortunately, the Southeastern Underwriters decision of 1944 had declared insurance to be interstate commerce and hence subject to antitrust statues. So a joint effort per se was illegal.

The matter stood at this impasse until one evening when George Light, an attorney for the Travelers, and I were returning to Hartford by train from an industry meeting in New York City. He said, "Look, we could do something for the aged population in Connecticut if we could get permission from the state for the companies to cooperate and to underwrite the coverage as a single pool." So the next day we went to our respective presidents and got permission to draft and seek passage of the necessary legislation.

That legislation did pass. As a result, we established the Connecticut 65 Plan, which offered reasonable benefits to persons age 65 and older residing in Connecticut. Connecticut 65 kept its expenses low but still had to charge a fairly high premium rate in order to cover its claims experience. Employers were encouraged to help pay the premium for their retirees, but few did so.

Connecticut, being a small state, did have difficulty getting the volume of coverage sold that was needed to make the pool self-supporting. But the idea caught on and, although I think there were only seven insurance companies that participated in the Connecticut pool, we were able to persuade the industry to set up similar pools in other states. I believe Massachusetts was next, followed by New York, California, and Ohio.

These state 65 Plans were just getting rolling when Lyndon Johnson's 1964 landslide election occurred. Johnson, with his mandate, was bound and determined to have a federal program for the aged. So the fact that the insurance industry was doing something constructive for the elderly was just lost on the Congress.

As a matter of fact, in late November 1964, following the election but before the new Congress started in the subsequent January, I talked with Wilbur Mills, who was then chairman of the House Ways and Means Committee. Mills said, "Dan, President-elect Johnson has called me and said we are to have a bill for the aged in the hopper as soon as Congress convenes, and it is going to go through."

Hearings in the Ways and Means Committee on King-Anderson began in July 1961 and extended into August. It soon became apparent that there would not be enough favorable votes in the committee to report the bill out.

Although the King-Anderson bill died in committee in 1961, President Kennedy maintained his support of the principle in speeches and in interviews with the press. Public sentiment was rising in favor of Medicare (some poll-sters reporting a 69 percent favorable response). Political conservatives were responding with reworked plans for federal subsidies of private insurance for the elderly. Even the AMA was beginning to think they might find accept-able some sort of federal subsidy for the needy among the aged. All of these swirls of action and proposed action climaxed (or anticlimaxed) in the spec-tacular event in Madison Square Garden on Sunday, May 20, 1962, when President Kennedy addressed a crowd of over 20,000 senior citizens. Nelson Cruikshank talked about his part in this event.

CRUIKSHANK:[14]

I had a very inglorious part in it. I was never much impressed by the effects of rallies. They were more of a CIO than an AF of L tradition. I came out of the AF of L side. I wasn't against them; however, if they weren't managed awfully well, they could do more harm than good. Also, if they are not a huge success, they are not a success at all.

I said OK. The people wanted to do it. I was certainly not going to try to stop it. I would play my part and do what I was told to do.

The idea was to have President Kennedy appear at Madison Square Garden. We would fill the Garden with labor people and senior citizen groups. Then we would have rallies all around the country in different cities. There would be a huge television screen at each of these local rallies, and at the right time President Kennedy would be wired in and we would fire up the whole thing.

At the actual rally, President Kennedy probably made the poorest speech he ever made. None of us ever quite knew why. He made a slip of the tongue; he said the cost of Medicare would be $12 a month instead of $12 a year.

On balance, the thing at Madison Square Garden, however, went all right. Then, you know, the American Medical Association came in and bought time on television to answer us. They made their famous speech to the empty chairs in Madison Square Garden.

The meetings out over the country were something else. There were about 20 of them set up. I was sent to Charleston, West Virginia. It was really something—the only time I made the front page of the AMA *News*, in a way I wasn't happy about.

As soon as I got in town Saturday night, I could smell defeat right away. There were no ads, no posters. The evening paper had no story on it. The thing was going to be a flop.

(The person who was supposed to be in charge had left town and turned it over to somebody else.)

The labor people had organized a luncheon. There were about 15 or 20 people at the luncheon, and then we went right over to this huge hall. When we got there, the AMA had doctors at every entrance of the hall handing out leaflets. Practically nobody showed up. We addressed this sea of empty chairs, whereupon the AMA had pictures of these empty chairs with me addressing them. They put that picture on the front page of the AMA *News* with the caption, "This Is the Kind of Support Cruikshank Has for His Program." It was a large piece of humble pie I had to chew on.

———————

As Nelson Cruikshank mentioned, Kennedy's speech in Madison Square Garden was one of the worst of his career. It has been said that he discarded the speech prepared for the occasion and attempted to write a new one on his way to the Garden in his limousine. Time was pressing, for the speech and ceremony at Madison Square Garden were to be on national television, so the President spoke extemporaneously—and badly.

His audience at the Garden was composed of elderly citizens. There was no need to impress them with the importance of health insurance for Social Security beneficiaries. However, out in the nation where a good impression was desired, the performance on television fell flat.

The AMA bought television time for a half-hour broadcast from Madison Square Garden two days later. The speaker for the AMA was Dr. Edward Annis of Miami, who became a spellbinding orator for the AMA in its fight against "socialized medicine." The contrast of Annis' speech with Kennedy's was pronounced.

One of the examples given by Annis of steps being taken to help the poor and indigent was the Kerr-Mills Act, which had been implemented just a year before. He pointed to the success of Kerr-Mills in 38 states. Actually, Kerr-Mills had only been approved in 24 states. Moreover, the Senate report on Kerr-Mills made shortly after the Annis speech showed that 90 percent of the federal funds were going to only four states, those which could afford to operate adequate Kerr-Mills programs.

A few weeks after the president's appearance at Madison Square Garden, an attempt was made to circumvent the usual practice of submitting a bill in Congress, having it reviewed in committee, and, if reported, having it voted on in the chamber where it was introduced.

With a few exceptions (including Kerr-Mills, total disability benefits under Social Security, military medicare) health bills had generally died in committee without a floor vote. The circumvention of normal procedures was the Anderson-Javits amendment, which was an attempt to attach an amendment to a Senate welfare bill which was under pressure for passage. The amendment, named for Anderson and Senator Jacob Javits (R–N.Y.), called for the main features of the King-Anderson Medicare bill plus some provisions for commercial insurance companies to participate.

It was a daring move, and it nearly succeeded in the Senate. However, the amendment was tabled on July 17, 1962, by the close vote of 52 to 48. Even had it passed in the Senate, it was thought unlikely to have passed in the House. [15]

Cruikshank talks about some maneuvering that went on in the attempt to attach the Anderson-Javits amendment to the welfare bill in the Senate.

CRUIKSHANK: [16]

In 1962 Mills said to us, "Take your bill over to the Senate." At that time we were within one vote of it in the Ways and Means Committee. Mills didn't want to give his vote, which would have broken the deadlock in the House. Of course, under the constitution that kind of act must originate in the House; it was technically a revenue tax act. "Take it over to the Senate and hook it onto something over there. Come back and we'll see what we can do."

We knew Wilbur Mills pretty well. This wasn't a definite promise; however, it was worth trying. So we hooked it onto something over in the Senate.

This became the Anderson-Javits amendment?

CRUIKSHANK: [17]

Yes. Javits came to us and said if there was a role for the insurance companies there were eight Republicans he had who would support it. We knew who a couple of them were. We weren't sure of Javits' comment, but he was an honest man. . . . We didn't know just what he meant by the role of insurance.

Once it was decided to go ahead with the amendment, a great deal of activity went into designing an amendment that would be satisfactory to Republicans and Democrats. Cruikshank tells of a night meeting suddenly called in the office of HEW secretary Abraham Ribicoff and attended by Wilbur Cohen, Senator Javits, and Cruikshank and Leonard Lesser representing the AFL-CIO. The key question was defining the role of insurance companies. The union representatives were restricted by instructions from George Meany, who, according to Cruikshank, had said, "Don't let the insurance companies in."

Meanwhile Meany had gone to Europe to an international union meeting, so it was difficult at times to reach him for advice as negotiations developed. Meany evidently was afraid the insurance companies would secure an underwriting role.

CRUIKSHANK:[18]

When the insurance companies are in an underwriting role, every claim for benefits is in competition with profits. We had seen that in workman's compensation. We had seen the corrosive effect of commercial insurance.

The union representatives were not able to get a clear definition of what Javits wanted for the insurance companies, so Cruikshank took the initiative and called a Sunday meeting of insurance and legislative experts from the union. Together they wrote a suggested amendment to attach to a Senate bill and presented it to Javits; he agreed to go along with it.

CRUIKSHANK:[19]

We didn't think he would . . . but Javits was a different kind of Republican, always had been.

Cruikshank and Andrew Biemiller, the legislative expert for the AFL-CIO, telephoned Meany in Europe. Meany told them to do the best they could without giving the insurance companies an underwriting role.

The year 1963 began as many others had in the history of the evolution of Medicare. On February 21 President Kennedy sent a special message to Congress on the problems of the aged. On the same day a slightly revised King-Anderson bill was introduced in Congress. Hearings on the bill in the Ways and Means Committee were interrupted on November 22, the day President Kennedy was assassinated.

The death of the president aroused tremendous sympathy for Kennedy, for his family—and for his legislative goals. Lyndon B. Johnson, his successor, moved quickly on that wave of sympathy and pledged himself to carry out Kennedy's programs. Johnson put Medicare high on his list of priorities, a fact he mentioned in his first speech to Congress.

The Johnson Years

During those early months of Johnson's administration, public sentiment was rising for Medicare. Proponents of the measure thought the necessary votes might now be available in the Ways and Means Committee to report the King-Anderson bill out. Wilbur Mills was keeping a tight hand on the Ways and Means Committee, however, and the bill was not reported.

Another bill (H.R. 11865) was reported, but it authorized only an increase in Social Security benefits—no health insurance. This bill was passed in the House and was sent to the Senate. In the meantime, the King-Anderson bill had failed to gain approval in the Senate Finance Committee, but there were enough votes in the Senate to attach it as an amendment to H.R. 11865, thus circumventing the finance committee.

Because of the amendment, the bill went to a conference committee of the House and Senate to work out compromises. To expedite matters, the Johnson administration proposed that a vote of the full House instruct the House conference committee members to vote for Medicare. This move was rather high-handed in the minds of many House members, and it failed. The committee was deadlocked; no compromise could be reached, so both the health insurance and the increase in Social Security benefits failed.

The failure of H.R. 11865 in the conference committee occurred in October 1964. The elections that took place in November of that year changed the nation's political complexion. Johnson was elected by the largest plurality ever registered up to that time. The House and the Senate both showed a two-to-one margin in favor of the Democrats. Several persons active in promoting Medicare at that time comment:

MILLS:[20]

Lyndon Johnson ran in '64 and was reelected in his own right. Then he announced to the Congress his desire to pass everything President Kennedy had advocated. Had President Kennedy lived, I don't know if Medicare would have passed. I don't think President Kennedy would have pushed it like President Johnson did. They were two different kinds of people. Not that Kennedy wasn't for it, it was just that President Johnson was far more tenacious about things.

CRUIKSHANK:[21]

It wasn't until the Democratic landslide of '64 that you had enough Northern Democrats to override the Southern Democrats. As a result, when '65 came around, President Johnson ordered Wilbur Mills to enlarge the House Ways and Means Committee and told him who to put on the committee, because, he said, "We are going to have a majority of your committee for Medicare."

PETTENGILL:[22]

Whenever a party gets a substantial increase in the number of their members in Congress, that party is entitled to take the committees and re-ratio the ratio of Democrats and Republicans. Because Lyndon's victory was a landslide, the Ways and Means Committee was enlarged. In making that enlargement, President Johnson was very careful to be sure that the House leadership chose people who would be supportive of Medicare.

The Passage of Medicare

Events of 1965 moved along swiftly but in the familiar pattern. The president made his State of the Union speech to Congress in January and stressed his determination to see the King-Anderson Medicare bill passed. Almost simultaneously the bill was introduced in Congress as H.R. 1 and S. 1, which seemed to indicate the party's estimation of its importance. In addition, Wilbur Mills was speaking in early 1965 as though the passage of the bill were certain and imminent.

The AMA again gathered its forces to resist. This time the resistance took the form of an AMA-supported bill called "eldercare." Eldercare would subsidize private health insurance for the elderly through federal and state grants. The bill was introduced in the House the day hearings began on King-Anderson.

Another alternative to Medicare was a bill introduced in the House by Representative John Byrnes (R–Wisc.). This bill called for federal subsidies for private health insurance for Social Security beneficiaries. The financing was to come two-thirds from the federal government and one-third from deductions from Social Security checks.

In the spring of 1965 there was a general feeling that some sort of Medicare legislation would pass in the current Congress. Public opinion polls showed that two-thirds of the respondents favored Medicare.

The tempo for moving the King-Anderson bill to the floor of the House for a vote picked up. Wilbur Mills now had a clear majority on his committee in support of a Medicare bill.

Mills was a superb politician who did not move until he had a situation under control. He knew Medicare was very likely to pass: he had found a way to pacify physicians (through Part B, which will be discussed later), and he had the Democratic majority in Congress necessary to pass the bill.

Mills, however, was faced with a wide spectrum of bills and amendments out of which the Ways and Means Committee had to write a bill. In order to clarify the situation, he asked Wilbur Cohen to appear before the committee and outline and discuss the various proposals, as well as the options that should be considered.

MILLS:[23]

Wilbur Cohen felt, as I did, that the program the administration espoused had to be improved.

I started off with the basic thought that the American people would feel that we misled them; and they'd be highly resentful if we did nothing more than just what President Johnson had initially recommended.

The administration's program would only take care of about a fourth of the total cost. People thought it was going to take care of it all. If we did no more than that, and they found out we were only taking care of a fourth, all of us would be in trouble. We had to find some way to take care of more of the cost.

I talked to the president about it and he agreed.

He didn't take the time to develop the ideas himself, but we had at our disposal all the ability of the members of the committee. Together we developed what was later called the "three-layer approach." We wanted to take care of the medical needs, fully, of those who were on welfare—everything— and we wanted to take care of the major portion of the needs of people on Social Security and Railroad Retirement.

After Cohen had finished describing the various bills and proposals on health insurance for the aged—the last plan discussed was the Byrnes "bettercare" bill—Mills said to Byrnes that he really liked Byrnes' idea of co-payment out of Social Security checks. He said he saw this as a supplement to Medicare to help pay the cost of physicians' services.

In fact Mills, to the surprise of all the committee members, then suggested a three-layer approach. The top layer was the Byrnes payment plan for the physicians. The middle layer was for hospital care, financed by payroll taxes and employer taxes. The bottom layer represented an enhanced Kerr-Mills program for the low-income and indigent, or Medicaid, as it became known.

Cohen speaks about that third layer, which became Medicaid, as does Kenneth Williamson.

COHEN:[24]

While Medicare was being fought in the frontline trenches between those who favored it and those who opposed it, there was also the entire issue of what to do about people who were either not covered by Medicare or not adequately covered.

Medicaid came about because the welfare system for low-income and indigent persons was not adequate in the United States. However, since the welfare program was primarily related to the state operations, financed partially by federal funds and with federal standards, the Medicaid program became a federal-state system, whereas Medicare became primarily a federal system. That's how these two programs evolved.

However, the most unusual aspect of the Medicare program was the fact that in the congressional consideration in the House Ways and Means Committee, a result of certain discussions between Wilbur D. Mills and John W. Byrnes (the Republican minority member of the Ways and Means Committee from Wisconsin), the entire idea of covering physicians' services on a voluntary basis was added to the program. This we now call part B, whereas the hospitalization insurance, which was compulsory in its coverage, was called part A.

This was rather unexpected on everyone's part and thus led to a good deal of interest. The most interesting aspect of that is that the part B was financed initially about half from general revenues and half from the beneficiaries, and today the general revenues portion has reached about 70 percent. As a result, we have general revenue financing a part of the Social Security and Medicare programs.

———

WILLIAMSON:[25]

One afternoon Congressman Wilbur Mills called me and told me about Medicaid. They had had the Kerr–Mills bill, which had preceded Medicaid. Mills and Senator Kerr drafted it, and it flopped. The states didn't support it. I was serving then as kind of a consultant to Mills. He would call me, and I would go over and talk to him about why the thing was a failure.

Anyway, he called me this one afternoon and said he would like to see me. I went up there. He had John Martin, his staff director, with him. Mills said, "We are drafting this program, Medicaid, for the poor. It will be a whole new thing." He sketched it out, and he said, "John will tell you the details. You can't talk about this, it is confidential at this stage. But," he said, "you have talked to me about hospitals and the way they should be handled, reimbursement and all." Then he said, "if you could put one thing in this bill in behalf of the hospitals, what would it be?"

I said, "That would be very simple. It would be to say that the states can't pay hospitals any less for care than Medicare pays. In other words, they must pay reasonable costs."

Mr. Mills accepted the idea and put it in the bill.

That has meant billions—not millions, billions—of dollars to hospitals. They have to fight for it now, they have had to go to court to justify it, but that wording raised the level of payment to hospitals enormously.

Anyway, Mills bought the idea. I often think that, in terms of money, there probably isn't anything I ever did that earned my pay more than that one day's work.

———

Mills gave the Republicans full credit for their contribution of the top layer of the three-layer cake.

MILLS:[26]

We finally worked out part B. Representative John Byrnes offered it. It was good that he did it. I was hoping that John would, because that meant it brought in Republican support. He brought them all with him. He brought them all in when he did it. John is entitled to an awful lot of credit in connection with the establishment of Medicare.

The basic thing was how to pay the doctors. The way Byrnes worked it out in his motion was that they (the beneficiaries) would be charged so much a month, and the federal government would put up a like amount [originally $3.00 per beneficiary per month from each source]. The Department of Health, Education, and Welfare came up with their estimates of what that premium should be. We tested it and found general acceptance of it.

The Republicans were astounded. Mills had stolen their thunder with his three-layer compromise program. The Ways and Means Committee approved the bill, 17–8, on a strict party-line vote.

President Johnson was delighted with the move and went on television the next day to tell the country the good news. Cohen had told him the three-layer approach might increase costs $500 million a year over the original plan, but Johnson did not seem concerned with the added costs.

PETTENGILL:[27]

Part B was the compromise which Mills gave to the Republicans who wanted an all-private plan. John Byrnes, from Wisconsin, was pushing this. And so Wilbur pulled a real coup by turning to Byrnes one day late in the discussion and saying to him, "OK, part A is going to be what we Democrats have been talking about, but we'll take your plan and limit it to just physician services. We'll insure it, and we'll hire the insurance companies and the Blues to be the carriers."

Byrnes was caught flatfooted. What was he to say? Here was the perfect political compromise. Part A was Lyndon Johnson's, part B was Johnny Byrnes', Republican. So, unfortunately, they agreed. It went so fast that neither one of them worried about cost.

MILLS:[28]

The AMA still opposed it [part B]. They met, they weren't going to participate, and some of the doctors didn't participate. They didn't want to get any payment from any source that had anything like the meaning of socialized medicine. Now I think they realize it's a gold mine. They can get things paid for that never otherwise would have been paid. They would have rendered the services and not been paid.

Nelson Cruikshank, of the AFL-CIO, commented on the Mills maneuver to bring out a bill that would provide for doctors' services as well as for hospital care.

CRUIKSHANK:[29]

He [Mills] worked out this compromise with the AMA. He didn't give the AMA very much, actually. He kind of took them at their word. He said that, "You talk about aid to the needy not the greedy. OK, we'll take care of the needy. We'll have a Medicaid bill and do that on a means test basis. The other people we'll handle on an insurance basis." You see, the AMA didn't want that part of it at all. He was able to kind of turn their propaganda against them and say that he was doing what they were asking. Of course he was doing a lot more. How could they object to that? They did object, but it didn't get anywhere.

The bill, with its compromises and a piece for everybody, passed the House on April 8, 1965. It was then sent to the Senate Finance Committee.

The passage in the House was nearly uneventful. One incident, however, showed that, without the new Democratic and Republican members favoring Medicare, the bill might have failed. A motion was made to send the Mills bill back to committee and substitute the original Byrnes bill. That motion lost by 45 votes, or one more than the number of new members favoring Medicare. Mills had been right: Medicare never would have passed in the 1963 session.

The Senate Finance Committee hearings on Medicare began in late April and were completed on May 19. The AMA's opposition was outspoken during those hearings, and the committee's response at times was acerbic. Furthermore, during the executive sessions of the committee, in which the Senate version of the House bill was being written, a major problem developed. Senator Russell B. Long (D–La.) announced a planned amendment to the bill. (This amendment certainly was known to the AMA, because one of its publications was in press with the news at the time.) The amendment called for unlimited hospital stays for persons age 65 and over. This was to be financed by a graduated scale of deductions based on income, ranging from 5 percent of the first $1,000 of income and 6 percent of the second, to 7 percent of any amount above that.

This maneuver by Long threw Anderson and others off balance, because it would load the bill with indeterminable added costs and would introduce a means test, which was anathema to most of the members.

Long's announcement came as a surprise, as did his request for a quick vote. The amendment carried in committee. The incident was darkened by

Long's misuse of a proxy from Senator J.W. Fulbright (D–Ark.). Further, Senator Paul Douglas (D–Ill.), a leading liberal, was misled into believing that this was the right thing to do until he began calculating cost and benefit figures. He was dismayed at how he had miscast his vote.[30]

Nelson Cruikshank was on the scene trying to help get the Medicare bill passed. He sat in on meetings in which the Democrats tried to plan a strategy to circumvent Long and get the Senate bill written so it would get out of committee and receive a favorable vote on the floor. He was asked what motivated Long.

CRUIKSHANK:[31]

It was awfully hard to tell what motivated him.

Senator Long was joined by Senator Abraham Ribicoff [D–Conn.]. The Long-Ribicoff amendments would have made Medicare a catastrophic insurance thing. When Long and Ribicoff came up with their amendments, Paul Douglas supported it. Then Douglas' conscience started working on him—not only his conscience, but his brain. He was a trained economist, you know. He called me over and he said, "Here's what I have done, and I feel unsure of myself."

I said, "I am glad you do, because I think you have undercut the whole thing. Our whole long battle is lost. We can't support this kind of thing."

"Well," he said, "how can we reverse it?"

I said, "You voted for it, didn't you?"

He said, "Yes."

I said, "That puts you in a parliamentary position to ask for a reconsideration in the finance committee."

"But that's very hard to do. That's never done," he said.

"Well, Senator, it's a matter of principle." (You could talk principle to Paul Douglas.)

Then in that milieu emerged Senator Vance Hartke of Indiana, who also was a member of the Senate Finance Committee. He came up with a compromise. I forget just what it was, but both Long and Ribicoff could support it. It went a long way toward the Long-Ribicoff proposal.

As I said, Hartke came up with a proposal, a compromise proposal. He called me over to his office.

He said, "I can pass this. I have got enough assurance that I can pass this compromise. You can't pass the House version in this committee."

I said, "I don't know whether we can or not."

At that point I didn't want to close the door entirely. I said we would think it over. I went to Senator Clinton Anderson. That was the Anderson bill in the Senate, you know. I said, "Where do we stand on this?"

Now Anderson was an insurance man himself. He made his money in insurance. He ran a big insurance company in New Mexico—workmen's compensation. He knew the insurance business. He used to tell his insurance colleagues, "You are crazy to oppose this. This is sound insurance."

Unfortunately, Anderson was not well. He was sick half the time. It was a heroic thing for him to even be on the floor during these battles. Anderson said that he would sound out the committee to see how many would stand by a vote to reconsider. Then, if they passed the vote to reconsider, he would put his original proposal forward for endorsement again by the Senate Finance Committee.

I said, "OK. See where you land, count your noses."

The meeting of the committee was to be held on Monday morning at 10 o'clock. I was in Anderson's office at 9 o'clock. He came out. He had worked over the weekend with his colleagues. There were 17 members on the committee.

I said, "Where do we stand, Senator?"

He said, "We've got nine people in favor of the original bill."

I said, "That's a majority of one."

He said, "That's right."

I said, "Who are they?"

He read them off. One was Senator Harry Byrd of Virginia, a conservative old character, you know.

I said, "My God, Clint, that's a weak reed to lean on. Maybe we've got to think of the Hartke proposal."

"Well," he said, "Senator Byrd said he would stand with me." And Anderson looked at me and said, "What do we do?"

I said, "Let's go for broke. We have compromised enough."

I'll never forget. He held on to my hand and said, "I hoped you would say that."

Later he told me that Senator Byrd voted with him and then in the committee he said, "I cast this vote this way, and I want to tell you why. I am going to vote against Medicare when it gets to the floor. I am against it on principle but I don't think the way to kill a bill is to load it up with ridiculous amendments. I think the bill ought to go before the Senate with a clean choice."

That was conservative old Byrd from Virginia. But that was touch and go. Years and years of work hung on that one vote.

=====

The Anderson forces won in the next Senate Finance Committee vote against the proposed Long amendments. The bill was reported out, and on July 9 the Senate passed the Medicare bill. Because of the differences in the House and Senate versions, the two bills were sent to a joint conference committee. The bill had originated in the House, so the committee was under the chairmanship of Wilbur Mills.

The joint conference committee took a week to complete proceedings and compromise on the differences in the bills. Both houses passed the compromise bill, which became part of the Social Security Amendments of 1965, by July 28, 1965. Two days later, President Johnson went to Independence, Missouri, for a ceremonial signing in the presence of former President Harry S. Truman. Several congressmen and others active in the writing and passing of Medicare and Medicaid were on the scene as witnesses. The event received wide television and press coverage.

Several persons have looked back at the legislative process of establishing, and the administrative process for implementing, Medicare and Medicaid. Walter McNerney, for 20 years president of the Blue Cross Association, commented on the compromises, the giving and taking, that went into the process of passing the legislation for Medicare.

McNERNEY:[32]

In the nature of compromise, under the general banner of pragmatism, there were arguments about whether there should be deductibles or copayments when planning Medicare. Some felt they should be included for no other reason than to keep the program financially sound.

It's wonderful to watch the government in action in this regard. I don't say this with disrespect, it's simply factual. When legislators and members of the administration saw the figures, they became concerned about the impact on the trust funds and on general tax revenues and began to talk deductibles and copayments. Evangelists for comprehensive coverage suddenly got very practical about matters and forgot the bad things they had said about indemnity or other forms of "inadequate" coverage.

The big issue over deductibles and copayments, aside from the precise design and amount, was could these be filled by private carrier coverages in the public market? Wilbur Mills tested the water on this issue and found out very fast, from other members of Congress and from the general public, that the public didn't want anybody stepping in the way. If they, the public, wanted to buy insurance to fill the gaps in Medicare, then they would fill them and to hell with the doctrine of whether deductibles and copayments would, could, or should be used. That water hasn't been tested since, because it came back so emphatically clear what the results would be.

I'd like to make one comment here.

It's very popular these days to point out that part of the bargain under the Medicare and Medicaid acts was that very little would be done to interfere with the practice of medicine or the operation of hospitals. You can point to it in the bill and in the committee reports. The implication is that, in order to get the deal swung, it had to be largely a financing operation, so hands off medicine and hospitals. It becomes very convenient to say that's why we ran into inflationary problems, that's why in the seventies we have so many beds, etc., etc. I want to offer this small historical note.

There was a fair amount of discussion about controls—not with the sophistication we do it today, but still there was a fair amount of discussion. The state of the art differed. We didn't know as much about how to exercise control. But don't let anybody kid you, the questions of how to negotiate formulas, of how to define qualified hospitals, of the desirability of strengthening areawide planning were all discussed at that point in the sixties.

The polite language for the sake of the health establishment, that things wouldn't be touched, was a front piece. There was already concern about how to shape things so this program wouldn't get out of hand. In fact, if you read the bills closely, you can see that certain controls were actually instituted. However, the action was along an evolutionary path.

———

Nelson Cruikshank also gives his observation of Medicare in action.

———

CRUIKSHANK:[33]

I have often said I have been talking about hospitals and health care all my life but have never been hospitalized. But last winter I spent 16 days in the hospital. I had a $12,000 hospital bill. Medicare paid almost all of it. You see, it is a damned good program in circumstances like that. Now, if I had a bad nosebleed or an ingrown toenail or something like that, Medicare probably wouldn't even cover it. Those things go into the average. That also says something about the nature of a health program. The health program ought to take care of minor things as well as major things. Medicare is a better program than people give it credit for. Fourteen of $15 billion worth of health bills for older people are paid for out of the system. As I say, the big bills are pretty well taken care of.

———

Implementation of Medicare

A frequent topic of conversation about Medicare is the role of the private sector in administering it.

One factor should be stressed: the insurance companies had a claims-processing apparatus in use and experienced personnel to operate it. The federal government passed the Medicare law and specified it would go into effect within 11 months. Could they buy equipment and set up a system to handle millions of claims monthly within that short time?

Another question was asked: Were the fiscal intermediaries for Medicare part A and the carriers for part B set up as a sop to the insurance companies, or could the claims services of insurance companies handle Medicare claims better than the government?

Wilbur Mills had no question about the need to use insurance companies. He saw them as fulfilling a need and also as a buffer mechanism.

MILLS:[34]

The use of private insurance was a means of softening the relationship between the doctor and the government. Get somebody in between you and the agency you deal with in the government. A provider's organization, primarily Blue Cross and Blue Shield, something they set up themselves— that could be the intermediary.

The whole theory that we had was the more services you make available, the more people you're going to need to provide those services. You don't want to rule any of them out, nor wipe them out. But, no, this was not done as a sop to anybody. Rather, it was the recognition of what we thought was a fact. They're all going to be needed. So you have got to work it out on the basis that they will participate.

Wilbur Cohen saw the use of an intermediary as a way of building the relationship between the public and private sectors.

COHEN:[35]

I have strongly taken the position that, under any kind of national health insurance plan, whether a partial one like Medicare or a comprehensive one, the payment process should be handled by fiscal intermediaries such as Blue Cross, Blue Shield, and commercial insurance companies. I believe that this is a very practical way of both handling some of the day-to-day administrative problems and of forging an effective relationship between the public and the private sectors.

James Hague, former director of publications and corporate secretary of the AHA, and Kenneth Williamson, former director of the Washington Service Bureau of the AHA, speak about intermediaries.

HAGUE:[36]

The American Hospital Association didn't want the Social Security Administration to administer the Medicare program. The AHA by and large prevailed, removing Social Security from the active administration of Medicare—through the intermediaries.

We fought for them and won. The AHA staff did the scut work that led to the nomination by an overwhelming majority of hospitals of the Blue

Cross Association as the intermediary. First, saying there had to be an intermediary; and then, second, naming Blue Cross Association as the intermediary. By and large, it's worked quite well, I think.

<hr/>

WILLIAMSON:[37]

In the writing of Medicare there has been a lot of discussion, some of which is amusing to me, about the Blue Cross role. I can tell you one thing flatly, no "if" or "and," the role Blue Cross had in Medicare *I* negotiated. The intermediary was *my* idea. If Ed Crosby [executive director of AHA] were alive, I am sure he would say this. I talked with him about it at the time we got to the bill-drafting stages.

The hospitals needed protection. They needed somebody they trusted between themselves and the government. The House Ways and Means Committee was discussing how to administer Medicare as they drafted the bill. The first thought was to go to the states. However, most of the states had had no experience, no ability to organize a health program or to administer one. Private insurance? No. There was nothing in the government field with sufficient ability. The biggest supporting argument I had is that, with Blue Cross, you have the one entity organized in the field at the state level and coordinated nationally with the support of the people you must have, the hospitals—a voluntary approach, with all the strengths of that and the goodwill that would come from it.

The intermediary role had the strengths I have mentioned. Ed Crosby agreed with me. We needed to do something; there was no time to stop and talk and ask Blue Cross if they wanted it. As a matter of fact, I said that it was for their best interest if we decide this and just put it in. We decided, and we put it in, and they have suffered the benefit. Interestingly enough, over the years I have heard all sorts of talk about how Blue Cross worked in developing this role. Hell's bells, they had nothing to do with it!

I read that book Odin Anderson wrote about two years ago about Blue Cross. I was amused by Odin's discussion of the Blue Cross role. Well, Blue Cross picked it up and did a great job. However, during those times (of planning Medicare) I never remember Blue Cross being considered, or talked to, or having anything to do with the intermediary role in advance. It came about because the government at a point in these discussions said, "How are we going to administer Medicare?"

The arguments favored Blue Cross, fit the times, and I was able to sell it. Nelson Cruikshank and Wilbur Cohen and others bought it. Blue Cross didn't come to them with the idea at all. When it was an accomplished fact, Blue Cross Association had to go and sell their field on what to do about it.

Once the concept of the intermediary became a part of the bill, Daniel Pettengill of Aetna sought out Wilbur Cohen to get clarification of how the insurance company might participate. Pettengill speaks of this conversation.

PETTENGILL:[38]

When it became obvious that Medicare was going to go through, I went to Wilbur Cohen, who was then the assistant secretary of the Department of Health, Education, and Welfare, and said to him, "I realize that the nation is going to have this Medicare program. But there is a provision in the proposed legislation that Medicare shall be administered by the private sector, unless you find the private sector unable to do it."

Wilbur, who is a very pleasant individual even though he was not exactly in my corner, smiled at me and said, "Dan, I've been planning on this ever since the Great Depression. Because, you know, they tried to get this into the original Social Security Act and just missed by the skin of their teeth because President Roosevelt had a change of heart at the last minute."

Then Wilbur said, "I could do this all with my own hand, but you're right, Congress is putting that feature in, so I appreciate your coming and telling me that you are willing to participate."

I was able to persuade a number of other commercial insurance companies to participate. Walter McNerney, as president of the Blue Cross Association, was also in Washington saying that the Blues would be very happy to do it all.

So there was considerable competition between the Blues and the insurance companies over the administration of Medicare. I must confess, the Blues got a much larger share than we did.

Walter J. McNerney discusses the process of choice of intermediaries. (Blue Cross Association, through a subcontracting arrangement with individual Blue Cross plans, was chosen intermediary in a large majority of instances.)

McNERNEY:[39]

The particular design of the nomination process for choosing fiscal intermediaries to administer Medicare part A and the prime contract involving the Blue Cross Association, as intermediary, had this negotiation factor as a backdrop.

It was a very good way of getting the cooperation of the American hospitals—giving them the right of some say over the intermediary. The intermediary position itself was a compromise between those who wanted HEW to pay claims versus those who wanted private carriers to do it on an underwritten basis. Once that pragmatic compromise was resolved, the hospitals said, quite rightly, that the use of intermediaries suggests that there are two ends. You have one end, we want the other. If you are going to have the right to administer the program, we want some say over who the intermediary is. It's a two-way street. The intermediary is almost a natural outgrowth of this realization.

Some of us put it in more concrete terms than others. At any rate, it became an attractive way of eliciting the support of hospitals and easing the interface between the public and private sectors, while capitalizing on existing and in-place institutions and expertise.

Blue Cross represented an attractive candidate for the intermediaryship. There were no profits to inure to individuals or groups of individuals. It made sense that intermediaries be largely community-oriented institutions. The fact that Blue Cross was there in that mold made it more or less a natural to get a lot of the nominations. The other side of the coin was that the nomination process became realistic because Blue Cross existed.

There are a lot of details about who felt how about what. I was impressed that Wilbur Mills, who at that point was playing a very prominent role, was simply trying to sift through a series of ideas that could be put into a workable framework, not trying to moralize on any perfect arrangement.

The Medicare part B side reflected a slightly different situation. A distinction was made between the carriers under part B and the intermediary under part A. It is interesting that the carrier had an extra function or two. Therefore, the buffer zone between the doctor and the government was presumably a little broader.

It didn't take a lot of intelligence to see that didn't mean anything extra special, because, whereas there might have been an extra function in the report, and bill language seemed to give the carrier a slightly more independent status, the secretary of HEW was empowered to designate the carriers by state and the physicians were not in the position to nominate by state. So it was about equal: what you lost in one variable you gained in another.

There were some interesting byplays in the nominations that the secretary made. For example, the number of states that went to Blue Shield as carrier was roughly proportionate to their percentage of population enrolled. It is interesting that the nomination design reflected in a way the history of hospitals versus doctors vis-a-vis the government.

========

McNerney also talks about the tremendous amount of work that had to be done by both government officials and Blue Cross, as the principal intermediary, in preparing to implement Medicare and Medicaid on July 1, 1966.

McNERNEY:[40]

The implementation of Medicare and Medicaid led to a lot of work.

Here it was, it had to be made to go as of July 1. I spent a tremendous amount of time with Robert Ball (commissioner of the Social Security Administration) and Art Hess (deputy commissioner of the Social Security Administration) ironing out what our relationships, our relative roles, would be. That led to a lot of gutsy, protracted discussions. Obviously, there were differences. The Social Security Administration, as far as this program was concerned, envisioned itself as the administrator and Blue Cross as an agent for getting the thing done.

We at Blue Cross, as intermediaries, thought of ourselves in little grander terms than that. Because we were nominated by the hospitals, for example, we felt we had a dual accountability. Also, we thought that we could be quite useful in shaping the destiny and the goals of the program, as well as carrying out its administrative provisions.

Bob and Art are highly capable people. Whereas this tension existed, they were bright enough, and I trust we were too, to overlook it and get down to practicalities of getting Medicare off the ground. I don't think there is a serious doubt that the program couldn't have gotten off the ground as it did if it hadn't been for Blue Cross and others in the private sector. I am very proud of the fact that, with 90 percent of the business on the part A side, we were able to move in and get it going with little friction as far as the American public was concerned. Not that everything went totally well, but, my God, it was impressive!

We had some trouble, for example, with some of our elderly subscribers who didn't want to give up their Blue Cross coverage because they trusted us more than they did the government. We finally talked them into that and developed some supplementary coverages. We eased the transition into Medicare the best we could. What has followed in the operation of the program since 1965 has been a series of encounters, contracts negotiated and renegotiated—a perfecting and a honing of relative roles.

Before I get off 1965, I want to remark that the negotiation as to who would do what (HEW vis-a-vis Blue Cross and the hospitals) often involved many HEW lawyers, six or seven or eight staff members from HEW, and a lesser, but nevertheless large, number from Blue Cross and other private institutions sitting and talking. On a few occasions I would call Bob Ball and say, "How about you and I going into a room alone?"

To his credit, he would join me. We'd shut the door and decide things. It took that because many were watching their territory and rationalizing their sentiments and so forth. There just had to be some gut decisions made.

I never felt uncomfortable making them with him, because his eye was on performance and he had a concern that the aged not get lost in the process.

I have no qualms at all about whether it was a good thing to do in 1965 or 1966. I think it was a very effective way of getting Medicare going, both on the part A and B sides. It was the best compromise. Even in retrospect I think it was the best compromise.

For the first five or ten years of the program, the intermediary relationship, I think, was viewed pretty congenially by all parties. HEW could not have started the program without the intermediary. The hospitals and doctors were relieved to have an intermediary versus dealing directly with HEW. Somewhere in the early seventies, however, Blue Cross–Blue Shield was increasingly put in the position of being the messenger of bad news. The intermediary role got tarnished by the field's frustration over excessive regulation, excessive this, excessive that.

As a result, the intermediary relationship became a source of strain between doctors, hospitals, and HEW. In the last year or so I think the intermediary is beginning to move back to a more treasured and appreciated relationship.

It's important to realize that over the years the Medicare contract has changed. You could guess what would happen. As government has become increasingly informed, they have felt they should have more direct control over the program and that the intermediary role should be lessened. So each year the contract negotiation revolves more around this basic point of relative roles.

In recent years we even hear, "Thank you so much for helping us get this started, but now that we have got it established in Washington and in regional offices around the country, outside of a few inconveniences, we can handle it." That isn't said publicly, because it would be politically inflammatory, but in a sense it's an unspoken word behind contract negotiations. Things haven't come to that, and they won't. I think we have too much to offer for that. There is no question our performance is better than anybody else's, both from a cost point of view and a quality point of view.

═══════

The implementation of the part B portion of Medicare, physician services, represented a different kind of problem. Daniel Pettengill and Nelson Cruikshank discuss it.

═══════

PETTENGILL:[41]

Surgical schedules are another interesting story. When, in 1938, the first surgical benefit was written on a group basis, somebody designed the so-called $150 schedule. It paid up to $100 for an appendectomy, and for most procedures it paid considerably less than that, while for certain very rare procedures it paid up to $150. If more than one procedure was per-formed, the maximum benefit for all procedures combined was $150.

When I first came to the group division at Aetna, in some of the lower cost areas of the country (and there wasn't that much variation in fees in those days) you would find doctors who would accept what was in that $150 schedule as their full fee. It was a convenience to their patients and to some extent to themselves, because there was no hassle.

The surgeon knew what the scheduled maximum amount was, what the individual had, and that's what he was most likely to collect as a fee. But then what happened was that surgeons began to say the payment rate was unrelated to the skill required to perform the surgery and you insurers ought to do something. So in 1945 the Society of Actuaries made a schedule based on actual charges under claims received by several of the major insurers . . . that's one of the first things I worked on. This new schedule had a maximum benefit of $200 and better relativity among the scheduled amounts for the various procedures.

Then in 1956 the Society of Actuaries made another study and came out with a $300 schedule. There never was another schedule made, basically for two reasons. First, the California doctors came out with the California Relative Value Schedule, which covered far more procedures than the typical insurance company schedules. Second, such a spread in medical care costs had developed from one part of the country to another that large employers who had employees all over the country were saying, "Look, there is no schedule that does us any good. If we take your $300 schedule and double it, why that might be appropriate for New York City and Chicago, but it's too low for San Francisco and Los Angeles and it's too high for New Orleans."

So insurers were forced to write an unscheduled benefit which would pay the surgeon's actual charge, provided it was reasonable. This was the reason that, when Medicare came along, the government said that for part B it would pay for 80 percent of the physician's usual and customary charge, but not more than the prevailing fee in the area.

Unfortunately, the government overlooked two very important facts. First, most insurance plans then in force still provided surgical benefits on a scheduled basis, so that physicians generally were not accustomed to ben-efits based on a usual and customary charge. Second, few, if any, insurers knew what each physician charged and had only a rough idea of the pre-vailing charge—and then only in areas where it had many people covered for major medical benefits. (Most major medical and comprehensive plans require that the service be necessary and the charge reasonable.) With Med-icare saying that, "If you accept an assignment of benefits, you're going to get 80 percent of your usual and customary fee," many physicians in the country suddenly increased their usual and customary fees; but valid statistical proof of these increases was often lacking.

This was one of the many problems and changes caused by Medicare that affected all health insurance. Although I have no proof, I am reasonably sure that Secretary Cohen was instructed by President Lyndon Johnson to make the administration of part B of Medicare acceptable to organized medicine so that the physicians wouldn't strike and ruin the operation of the Medicare program.

Time and again I would say to Secretary Cohen, "Look, you don't want to do that. I know from personal experience it's going to cause all kinds of problems." But he would ignore my advice whenever the doctors would say, "We want it this way."

One of the best examples of sound advice ignored because of pressure from organized medicine was the handling of the charges for radiation therapy, diagnostic X rays, and pathology. Prior to Medicare, when a patient received one of these services in the hospital, the charge for it was considered as being a hospital charge. Indeed, the charge for the service normally came through on the hospital bill. There was not a separate bill from the physician involved. The physician generally had a separate arrangement with the hospital to pay him for his part in the service, but the hospital did not itemize this on its bill to the patient. So insurers paid the one charge as part of the hospital-ancillary service benefit.

The doctors came down and said, "Look, we don't want that. We want to bill the patient ourselves." And Secretary Cohen gave in to them, even after the hospitals said that they would continue to bill the patient for supplies and the use of equipment and hospital employees. What Secretary Cohen finally did was to permit the physician to charge for the professional component of the service and the hospital to charge for the nonprofessional component, the former to be covered under part B and the latter under part A of Medicare. [Wilbur Cohen says Congress did this against the administration's wishes.]

So overnight the cost of these services was virtually doubled, not just for Medicare, but for everyone, because physicians very quickly did this for all their patients, not just their Medicare patients. The result was a tragic increase in costs.

That was a battle, it was a bitter battle, but it was lost because Secretary Cohen, I believe, was under instructions from President Johnson to give in to the extent necessary to keep peace with the doctors. [Cohen says Pettengill is "absolutely wrong; L.B.J. was opposed."]

CRUIKSHANK:[42]

I was against Medicare B [he had expressed opposition to Medicaid]. Not on principle, but on tactics Leonard Lesser and I teamed up and appeared before the committees and talked to our friends in the Ways and Means Committee, saying that our experience with negotiated health plans was that these doctors' services are the things that give us the most trouble. "Pass the hospital part, run that for a few years and digest it. Sure, the older people need the doctors' thing that's set up in part B, but let's not clog the machinery. Let's make this a bite at a time."

Our strongest friends on the Ways and Means said, "Aw, come on, fellows, you got what you want. Let's not be picayune. The hell with it. This is going to ride through. Don't try to stop it." So we had to ride with the punch. The fact is that our trouble with Medicare is in part B to this day.

On balance, Medicare has been a good program that has brought needed care to many elderly persons who might otherwise have gone without it. Billions of dollars have been paid in benefits, and the entire practice of medicine has been changed.

Many aspects of the Medicare program have developed differently than expected. For example, actuaries, both government and private, were unable to estimate accurately what the costs of the program would be. Their estimates were a fraction of actual costs. Now the nation is struggling to make adjustments in order to avoid bankruptcy for Medicare. Total expenditures are uncontrollable, and politically it is impossible to cut benefits.

Medicare B has been unsatisfactory in other ways. Doctors generally have not accepted the schedule of fees posted under Medicare, so in many cases patients have had to pay an additional fee. The copayment feature for financing part B began at $3.00 per month, deducted from the monthly Social Security check. The federal government matched this. The copayment fee has had to be raised nearly every year in order to meet expenses. Now, instead of being $3.00 per month, it is nearly five times that. Also, the government has increased its contribution from 50 percent to 75 percent.

Medicaid has not worked well either. It is still not a program of uniform benefits in all the states, and it has been a tremendous financial burden in many states.

All in all, however, Medicare and Medicaid have been steps forward. Practically no one would wish to return to the conditions that existed before 1966. Adjustments and changes will come, and obstacles will be overcome. Medicare and Medicaid will prevail, even if altered in a form to adjust to changing political and economic realities.

Notes

(Transcripts of the oral histories cited here are housed in the library of the American Hospital Association, 840 North Lake Shore Drive, Chicago, Illinois 60611. The Oral History Collection is a joint project of the Hospital Research and Educational Trust and the AHA.)

1. See Profiles of Participants, in the center of this book, for biographical information.

2. *Nelson Cruikshank, In the First Person: An Oral History.*

3. *Cruikshank, Oral History.*

4. Ibid.

5. Marion Folsom and Arthur Larson, both prominent Republicans, privately favored Medicare.

6. *Cruikshank, Oral History.*

7. See Profiles of Participants for biographical information.

8. *Wilbur Cohen, in the First Person: An Oral History.*

9. *Walter J. McNerney, In the First Person: An Oral History.* See Profiles of Participants for biographical information.

10. See Profiles of Participants for biographical information.

11. *John R. Mannix, In the First Person: An Oral History.*

12. See Profiles of Participants for biographical information.

13. *Daniel W. Pettengill, In the First Person: An Oral History.*

14. *Cruikshank, Oral History.*

15. For a detailed account of the attempted Anderson-Javits amendment, see the monograph by Gary L. Filerman, *The Senate Rejects Health Insurance for the Aged,* available from University Microfilms, 300 N. Zeeb Road, Ann Arbor, Mich. 48107.

16. *Cruikshank, Oral History.*

17. Ibid.

18. Ibid.

19. Ibid.

20. *Wilbur D. Mills, In the First Person: An Oral History.* See Profiles of Participants for biographical information.

21. *Cruikshank, Oral History.*

22. *Pettengill, Oral History.*

23. *Mills, Oral History.*

24. *Cohen, Oral History.*

25. *Kenneth Williamson, In the First Person: An Oral History.* See Profiles of Participants for biographical information.

26. *Mills, Oral History.*

27. *Pettengill, Oral History.*

28. *Mills, Oral History.*

29. *Cruikshank, Oral History.*

30. Douglas' account of his activities during the passage of Medicare can be found in his autobiography, *In the Fullness of Time* (New York: Harcourt Brace Jovanovich, 1972), pp. 394–96.

31. *Cruikshank, Oral History.*

32. *McNerney, Oral History.*

33. *Cruikshank, Oral History.*

34. *Mills, Oral History.*

35. *Cohen, Oral History.*

36. *James Hague, In the First Person: An Oral History.* See Profiles of Participants for biographical information.

37. *Williamson, Oral History.*
38. *Pettengill, Oral History.*
39. *McNerney, Oral History.*
40. Ibid.
41. *Pettengill, Oral History.*
42. *Cruikshank, Oral History.*

Profiles of Participants

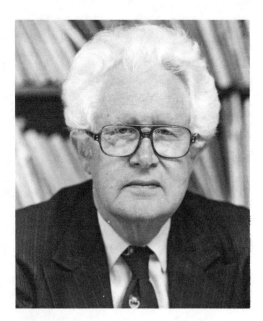

Odin W. Anderson

Odin W. Anderson was born in Minneapolis on July 5, 1914. He was orphaned at the age of three and grew up in a rural Norwegian community in Wisconsin in the home of an uncle. Anderson said that it was a "given" in that home that he would get an education. He earned a bachelor's degree (1937) and a master's degree (1938) in sociology at the University of Wisconsin and a bachelor's degree (1940) in library science and a doctorate (1948) in sociology at the University of Michigan.

He taught what later became known as medical sociology at the University of Western Ontario (1949–1952) before moving to the Health Information Foundation in New York City as research director. At HIF (1952–1962) he developed a new dimension of the household interview survey methodology, which had originally been designed in the early 1930s by his mentor at the University of Michigan, Nathan Sinai, for the Committee on the Costs of Medical Care.

Anderson left HIF in 1962 to join the faculty of the University of Chicago as research director for the Center for Health Administration Studies and as associate professor in the Graduate School of Business and the department of sociology. (He became a full professor in 1964.) In 1967 Anderson became associate director of the center, and in 1972, director. In addition, he was appointed director of the Graduate Program in Health Administration and served in that post from 1978 to 1980.

On receiving emeritus status in 1980, Anderson accepted part-time appointments at both the University of Chicago and the University of Wisconsin.

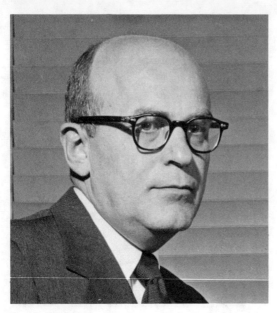

George Bugbee

George Bugbee was born in Waukesha, Wisconsin, in 1904. He was graduated from the University of Michigan in 1926 and was a member of Phi Beta Kappa. He immediately went to work at the University of Michigan's new hospital as an accountant. By 1938, he was assistant director. Bugbee left the hospital to become superintendent of Cleveland City Hospital. He remained there until 1943, when he accepted the position of executive director of the American Hospital Association. His job was to transform the AHA into an association capable of assuming broad responsibilities in the hospital field: representing members before government and other bodies and the public in general; carrying out research and standardizing practice in hospitals; and undertaking educational projects. During Bugbee's tenure (1943–1954), the AHA grew stronger and its educational and research activities were enhanced. A study commission on hospital care was encouraged; this led to the Hospital Survey and Construction (Hill-Burton) Act, which aided in the construction of hospitals. Also at this time, the AHA became a founder and participant in the Joint Commission on Accreditation of Hospitals.

Bugbee left the AHA in 1954 to head the Health Information Foundation, which was created to do research in health care. When the HIF decided to disband in 1962, Bugbee moved to the University of Chicago with the remainder of the HIF grant. There he established the Center for Health Administration Studies and became director of the university's program in hospital administration. He retired to emeritus status in 1970 but continues to work as a consultant and, until recently, as director of the Veterans Administration Forum.

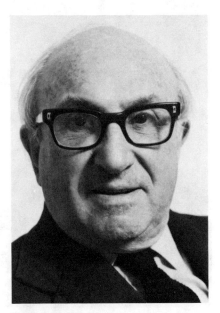

Wilbur J. Cohen

Wilbur J. Cohen was born in Milwaukee on June 10, 1913. He was graduated from the University of Wisconsin with a bachelor's degree in economics in 1936 and went to Washington, D.C., later that year as assistant to the director of the cabinet-level Committee on Economic Security. (The director was Edwin Witte, under whom Cohen had studied at Wisconsin.) That committee's report formed the basis of the Social Security Act. After the Social Security Act was passed, Cohen joined the staff of the Social Security Administration as technical adviser to the commissioner. Cohen worked there from 1936 to 1955, and at the time of his resignation he was the director of the Division of Research and Statistics.

Cohen became professor of public welfare at the University of Michigan School of Social Work in 1956. He remained at Michigan until 1961. During that time, he was sought after as a consultant by many federal and state councils, commissions, and task forces.

The administration of John F. Kennedy called Cohen back to government service in 1961. He was first appointed assistant secretary of health, education, and welfare, then under secretary in 1965, and finally secretary, in which post he served from 1968 to 1969.

Cohen returned to the Michigan campus as dean of the School of Education; he took emeritus status in 1978. In 1980 Wilbur Cohen was appointed Sid W. Richardson Professor of Public Affairs at the Lyndon Baines Johnson School of Public Affairs, University of Texas, Austin.

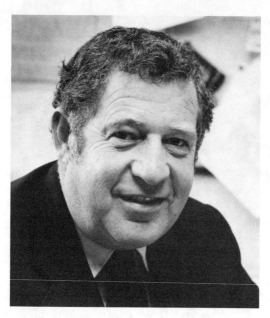

Edward J. Connors

Edward J. Connors was born in Sioux City, Iowa, on February 23, 1929. He was graduated from the University of South Dakota with a B.S. in mathematics in 1951. He originally intended to be a teacher or a school administrator, but his career plans were interrupted by the Korean war. Connors served as an army infantry officer from 1951 to 1953. On his return to civilian life, Connors enrolled in the graduate program in hospital adminis-tration at the University of Minnesota under James Hamilton. He served his residency with O.G. Pratt at Rhode Island Hospital and stayed on an extra year as an administrative assistant (1954–1955). In 1956 Walter J. McNerney, a former Rhode Island Hospital resident, invited Connors to join him as assistant director of a program in hospital administration that he was starting at the University of Michigan. Connors taught in the program, directed community surveys for hospitals, and worked on the Michigan study of hospital and medical economics.

In 1960, at the age of 31, Connors became superintendent of the University of Wisconsin hospital. He held this position from 1963 to 1969, also serving during this time as assistant director of the University Medical Center. He took a sabbatical (1968–1969) to serve as a consultant to the Department of Health, Education, and Welfare. In 1969 he was invited to return to Michigan as director of the university hospital. In 1974 Connors left the hospital and acted as a consultant to the Sisters of Mercy Health Corporation, a multi-institutional health corporation. In 1976 he became president of the corporation.

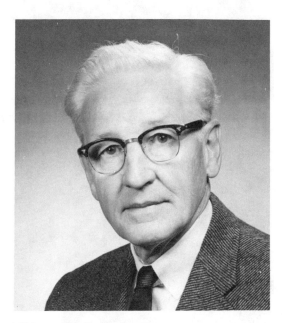

Nelson H. Cruikshank

Nelson H. Cruikshank entered the health field indirectly, through the American Federation of Labor (AFL). He was born on June 21, 1902, in Bradford, Ohio, where his father was a grain merchant. He was graduated in 1925 from Ohio Wesleyan University and in 1929 from Union Theological Seminary, where he prepared for the ministry. Cruikshank became interested in the labor movement during summer vacations from school, when he worked on Great Lakes freighters and was a member of the Seafarers' Union. After ordination, he divided his time between church work and labor organizing in Brooklyn and New Haven (1931–1935). He worked for the Works Progress Administration and then became the New England director of the Farm Security Administration (1935–1942). From 1943 to 1944, Cruikshank worked with another government agency, the War Manpower Commission.

As the war ended, Cruikshank joined the AF of L as director of social insurance activities (1944–1950). During this period he served on several national and international commissions for UNESCO (the United Nations Economic, Social, and Cultural Organization), the World Health Organization, the U.S. Public Health Service, the Department of Labor, and other organizations. He went back to the AF of L from 1953 to 1955, when its merger with the Congress of Industrial Organizations (CIO) took place. He became director of the department of social security, AFL-CIO, between 1955 and 1965, when he played a great part in helping develop Medicare. Cruikshank served on HIBAC (Health Insurance Benefits Council), the Medicare advisory council, from 1965 to 1972. Between 1965 and 1969 he was a visiting professor or lecturer at several universities. He served as president of the National Council of Senior Citizens (1969–1977) and as counselor on aging to President Carter (1977–1980).

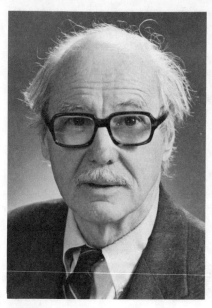

Robert M. Cunningham, Jr.

Robert M. Cunningham, Jr., was born in Chicago on May 28, 1909, and was graduated from the University of Chicago in 1931. His first job after college was with Perry Addleman, a fund raiser for the Armour Institute of Technology. Cunningham subsequently became assistant to the president of the institute. Through a recommendation from Addleman, Cunningham in 1937 moved to the position of assistant to the superintendent of Evanston (Illinois) Hospital. The hospital was planning a fund-raising campaign and needed a public relations person. After a few months' work, the fund-raising plan was postponed.

In 1938 Addleman invited Cunningham to join him at a Chicago group hospitalization prepayment plan called the Plan for Hospital Care (later the Chicago Blue Cross). Cunningham was hired to do public relations and general staff work.

In 1941 Cunningham left the plan to become associate editor of *Hygeia,* a magazine published by the American Medical Association. There he worked under the tutelage of Morris Fishbein, editor of the *Journal of the American Medical Association* and a spokesman for the AMA.

In 1945 Cunningham was employed by Otho Ball to be managing editor of *Modern Hospital.* He served as editor of the journal from 1951 to 1974. During that time, the magazine had several owners, including the F. W. Dodge Corporation and McGraw-Hill.

Since retirement in 1974, Cunningham has worked as consulting or contributing editor to the Blue Cross Association, *Hospitals, Trustee, Inquiry,* and McGraw-Hill's *Washington Newsletter on Health.*

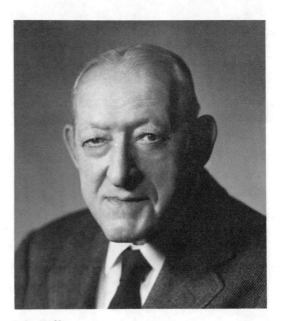

I.S. Falk

I.S. Falk was born in Brooklyn on September 30, 1899. He was graduated from a local high school at age 14 but was considered too young to enter college. This was fortunate, because Falk became the lab boy for Charles-Edward Amory Winslow, one of the greats in public health education. Winslow moved from New York City to Yale University to set up a new department in public health, and he took Falk with him. Winslow made Falk his protege and supervised his education before and after his matriculation at Yale. Falk received his Ph.B. from Yale in 1920 and his Ph.D. in 1923.

Falk became an assistant professor of bacteriology at the University of Chicago in 1923. He became associate professor in 1926 and full professor in 1929, at age 30. He became discouraged when construction of a school of public health at Chicago was postponed; he left the university to become director of research for the Committee on the Costs of Medical Care (CCMC) in 1929. This was midway in the life of CCMC, and research was behind schedule. Under Falk, studies were completed on schedule. In 1934, while he was on leave from the Milbank Foundation, Falk worked with the cabinet-level Committee on Economic Security, whose report became the basis for the Social Security Act. From 1936 to 1954, Falk worked in the Division of Research and Statistics of the Social Security Administration, the last years as director. Falk later worked as a consultant for the World Bank and other organizations. In 1961 he went back to Yale as a professor of public health, but from 1968 to 1979 he had another career, as executive director of a health maintenance organization located in New Haven and connected with Yale. Falk died in New Haven in 1984.

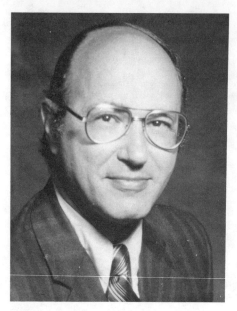

Gary L. Filerman

Gary L. Filerman was born in Minneapolis on November 16, 1936. As a student at the University of Minnesota, where he received his B.A. in 1958, he was interested in political and student activities. He began his health care career by working part-time at Mount Sinai Hospital in Minneapolis (1958–1959). He learned about administrative practice while serving as a fellow in the university president's office.

Filerman entered the graduate program in hospital administration at Minnesota and received his M.H.A. in 1960. He served his residency at the Johns Hopkins Hospital (1961–1962) under Dr. Russell Nelson. Concurrent with his work for the M.H.A., he had been working on a master's degree in political science, which he received in 1962. That summer he spent in Washington, D.C., at the Brookings Institution as a guest scholar. He studied the attempts to attach the proposed King-Anderson amendment to a Senate bill in an effort to keep alive an early version of the Medicare bill. The study resulted in a report by Filerman (with Frances Shattuck) titled "The Senate Rejects Health Insurance for the Aged."

Filerman returned to Minnesota for his Ph.D., which he received in 1964. The following weeks he spent studying health administration in Latin America. In 1965 he began his career with the Association of University Programs in Health Administration, first as director and then as president, with the goals of improving health administration teaching and education in the United States and improving ties with health administration programs in Latin America and Europe.

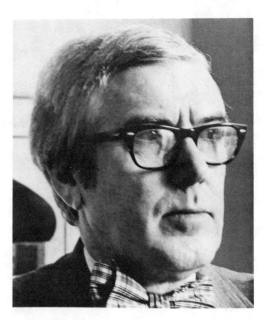

James E. Hague

James E. Hague was born on October 6, 1914, in Burnley, Lancashire, England, and came to the United States in 1924. His career in editing and publishing began as a newspaperman. He was a reporter for the Bridgeport *Times-Star* from 1933 to 1941. He then worked at the Hartford *Times* for a few months before joining the Associated Press in Baltimore as an editor and science writer. He served in the Pacific during World War II as a combat correspondent with the U.S. Marines.

After the war, Hague worked as director of public relations at the Johns Hopkins Hospital and as assistant to Dr. Edwin L. Crosby, the director of the hospital. Hague remained at Hopkins for four or five years, but had an urge to go back in the newspaper business. This led to his taking a job as assistant city editor of the Washington *Post* (1949–1953).

When George Bugbee had an opening at the American Hospital Association for a public relations person, Crosby recommended Hague. Thus began a long career for Hague at the AHA (1953–1977). In 1954 Crosby became executive director of the AHA. At this time, the editor of *Hospitals* wanted a change of duties, so Hague was appointed executive editor of the journal (1954–1959). Other positions at AHA followed for Hague: editor of *Trustee* (1957–1959); assistant director of the AHA (1957–1967); assistant corporate secretary of the AHA (1958–1962); editor-in-chief of the AHA (1959–1974); corporate secretary of the AHA (1962–1977); associate director of the AHA (1967–1974); and secretary emeritus of the AHA (1977).

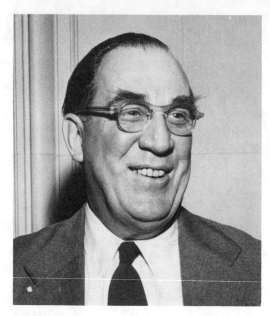

James A. Hamilton

James A. Hamilton was born in Brighton, Michigan, on July 14, 1899, but spent most of his boyhood in Lawrence, Massachusetts. His family was poor, but he worked his way through Dartmouth College, earning a bachelor's degree in science in 1922 and a master's in 1923. He stayed on at Dartmouth as an instructor and then an assistant professor in industrial engineering in the Amos Tuck School of Business (1923–1936). During his teaching years at Dartmouth he was very active in other activities: consultant in industrial engineering (1923–1936); assistant graduate manager of athletics of the college (1923–1936); superintendent of the Mary Hitchcock Memorial Hospital (1926–1936); and president of the New England Hospital Association (1930).

In 1936 Hamilton became superintendent of the Cleveland City Hospital. At about that time he began doing consulting work in hospital administration. In 1938 he returned to New England as director of the New Haven Hospital and as associate professor, and later professor, of hospital administration at Yale University. He remained there until 1946.

During this time, characteristically, he was also busy doing other things, including serving as president of the American College of Hospital Administrators (1939), a member of the secretary of war's Medical Service Commission (1942–1944), and president of the American Hospital Association (1943).

Hamilton was the founding director of the graduate program in hospital administration at the University of Minnesota in 1946. That same year he founded the consulting firm James A. Hamilton Associates. He served in both positions until his retirement in 1966.

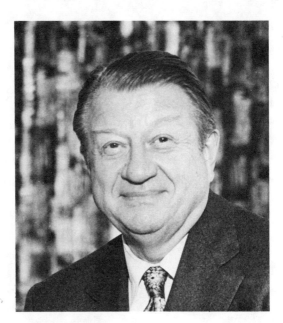

Gerhard Hartman

Gerhard Hartman was born in Buffalo on April 21, 1911, and received his bachelor's degree from the University of Buffalo in 1932, with a major in statistics. While there, he assisted in a study of a workers' prepayment health plan at Endicott Shoe Co. for the Committee on the Costs of Medical Care.

Hartman was under family pressure to choose a career as a violinist, physician, or business manager. With the idea of choosing in mind, he took a course at the university medical school to learn about the health care field. He also interviewed several leaders of the health field about training for hospital administration. After graduating from Buffalo, Hartman became an administrative statistician at Presbyterian Hospital in New York (1932–1934) while finishing his master's at Buffalo in business administration (1935). He then went on to the University of Chicago to study hospital administration and work on his doctorate under Arthur Bachmeyer.

Hartman became an instructor in hospital administration at Chicago (1937–1939) and executive secretary of the American College of Hospital Administrators (1937–1942). He received his doctorate in 1942, after he had begun working as director of Newton-Wellesley Hospital in Massachusetts (1942–1946). In 1946 he accepted a dual post at the State University of Iowa, where he remained the rest of his academic career (1946–1979). He became director of the university hospitals and professor (1946–1979) and chairman (1946–1977) of the graduate program in hospital administration.

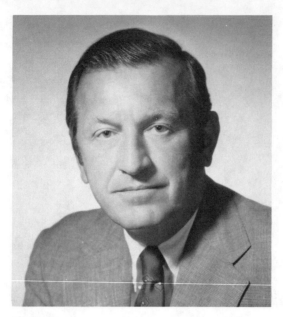

Walter J. McNerney

Walter J. McNerney was born on June 8, 1925, in New Haven, Connecticut, and was graduated from Yale University in 1947. While at Yale, he worked as a research assistant in the Labor-Management Center. After leaving Yale, he became an instructor in higher mathematics at Hopkins Preparatory School (1947–1948). McNerney entered the health field by completing the master's degree program in hospital administration at the University of Minnesota (1949–1950). He served his administrative residency under O.G. Pratt at Rhode Island Hospital. The next five years were spent at the University of Pittsburgh, as a teacher of hospital administration, an assistant to the coordinator of hospitals and clinics, and an administrator of one of the medical center hospitals. In 1955 McNerney was selected to be the first director of the program in hospital administration at the University of Michigan. While at Michigan, he directed an important study of the hospital and medical economics of the state. This study received national attention and undoubtedly led to his being offered the presidency of the Blue Cross Association in 1961. For the next 20 years McNerney built BCA into a strong national organization of Blue Cross plans. One notable result was the establishment of the Blue Cross Association in a dominant position among the fiscal intermediaries for Medicare. In 1977 the Blue Cross Association merged with the Blue Shield Association, with McNerney serving as president of the new corporation. McNerney is now Herman Smith Professor at the J.L. Kellogg Graduate School of Management at Northwestern University.

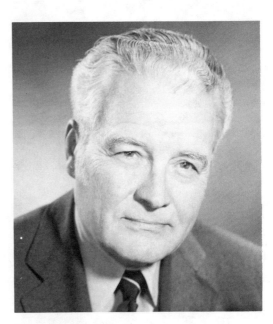

John Robert Mannix

John Mannix was born in Cleveland on June 4, 1902, and started working at Mount Sinai Hospital in that city while still in school. By 1926 he was supervisor of services under Frank E. Chapman, the administrator. At this time there grew up the idea that one uniform, inclusive hospital rate could pay for regular and ancillary services. Mannix developed the concept further as superintendent of Elyria (Ohio) Memorial Hospital (1926–1930). In 1930 he returned to Cleveland as assistant director, under Chapman, of the newly merged University Hospitals, and in 1932 the hospitals adopted the inclusive rate concept. During his years at University Hospitals (1930–1939), Mannix worked with others planning a group hospitalization prepayment plan for Cleveland. In 1939 he was asked to start and be chief executive of a Blue Cross plan for Michigan. In 1944 the Chicago plan invited Mannix to come there as chief executive officer. He stayed until 1946. One problem for Blue Cross plans was handling national accounts and claims for services across plan boundaries. Mannix suggested a national Blue Cross plan. When no interest was shown in the idea, he helped form the John Marshall Insurance Company to market health insurance nationally. The company did not survive in its original form and was sold. Mannix then became executive vice president of Cleveland Blue Cross (1948–1965) and later (1965–1972) vice president for research and planning. Mannix was also active in the American Hospital Association, particularly in the 1940s.

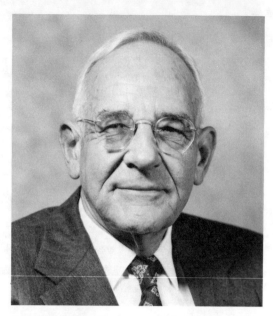

John S. Millis

John S. Millis was born on November 22, 1903, in Palo Alto, California, where his father was a professor at Stanford University. He studied physics at the University of Chicago under three Nobel laureates, Albert Michelson, Robert A. Millikan, and A.H. Compton. After being graduated from the University of Chicago in 1924, he was Master at Howe School (1924–1925). He returned to Chicago for his master's degree in 1927 and his doctorate in 1931. In the meantime, he spent the years between 1927 and 1941 at Lawrence College, Wisconsin (taking leave to finish his doctorate). At Lawrence he began as instructor and became professor of physics; he was also dean (1936–1941).

In 1939 Millis received a Carnegie Foundation Young Administrator's Grant, which allowed him to travel, visit, and study various colleges and educational systems. Through this experience he became known to Carnegie officials and was recommended for president of the University of Vermont, in which post he served from 1941 to 1949. He next became president of Western Reserve University (1949–1967). He was there when the Case-Western Reserve federation was effected, and he became chancellor in 1967. He took emeritus status in 1969.

Since retirement, Millis has served with many study groups on education, among them the AMA Citizens' Committee on Graduate Medical Education, the National Fund for Medical Education, the National Advisory Council for Dental Research, the National Board of Medical Examiners, the American Dietetic Study Commission, the Commission on Foreign Medical Graduates, the American Association of Colleges of Pharmacy study, and the Educational Commission on Foreign Medical Graduates.

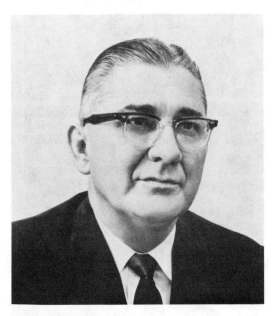

Wilbur D. Mills

Wilbur D. Mills is a native of Kensett, Arkansas, where he was born on May 14, 1909, the son of a banker. He was graduated from Hendricks College, in Conway, Arkansas, in 1930 and went on to Harvard Law School (1930–1933). He was admitted to the Arkansas bar and practiced for a short time in Searcy, Arkansas. Although his father was encouraging him to go into banking and other businesses, Mills was interested in law and politics. Years later Mills was to say that, if he had followed his father's advice, he might have become a wealthy man. Instead, after a four-year stint in his father's bank (1934–1938), he chose public service. Mills has said that his desire to serve in Congress, and especially on the Ways and Means Committee, dates back to boyhood.

Mills' political career began as a county and probate judge in White County, Arkansas. In 1939 he was elected to Congress, and he served in the House of Representatives with distinction until 1976. In 1942 Mills was appointed to the Ways and Means Committee. He was determined to be a knowledgeable member of that committee, so he reputedly memorized the Internal Revenue Code as well as studying the other laws affecting the work of the committee. Mills became chairman of the Ways and Means Committee in 1958, thus fulfilling a boyhood dream. Mills is remembered in the health field for his part in writing the Kerr-Mills, Medicare, and Medicaid legislation.

Since leaving Congress, he has been associated with Shea & Gould, a Washington, D.C., law firm, as a tax counsel.

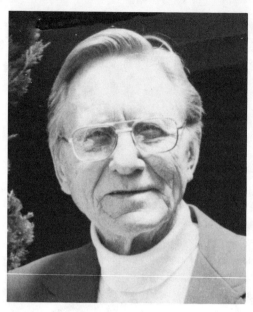

Maurice J. Norby

Maurice Norby was born in Le Center, Minnesota, on May 21, 1908, and was graduated from St. Olaf College, in Northfield, Minnesota, in 1930. He began teaching high school science but worked on his master's degree during vacations. He received his M.A. from the University of Minnesota in 1934 and continued teaching until 1937.

Through his father, Joseph, a hospital administrator, Maurice met E.A. van Steenwyk, the promoter of a forerunner of Blue Cross in Minneapolis. Young Norby worked for van Steenwyk during the summers and, for a few months, with Rufus Rorem at the Hospital Services Plan Commission (known later as the Blue Cross Commission) at the American Hospital Association (1937–1938). Because of this experience, Norby was appointed director of a new Blue Cross plan in Pittsburgh (1939).

Norby left Pittsburgh to join Rorem at the Blue Cross Commission as director of research (1941–1945). On a leave of absence, Norby became associate director of the Commission on Hospital Care (1946–1948). The commission's findings were of great value in writing the Hospital Survey and Construction (Hill-Burton) Act.

After the work of the commission was finished, Norby joined the AHA and stayed until his retirement (1948–1973). At the AHA he was deputy director (1953–1962), secretary (1959–1964), director of the western office (1964–1966), and staff consultant (1967–1973).

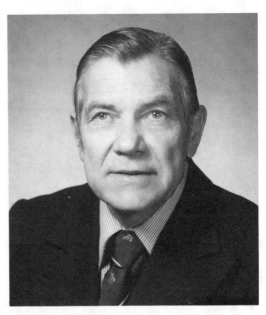

Andrew Pattullo

Andrew Pattullo was born in Omaha on February 12, 1917, and was graduated from the University of Nebraska in 1941. He was in one of the early classes in hospital administration at the University of Chicago, under Arthur Bachmeyer, and received his master's degree in 1943.

He applied for and received a one-year W.K. Kellogg Foundation Fellowship to work with hospitals in the Battle Creek area (1943–1944). At the end of the year he was invited to stay on with the foundation as associate director of the Division of Hospitals under Graham Davis, an invitation he accepted. Pattullo succeeded Davis in 1951 and served as director of the division until 1967. In that year, Pattullo was made program director of the foundation; this was followed by promotion to vice president for programs (1971–1975). In the meantime, Pattullo was made a trustee of the foundation in 1972. In 1975 he was appointed vice president of the W.K. Kellogg Foundation; he became senior vice president in 1978 and served in that position until his retirement in 1982.

Pattullo served with the foundation during most of its existence. He saw it change from a body that mainly built schools and hospitals in southeastern Michigan to one that supported competent institutions in testing innovative and experimental concepts in health care, education, and agriculture throughout the world. During his career, Pattullo served on the Federal Hospital Council and on various health care advisory bodies, governmental commissions, and educational boards.

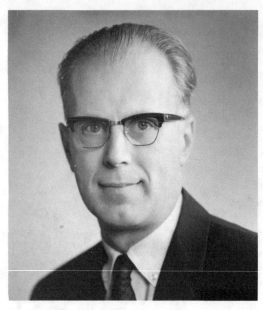

Daniel W. Pettengill

Daniel Pettengill was born on March 4, 1916, in Cambridge, Massachusetts. He received his bachelor's degree from Bowdoin College in 1937. That same year he joined the Aetna Life and Casualty Company, where he spent the next 41 years. Pettengill was a vice president of the company from 1964 to 1978. He has worked as a consultant since his retirement.

Aetna wrote its first group hospital expense benefit policy in 1937. It provided a $3.00 daily room and board benefit and a $15.00 maximum allowance for ancillary services. In Pettengill's first years with Aetna, the Blue Cross movement was developing and commercial insurance companies were attempting to adjust from indemnity payments to payments for services. He was there when the Federal Employees' Health Benefits Act was formulated.

Pettengill was one of the originators of the Connecticut 65 Plan, which, in those days before Medicare, was designed to furnish health insurance coverage to individuals age 65 or older. This plan was ready in 1965, when President Johnson, who had just been elected in his own right, insisted on the enactment of Medicare. There was a provision in Medicare that capable nongovernmental entities might be chosen by health care providers to be fiscal intermediaries to process and pay Medicare benefits claims. Pettengill took an active part in encouraging insurance companies to participate as intermediaries.

In his capacity as an insurance company actuary, Pettengill has been a consultant to insurance company associations and councils, government agencies, planning councils, and the Social Security Administration.

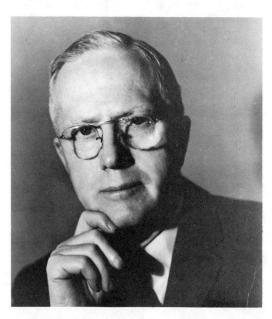

C. Rufus Rorem

    C. Rufus Rorem was born in Radcliffe, Iowa, in 1894. He was graduated from Oberlin College in 1916 and was a member of Phi Beta Kappa.
He worked for Goodyear Tire and Rubber Company as an apprentice in the
manufacturer's sales office from 1916 to 1917 and left to serve in the U.S.
Army. For a few months after the war, he worked as a reporter on an Iowa
newspaper. He then took a sales job with Goodyear from 1919 to 1922.
Rorem tired of traveling, however, so he decided to teach school. Earlham
College offered him a job as assistant professor, teaching various business
courses, including accounting. Since he had never studied accounting, he went
to summer school at the University of Chicago and then taught accounting
courses at Earlham, from 1922 to 1924. He qualified as a CPA in Indiana in
1923. Rorem went to the University of Chicago as an instructor in accounting
(1924–1927), and there he earned a master's degree (1925) and a doctorate
(1929). In 1928 he became an assistant professor and assistant dean of the
School of Commerce and Administration. He became an associate professor
in 1929. Later in 1929 Rorem left Chicago to join the Julius Rosenwald Fund
as associate director of medical services; through the fund, he took part in
the research and publications of the Committee on the Costs of Medical
Care. The fund gave Rorem, through the American Hospital Association,
a three-year grant to help develop group practice by physicians, uniform
hospital accounting, and group hospitalization. Through this work Rorem
set standards and approval programs for what became Blue Cross plans
(1937–1946). After his Blue Cross work he had two jobs: executive director
of the Hospital Council of Philadelphia (1947–1960) and director of the Hospital Planning Association of Allegheny County (1960–1964).

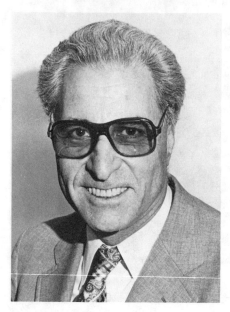

Robert M. Sigmond

Robert M. Sigmond considers Philadelphia his hometown even though he was born in Seattle on June 18, 1920. He is a graduate of Pennsylvania State University (1941) and served during World War II (1942–1945) in civilian assignments with the U.S. Air Force, War Department, and War Labor Board. After the war, he was a research associate with the Pennsylvania Governor's Commission on Hospital Facilities, Standards, and Organizations (1946–1950), which was formed to write a program to qualify for federal funds to operate a Hill-Burton agency.

Shortly after finishing the Hill-Burton project, Sigmond was hired by C. Rufus Rorem to work at the newly formed Hospital Council of Philadelphia (1946–1950). Sigmond felt the need of actual hospital experience, so he became assistant to the director of the Jewish Hospital (later a part of Philadelphia's merged Albert Einstein Medical Center) from 1950 to 1955. While there he took leave (1952–1954) to become director of fiscal studies for the national Commission on Financing of Hospital Care. About a year after completion of the study, Sigmond left Einstein to become director of the Hospital Council of Western Pennsylvania, in Pittsburgh (1955–1964). Between 1964 and 1968, he was director of the Hospital Planning Association of Allegheny County (Pittsburgh) (membership was made up of civic leaders of the county). Sigmond was invited back to Einstein Medical Center to be executive vice president for planning (1968–1970), then executive vice president of the center (1971–1975). In 1976, Sigmond became a consultant to Blue Cross–Blue Shield of Greater Philadelphia before moving to his next post in 1977 as special adviser to the national Blue Cross–Blue Shield Association.

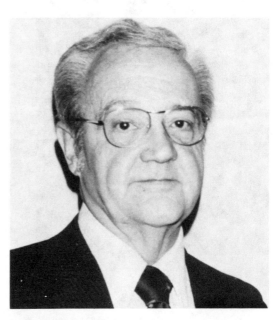

Richard J. Stull

Richard Stull was born in Washington, Pennsylvania, on September 17, 1916. He attended Duke University and, while hospitalized there with a football injury, became interested in hospital administration. He received a bachelor's degree in 1940 and a Certificate of Hospital Administration after a preceptor course at Duke University Hospital in 1942.

His first job as a hospital administrator was at Phoenixville (Pennsylvania) Hospital, from 1942–1944. There he undertook a building program, the first of many in his career. During World War II he became administrator of the Norfolk (Virginia) General Hospital (1944–1946).

His next move resulted from a recommendation of Graham Davis of the W.K. Kellogg Foundation. The Hospital Survey and Construction (Hill-Burton) Act was being put into effect, and each state needed a plan for proposed hospital construction in order to qualify for funds. California wanted someone to survey its needs, and Stull undertook the job (1946–1947). Afterwards, Stull became the western representative of James A. Hamilton Associates and did a survey of the hospital needs of metropolitan Los Angeles (1947–1948). This work led to a part in planning a new medical center for the University of California, San Francisco. Because of the state's tremendous population growth, the California university system needed other medical centers, and Stull worked on these (1948–1960). Before he completed his job in 1960, he had become a vice president and a full professor of the university. After taking jobs in industry between 1960 and 1965, Stull started work on his final accomplishment: the rebuilding, reorienting, and strengthening of the American College of Hospital Administrators as its chief executive (1965–1978). Stull died December 1, 1982.

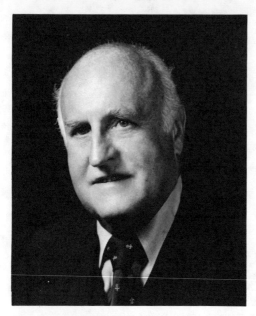

Kenneth Williamson

Kenneth Williamson was born in Hull, England, on March 31, 1912. His first experience in the health field was working in the pharmacy of the Methodist Hospital of Southern California (Los Angeles) after school. He was eager to learn administration and sought advice from national leaders. (In 1930 there were no formal university programs in hospital administration.) Dr. Malcolm MacEachern outlined a course of study. Williamson studied and worked up to the position of assistant director of Methodist Hospital (1930–1937). He then moved to Good Samaritan Hospital (Los Angeles) as business associate (1937–1939). Williamson next joined the Blue Cross of California as assistant director (1939–1941) and simultaneously became executive director of the California Hospital Association and of the Western Hospital Association (1941–1943). In 1943 George Bugbee, newly named executive secretary of the American Hospital Association, was looking for executive talent. He hired Williamson as assistant director and as secretary of the council on administrative practice, where he remained until 1950. That year he left and became executive vice president of the Health Information Foundation, a research group in New York City supported primarily by proprietary drug manufacturers. The titular head of the foundation was Admiral W.H.P. Blandy. Williamson ran the everyday operation and worked closely with Odin Anderson, the director of research. Bugbee appointed Williamson chief of the AHA Washington Service Bureau in 1954. Williamson remained there during the crucial years when Medicare and Medicaid were developed, giving valuable service to the industry. In 1972 he retired and opened a consulting firm, which ran until he again retired, in 1980.

PART II

Blue Cross: An Evolving Social Movement

6

In the Beginning of Blue Cross

Blue Cross is the term the average person associates with hospital insurance. From a few hundred in 1929, the number of Blue Cross subscribers has grown to more than 80 million. Blue Cross has been a social movement rather than just a means of insuring oneself and one's family against the costs of hospital care. The key has been the concept of prepayment for services.

Prepayment for hospital services was as attractive an idea as Social Security, and it drew the patient, the family, and the community hospital into a mutually secure relationship. This was true for the Dallas school teachers in 1929 paying 50¢ a month for up to 14 days of hospital care at Baylor University Hospital.

Prepaid health services were also available in 1933 for 5,000 workers building an aqueduct, canals, and dams to bring water across the desert of Southern California to Los Angeles. This plan cost 10¢ per worker per day— 5¢ a day from a commercial insurance carrier to cover accidents on the job, and 5¢ a day from the worker himself to cover illness off the job. The prepayment money for the aqueduct project was paid to a young physician named Sidney Garfield,[1] who was able to operate a small hospital on the desert job site and furnish hospital and medical care to the workers.

Thus early experiments with prepayment were generally localized and community-oriented.

Later, of course, under the Blue Cross plans, this changed. In the ensuing years, consumer demands forced the movement to spread from care at one hospital to several or all of the hospitals in a community, area, or state. Even national coverage was arranged eventually to accommodate travelers and employees of businesses operating in several communities throughout the country. Garfield's prepayment plan worked in the desert, it worked for employees and their families at Grand Coulee dam in the state of Washington, and it worked for employees in the Kaiser shipyards in California. Of all the prepayment mechanisms, however, the Blue Cross plans provided more people financial access to hospital services than any other system.

Blue Cross was not originally visualized as insurance. It was perceived as prepayment for hospital services rather than a cash benefit, as a communal approach to budgeting for the expenses of hospital care. Even today the Blue Cross approach to financing and paying for hospital care does not neatly fit the insurance mode. In many respects it is still an evolving social movement, struggling to adapt its fundamental principles to a changing political and economic environment.

There are many ways to tell the Blue Cross story. Perhaps the best, at least for our purposes, is to go directly to the sources and let them tell the story in their own words. In this and the following chapters in part II, the Blue Cross movement is told from the perspective of the people whose minds created it and whose hands shaped it.

To explain how Blue Cross started, what it is, its underlying philosophy, and its essential characteristics as a business entity, we turned to C. Rufus Rorem.[2] Rorem was the director of the AHA's Hospital Services Plan Commission in 1937. This commission evolved into the Blue Cross Commission, which Rorem headed until 1947.

In reviewing Rorem's reminiscences, the reader should note the continuity as well as the progression of his thinking from the days of his work on the Committee on the Costs of Medical Care (see chapter 2). Also, the close relationship between Blue Cross plans and hospitals should be recognized. To add flavor to this last point, the words of George Bugbee, Kenneth Williamson, James Hague, and John Mannix are included. Finally, to provide a sense of Rorem as a person, the observations of Maurice Norby and Robert Sigmond are included.

ROREM:[3]

In 1931, after about two years with the Committee on the Costs of Medical Care, I came back to Chicago to join the staff of the Julius Rosenwald Fund. Prior to joining the committee, I had been on the faculty of the University of Chicago.

I went to the committee to work on a specific study, funded by the

Rockefeller Foundation, with Michael Davis. Michael was the director of medical services for the Rosenwald Fund. I came back to Chicago to work under Michael, as the associate director of medical services.

I remained with the Julius Rosenwald Fund until December 1936, when the trustees of the fund liquidated their program in medical economics. During the five years [in] which I was on the staff of the fund, I conducted some research, but most of my time was devoted to the promotion of uniform accounting among hospitals, the development of clinical group practices, the development of group practice by physicians and at hospitals, and the development of "group hospitalization," which was the name originally given to the Blue Cross movement for the group payment of hospital and medical services. As you can see, much of my work was an outgrowth of the directions set by the Committee on the Costs of Medical Care. [See chapter 2 for a discussion of the Committee on the Costs of Medical Care.]

During this time, as you know from the committee's Minority Report Number One and the American Medical Association's response to the committee's final report, organized medicine was reluctant to accept group hospitalization. Their reluctance was grounded in the general principle that group hospitalization would result in socialized medicine and the removal of medical practice from control by the doctors.

Any sort of unified, explicit resistance, however, was relatively short-lived. The first formal recognition of group hospitalization by a medical group came from the American College of Surgeons in 1934. Surgeons, by that time, were providing almost all their services in hospitals. As a result, they saw in the Blue Cross movement a device by which they could either collect larger fees or find it easier to collect all of their fees, because there would be no hospital bills to compete for payment with, or perhaps take precedence over, the surgeon's charge.

The Creation of Blue Cross

Let me explain more carefully what group hospitalization—i.e., hospital care prepayment or hospital insurance—was thought to mean or be and how it came about.

Hospital care insurance originated as a device by which an individual hospital would be guaranteed specified revenue and would in turn assume responsibility for specific services for groups of people who paid money to the institution. These people—beneficiaries—were eligible to receive specified care at that institution without having to pay any extra fees at the time of their illness and use of the hospital.

The most publicized of the early hospital insurance programs was the one initiated in Dallas, Texas, by the Baylor University Hospital.

Many individually sponsored insurance programs had been established before. Baylor, however, was probably the first to start a program of health service benefits, as opposed to one of cash indemnities toward the hospital bill. The services benefit principle is the feature, and probably the only distinctive characteristic, which explains the rapid growth of the insurance principle in paying for hospital care.

One weakness of the Baylor Hospital plan was that the benefits were available in only one hospital, a Baptist hospital. Therefore, the plan was not widely acceptable to people of other religious beliefs.

During the time that Baylor Hospital was expanding its coverage from approximately 1,600 to 6,000 beneficiaries in the city of Dallas, two other hospitals established similar and competing programs. One was a Catholic hospital, the other a Methodist institution. Both of these hospitals ultimately enrolled approximately 5,000 beneficiaries. These beneficiaries paid 75¢ a month, through a promoter, for the same benefits as Baylor offered for 50¢ a month.

The hospitals received 50¢—of the total 75¢ monthly fee—for each person enrolled by the promoter. The enrollment in the Methodist and Catholic programs was not, however, deterred by the fact that their fee was $9.00 a year while the Baylor program was available at only $6.00 per year. Reluctance to participate, or at least what reluctance there was, arose from disbelief in these programs in their entirety, not from their price.

For example, I found out later, when interviewing business executives about enrollment of employees, that none of them objected on the grounds that family coverage was not worth, at that time, $24.00 a year. They doubted whether the contract was worth anything. They just did not believe in the program at all.

As originally organized, people were required to choose one hospital at the time they joined a group hospitalization plan. It soon became apparent that it was necessary to allow people to choose their hospital at the time of illness rather than at the time of enrollment. This meant, of course, that effective group insurance for hospital care should allow free choice among several alternative institutions. Interestingly, while being among the first to recognize the importance of group hospitalization, the state of Texas was among the last areas of the country to recognize and implement a free-choice, areawide plan. Ultimately, the single-hospital plans which had been formed in Dallas, Houston, and Fort Worth were merged into one plan, the Hospital Services Association of Texas.

The earliest plan to provide service benefits in several institutions appeared in New Orleans. There the Baptist Memorial Hospital joined with the Touro Infirmary to establish a citywide program with service benefits at the two institutions. Modest cash benefits were also provided for services in other hospitals.

The first full-blown, communitywide, free-choice, service benefit plan was developed in Newark, New Jersey. It was introduced in 1933 by Frank Van Dyk, who later moved to New York (1935) to become director of the New York City Plan. In Newark the areawide plan covered about 12 hospitals, each of which agreed to provide stated benefits for a stated amount expressed in terms of dollars per day.

Another important early citywide plan was developed in 1934 in St. Paul, Minnesota. Here Mr. E.A. van Steenwyk, a 29-year-old former real estate operator, conceived the idea of free-choice benefits among all the institutions in St. Paul. He also introduced for the first time the option of dependents' benefits. Up to that point, benefit coverage had emphasized just employed persons. No coverage was available for the wife or children of the employed individual. Van Steenwyk's idea was that, for an additional monthly premium charge, coverage could be purchased for that person's dependents.

As a footnote to van Steenwyk's idea, it's interesting to remember that initially it was the practice to charge an additional premium for each dependent who was covered. Within a few years, however, the data showed that it would be practicable, from a statistical point of view, to have a standard family rate, regardless of the size of the family. In other words, one rate for a one-person family, male or female, and one rate for a family of two or more persons, regardless of the number of dependents. So in time, pricing practices changed over to essentially what they are today.

―――――――

John Mannix was a contemporary of Rorem's, both in time and in his involvement in Blue Cross. Mannix describes the energy and spontaneity which characterized the beginning of the Blue Cross movement.

―――――――

MANNIX:[4]
The Blue Cross plan in Cleveland was started in 1934 and has been very successful. An interesting aspect to me when I review the history of Blue Cross is that I have always thought of several plans starting at about the same time: one in Newark, New Jersey; one in Washington, D.C.; the Cleveland plan; the St. Paul plan; and the plan at Sacramento, California. These plans were all started within about 18 months of each other. While I later got to know all of the individuals who took the leadership of these plans, none of us knew each other at that time. That was a perfect demonstration of an idea whose time had come.

I think the report of the Committee on the Costs of Medical Care accelerated this, but all of us were working on the idea without any particular knowledge of what the committee was doing or what they were likely to recommend. I do not believe that the people who were interested in developing these various initiatives had any more knowledge of the earlier history than I did. We all thought we had come up with a new, logical, and sound idea by independent actions in widely separated parts of the country.

ROREM:[5]

During this early period of Blue Cross' development, I was with the fund. My interest, however, was in this area. So, upon request, I visited over the course of several years at least 40 of the communities where prepaid, group hospitalization plans were being established. For several of these plans I had the opportunity to recommend the people who became the executive director of the plans. These directors were recruited from many fields: finance, industry, accounting, sales, hospital administration, social work, and education.

As I mentioned, the Rosenwald Fund decided in 1936 to discontinue its program in medical economics. I can only speculate as to the impetus for this decision. It was clear, however, that some board members of the fund were embarrassed by personal criticisms from their family physicians, who objected to changes in medical service organization which were being discussed and even taking place. As a result, early in 1936 they decided that the medical economics section of the fund should be discontinued at the end of the year.

The Rosenwald Fund faced the problem of what should become of the medical economics staff, Michael M. Davis and me. Their decision was to allocate, in effect, transition grants of $150,000 for Davis and $100,000 for me. These grants were to be paid out over four years in equal installments. The problem then was to find an organization which would accept and could receive these grants, since the fund was required to restrict its donations to eligible nonprofit organizations.

Michael decided to move to New York City. There he established a nonprofit corporation called the Committee for Research in Medical Economics. It was headquartered in New York City for several years, until he moved to Washington, D.C., to continue his interest in health economics on a personal basis.

My grant was offered to several agencies. My first suggestion was that the money be granted to the Twentieth Century Fund, which had an interest in medical economics. The Twentieth Century Fund decided not to accept the grant, since it would mean the addition of a "stranger" to their division of medical economics.

I then made the suggestion that the National Association of Community Chests might consider a program of this type. The director of that organization, however, considered this program as outside its sphere of interest, which was charity and public services to be financed by donations from individuals and groups. He recognized, quite accurately, that group hospitalization was a way by which people collected their own money for services for themselves. Furthermore, he foresaw that such programs could become areawide or even statewide and would not fit into the programs of local community chests and their charitable activities.

The third offer was made to the American Hospital Association, which promptly accepted the grant. The AHA, however, accepted the grant with the understanding that, while I would become a part of their staff, I would be paid from the money from the Rosenwald Fund.

Blue Cross and the AHA

The acceptance of the grant from the Rosenwald Fund was part of the AHA's continuing interest in hospital prepayment insurance.

In 1933 the AHA decided to undertake a special study of the trend toward hospital care insurance, with a view to recommending standards for insurance programs should they develop throughout the country. The AHA warned against the indiscriminate development of plans as panaceas for either the individual's problem of obtaining hospital services or the hospital's problem of securing adequate income. It officially endorsed the insurance principle for the purchase of hospital care.

The AHA and the hospital field's interest in hospital insurance continued, and in 1935, at its annual convention, the AHA passed the following resolution:

> Be it resolved that hospitals contemplating the establishment of, or participation in, group hospitalization plans bear in mind the recommendations of the Association and, before any active participation in such plans, consult with the officers of the Association for information and advice concerning individuals or agencies sponsoring periodic payment plans for the payment of hospital care.

Rorem continues his account of how he happened to join the AHA and to bring with him the grant from the Julius Rosenwald Fund.

ROREM:[6]

So beginning January 1, 1937, I moved my offices from the Julius Rosenwald Fund to the AHA headquarters at 18 East Division Street in Chicago. I became the third male employee of the AHA. The others were Dr. Bert W. Caldwell, executive secretary of the association, and an individual who served as the janitor. By the vote of the trustees, I was given the title of associate secretary of the AHA and executive secretary of the committee on hospital services of the AHA.

I assumed no duties or responsibilities for the activities of the association as a whole; I was not invited to the meetings of the AHA's board of trustees and was not dependent on the association for supporting travel expenses or any other costs of the committee on hospital services.

The committee on hospital services had two primary objectives. The first was improvement of hospitals through the development of uniform accounting. The emphasis of this effort was on promoting a standard program of uniform accounting. This program had been developed in 1933–1935 by a committee which I chaired while I was still with the Rosenwald Fund. The second objective was to continue the development of group hospital insurance for the payment of hospital bills on a community, state, and national basis.

I stayed at the AHA for ten years (January 1937 to December 1946). During this time the committee on hospital services changed its character in several ways.

During the second year (1938) an approval program for group hospitalization plans was developed, based on standards I had drafted. [See Appendixes I and J.] Also during the second year the name of the committee was changed to the Hospital Services Plan Commission. Later the term Blue Cross was introduced, and the committee was known as the Blue Cross Plan Commission. The commission was the forerunner of the Blue Cross Association.

As an historical anecdote, it might be of interest to comment on the origin of the term "Blue Cross," which was used to identify nonprofit hospital service plans which had gained the approval of the AHA. The term "Blue Cross" was first introduced by E.A. van Steenwyk, who used this title to identify his plan in St. Paul, both as a design on the literature and as a term to describe the organization, which was registered by the State of Minnesota not as an insurance organization, but as a hospital service plan association.

The Blue Cross name and mark were widely adopted, with or without permission, by various plans being formed throughout the United States. In the spring of 1949, a list of approved plans was issued. These plans were allowed to identify themselves by a blue cross on which the seal of the AHA was superimposed. This granting of the seal to indicate approval by AHA came about through formal action of the AHA's trustees, approved by the association's house of delegates and membership.

The relationship of the Blue Cross plans to the AHA also involved the plans' being members of the association. Each approved plan paid annual dues to the AHA based on the number of subscribers in the plan at the end of the calendar year. Each approved plan then became an associate member of the AHA. The dues paid by the plans were used in the main to support the activities and expenses of the Blue Cross Plan Commission.

Blue Cross, the AHA, and Hospitals: A Changing Relationship

Up to this point, the Blue Cross plans and the AHA had a close and productive relationship. In fact, in many instances it was hospitals that had the major role in both creating Blue Cross plans and in maintaining the early fiscal solvency of those plans. Many early Blue Cross plan–hospital contracts contained provisions requiring that the participating hospitals share in the plan's losses or guarantee the provision of services to the plan's subscribers, or both. The closeness of the plan-hospital relationship is illustrated by the following comments from two hospital leaders—George Bugbee and Kenneth Williamson. Bugbee was the executive director of the AHA from 1943 to 1954. Prior to that he was the chief executive of Cleveland City Hospital. Williamson was the executive director of the Association of California Hospitals and the Association of Western Hospitals. Later he was director of the AHA's Washington Service Bureau. In the late 1930s, however, he was the assistant director of the hospital service plan (Blue Cross) of Southern California.

———

BUGBEE:[7]

The connection between hospitals and Blue Cross has always been hand in glove.

Every so often I read that hospitals supported Blue Cross because it was a time of the Great Depression and people couldn't pay their bills. Well, I always thought that that was nonsense. Blue Cross went so slowly at first that it paid few bills in the depression.

I prefer a much more altruisitc description of the reason. I think in some degree it's true. In fact, for the people who went through it, I think it *is* true. They thought people ought to have protection against high-cost bills.

I think there was a great deal done to help Blue Cross get off the ground. Blue Cross needed hospital support. Hospitals were told it was a good thing by their leadership, over and over again.

The Blue Cross pioneers made a special point of being hand in glove with hospital leadership.

———

WILLIAMSON:[8]

I was appointed as the assistant director of the Blue Cross plan.

The experience was important to me because I went to every hospital in Southern California and met with their boards to sell them on the idea of joining Blue Cross. It was great experience, and it was a great test of whether I could put across ideas. These boards had to be willing to put up a kitty of $8.00 a bed and sign a contract that would make them responsible for guaranteeing services to the Blue Cross subscribers. Blue Cross was nothing but an idea with some hope and a lot of risk for hospitals.

The importance, in terms of their ongoing relationship, of hospitals' sharing the risk with their Blue Cross plan should not be underestimated. This risk sharing was the glue that held the two together, making voluntary hospitals and voluntary payment two sides of the same coin.

Over time, as the risk-sharing contract provisions fell by the wayside, it is understandable that Blue Cross and hospitals should drift apart. This separation becomes most obvious in the demands and expectations by hospitals that Blue Cross pay them at the same rate as any other private payer.

Rorem comments on the separation of the two voluntary movements.

ROREM:[9]

The change was probably inevitable as each side, Blue Cross and hospitals, organizationally and economically matured.

In my opinion the most important thing that happened in the relationships of the Blue Cross Association and the Blue Cross plans to the providers—hospitals and doctors—was the separation of BCA from AHA. I think it was long overdue.

The separation was a healthy thing. It wasn't a sign of anything bad. It wasn't going from bad to worse. I think they [AHA and BCA] were just recognizing human nature and the practice of medicine as it both was and was likely to continue.

It is unreal to assume that over the long run a buyer and a seller can act as partners in a capitalistic society.

Whereas Rorem viewed the separation as inevitable and healthy, there were also other, less enthusiastic viewpoints, including those of Robert Sigmond, John Mannix, and James Hague.

SIGMOND:[10]

It was necessary for them [AHA and BCA] to separate, but I think it was poorly handled.

The concept was, let's separate so that we can have a more effective working relationship. Let's separate so that we can pursue our common goals and objectives better. I say it was poorly handled, partly because the separation occurred just before the death of Edwin Crosby, executive director of the AHA.

As a result, I think the emphasis became, let's separate because we're too close. The positive aspects of it were never gotten at. The original documents, which were worked out between Ed Crosby and Walt McNerney, president of the Blue Cross Association, were interpreted as reflecting AHA and BCA moving away from each other, towards an adversary relationship. That was not the intention. However, that point was not communicated effectively, either among hospitals and Blue Cross plans or within the AHA.

MANNIX:[11]

There always were several plans that were not comfortable under the banner of the American Hospital Association. I always felt that their concerns were not justified and took a stand for a very strong AHA relationship. I felt that the plans were offering hospital services to the public on a monthly payment basis, and the success of this type of program necessitated cooperation between the plans and the hospitals.

In the very early 1940s, a group of plan leaders were interested in complete separation from the AHA. That resulted in a weekend meeting in about 1941 at the headquarters of the AHA. Nearly all the plan executives were present, along with a large representation from the AHA. The result of this meeting was a decision on the part of plans to continue under the aegis of the American Hospital Association, and probably a stronger interest than ever on the part of the AHA in prepayment for hospital care.

However, there continued among plan executives an interest in having their own separate organization and in having more autonomy. Actually, in my opinion the individual plans were separate corporations and had complete autonomy. The American Hospital Association activity was primarily strong support of the plans without any dictation about their operation.

Further discussions resulted in the establishment of a new type of AHA membership, called type IV. Types I, II, and III were institutional and personal memberships. Type IV membership was for Blue Cross plans.

Concern again flared up in the late 1960s and early 1970s regarding the AHA–Blue Cross relationship. This resulted in the establishment of the Blue Cross Association as a separate corporation: i.e., elimination of the interlocking board with AHA. This was promoted on the basis of a partnership between the Blue Cross Association and the American Hospital Association. Even though the term "partnership" was continually used, it meant further separation of the plans from the AHA, although the Blue Cross Association continued to occupy space in the AHA headquarters building until 1980, when BCA acquired separate building space.[12]

I always felt the Blue Cross program of financing hospital care would

be much more effective with a strong AHA relationship. While my background was in the hospital field, I do not think this had anything to do with
the way I felt.

A corollary to this is that I have always felt that the American Medical
Association would have been wise to maintain a strong relationship with the
Blue Shield plans. At one time the headquarters of the Blue Shield plans was
in the AMA building.

In the last few years people have raised antitrust questions in connection
with this relationship, but I have always believed that a maximum degree of
cooperation between Blue Cross and Blue Shield, on one hand, and hospitals
and the medical profession, on the other, was in the public interest. I agree
that there could be certain dangers in this, but after watching the development
of Blue Cross and Blue Shield for 50 years I think these programs have been
operating in the public interest, and the record shows that.

HAGUE:[13]

I thought Blue Cross divorced itself from the AHA because people
were complaining about the appearances of Blue Cross and hospitals being
in each other's back pockets. I didn't think they were. There was enough
evidence to indicate that they weren't. It seemed to me that the combination
of a very close working relationship between the purse and the provider was
very good for the patient. I don't think any one of the insurance commissioners or politicians has ever proven any evil results.

Anyone who believes in the voluntary aspects of society could not say
anything but that the relationship between hospitals and Blue Cross contributed significantly to the success of the Blue Cross movement and its benefits
to the American people. I don't think that's a very arguable point of view.
If this were the result, and I believe it was, then before you divorce yourself,
before you sunder that relationship, it seems to me you have to show some
malignancy, some malevolence. I have never been persuaded that any such
showing was ever made.

In spite of the differences of opinion about the Blue Cross–AHA relationship, it is important to recognize that hospitals had a major role in both
founding many Blue Cross plans and in maintaining the early fiscal solvency
of those plans. Many early Blue Cross–hospital contracts contained provisions requiring that the participating hospitals share in plan losses and/or
guarantee the provision of services to plan subscribers. The importance, in
terms of their ongoing relationship, of hospitals' sharing risk with plans
should not be underemphasized.

Over time, as these contract provisions have been eliminated, it is also
understandable that hospitals and plans, from a business perspective, would
drift apart. This drift becomes more obvious in the demands–expectations by

hospitals that Blue Cross pay them at the same rate as other private payers do.

Moving On

Rorem stayed with the Blue Cross Plan Commission until 1947. During his tenure tremendous accomplishments were achieved (Appendix K), yet, when the group hospitalization movement was about to reap the benefits of his pioneering work, he moved on to another position outside of Blue Cross. Rorem comments on his leaving.

ROREM:[14]

In January of 1947 I resigned from the Blue Cross Plan Commission to accept the job of executive director of the Hospital Council of Greater Philadelphia.

Possibly I haven't explained well enough why I decided at that point in time to leave.

The first reason was to stop traveling a hundred nights a year all over the United States. The second was that I had an offer of a job which sounded interesting. The offer came from a place that would allow me to work in one neighborhood and sleep in my own bed every night. Also, I felt the battle for health insurance was over. It was just a question of when it was going to come, and in what form, and how broadly it would be expanded. The concept, the principle was not debatable any more.

There was still much work to be done in the coordination of care: in planning for hospitals, in group practice of medicine, and in the development of ambulatory care throughout the communities—now called primary care. In working along those lines, I thought the new job would be more interesting.

So, I left. I left essentially to take on what I felt would be a new and exciting challenge. A challenge as exciting as the one I had taken on in 1936.

To help complete a picture of Rorem, the following anecdotes are provided by two of his former staff members, Maurice Norby and Robert Sigmond. Norby worked with Rorem in the 1930s and 1940s. Sigmond worked with him in Philadelphia in the 1940s.

NORBY:[15]

Rufus once brought me a manuscript of a speech he was to make some place soon and asked me to edit it for him. I read it and thought this was just fine, just great. I may have taken out a word or two, not more than ten from this whole 20-minute speech. I brought it back to him.

I still remember. He said, "I wanted you to edit it."

I said, "I did. It's great. It is just fine."

"Oh, OK."

He took it and went through the whole thing again. I finally saw the secretary typing it again. I could hardly find the original words in it.

In a week or so I had to make a speech some place. So I had my speech typed up. I thought out of courtesy I would give it to Rufus.

I said, "How about editing mine for me?"

It came back just black. I read it and it did sound a lot better.

I went back in to Rufus' office and said, "I think I had better leave."

He said, "What's the matter?"

I said, "Obviously I can't meet the quality of work that you are used to and that you demand."

He said, "What's the matter?"

I said, "The speech I gave you."

He said, "You had some good ideas in there."

"But," I said, "they are lost."

"No, no. Every idea is there. All I did was change the words around."

That's the kind of fellow he was. He didn't mean to hurt you at all.

*   *   *

As time went on, there was a lot of nitpicking among the Blue Cross plans. There was infighting to become members of the Blue Cross Commission. It was done by election of the peers. There was a lot of twisting and struggling. Rufus didn't care for that, but he was forced into managing it. He wasn't too good a political manager. He was direct. He said exactly what he meant and wanted to say. I think he finally decided that life was too short to fight political situations.

SIGMOND:[16]

I went to work for Rufus at the Hospital Council of Philadelphia. Rufus had just left the Blue Cross Plan Commission. He decided that that job had gotten beyond the promotional stage, it was a management job. He wanted to work at the community level and he thought the Philadelphia position would be a good opportunity.

Rufus has been the single strongest influence in the health field on my life—still is. I talk to him at least twice a week, and I think I probably have all my life from the time I went to work for him. If you're interested in some anecdotes, I could probably give you an hour or two.

Matter of fact, just yesterday I was talking to him and he says, "You know, when it comes to this HMO idea it looks like all these folks are rediscovering the wheel." He said, "You know, if they lost it, there's nothing wrong with them rediscovering it." That's kind of a typical Roremism.

*   *   *

I think that I've come to appreciate the impact that Rufus had on me in those early days more as I've thought about it. I mean, it wasn't something I was glorying in, I was just doing my job. As a matter of fact, I'll never forget an event that happened the second or third week I was working for him. Some issue had come up: the organization was very new and they were forming a retirement plan. As it was getting developed, it looked like the secretaries were going to be left out. I thought that was wrong. We were having a little staff meeting—there were only four of us—and I spoke up pretty vigorously. Rufus was obviously upset about how aggressive I was being on this point, so a couple of weeks later he called me into his office and he said, "You know, I really want to sit down and talk to you because I was surprised at your behavior in that discussion the other day. I always thought I'd like to have an organization that was a nice, big, happy family. Let's talk about that. It didn't seem to me you were behaving like a member of a happy family."

I said to Rufus, "I don't know very much about your family, but I was behaving just like I do with my happy family. If there's some kind of issue, we're screaming and shouting."

Then he sat back and laughed. "You're right," he said, "you're right. In a Quaker family you don't do things that way."

I said, "Well, in a Jewish family that's the way you do things." We were both agreeing that we ought to be a good, happy family, it's just a whole different cultural background.

Working for Rufus I think gave me maybe three things. First, he gave me appreciation of the potential of the hospital as a community institution. He didn't believe that everything that hospitals did was right, but he gave me a sense of the importance of the organizational form that the hospital represents in American society. Secondly, he gave me a sense of the importance of keeping the financing as close to the management as possible at the community level. And third, he really hooked me on Blue Cross. It's important to recognize that, when Rufus left the Blue Cross Plan Commision, there was no strong leadership at the commission or its successor organization [BCA] until Walt McNerney came along 15 years later.

Immediately after Rufus left the Blue Cross Commission, if there was an individual running one of the plans who wanted to talk to somebody about a basic issue, a basic problem, he had always called Rufus, and so he did. Of course Rufus helped most of those folks not only to get their job, but to get organized.

I would say, in the early days when I went to work for Rufus, he was quite free in giving advice to Blue Cross people—and I mean literally free. He didn't set up a consulting business, and the office was involved with whatever Rufus was doing. So I got involved. In effect, we were running an unofficial, informal Blue Cross Plan Commission. So I got to know a lot of those Blue Cross folks and their problems. Rufus wasn't doing anything that could be interpreted as undermining the Blue Cross Commission. He just tried to help people.

Notes

(Transcripts of the oral histories cited here are housed in the library of the American Hospital Association, 840 North Lake Shore Drive, Chicago, Illinois 60611. The Oral History Collection is a joint project of the Hospital Research and Educational Trust and the AHA.)

1. Until his death in December 1984, Sidney Garfield was an administrator of the Total Health Program of the Permanente Medical Group in Oakland, California.

2. See Profiles of Participants, in the center of this book, for biographical information.

3. *C. Rufus Rorem, In the First Person: An Oral History.*

4. *John R. Mannix, In the First Person: An Oral History.* See Profiles of Participants for biographical information.

5. *Rorem, Oral History.*

6. *Rorem, Oral History.*

7. *George Bugbee, In the First Person: An Oral History.* See Profiles of Participants for biographical information.

8. *Kenneth Williamson, In the First Person: An Oral History.* See Profiles of Participants for biographical information.

9. *Rorem, Oral History.*

10. *Robert M. Sigmond, In the First Person: An Oral History.* See Profiles of Participants for biographical information.

11. *Mannix, Oral History.*

12. Robert M. Sigmond, on this point, mentioned that the BCA was originally set up by some of the plans in New York City to help in national marketing and that it was always separate from AHA and the Blue Cross Commission. The Blue Cross Commission and the AHA merged in 1961, when McNerney became president of the Blue Cross Association.

13. *James E. Hague, In the First Person: An Oral History.* See Profiles of Participants for biographical information.

14. *Rorem, Oral History.*

15. *Maurice J. Norby, In the First Person: An Oral History.* See Profiles of Participants for biographical information about Mr. Norby.

16. *Sigmond, Oral History.*

7

Building the Movement

The national growth of the Blue Cross movement resulted from hundreds—thousands—of persons contributing ideas and devoting a great deal of time, both off and on the job, to its development. Many of these ideas occurred at the same time, but independently of each other. John R. Mannix,[1] for example, worked independently developing the Cleveland plan at a time when six other plans were being developed.

Unfortunately, some of these pioneers are no longer alive to converse with. One was E.A. van Steenwyk, the ingenious young builder and financer of houses before the depression who started the St. Paul plan. Mannix, however, is available to tell his story.

———————

MANNIX:[2]

My involvement in Blue Cross began probably before I realized it.

In July of 1932 I established an all-inclusive rate system at University Hospitals of Cleveland, eliminating all separate charges for ancillary services. We had one rate, which varied only by the type of accommodation, whether it was a private room, semiprivate, or ward accommodation. At the start, we offered the patients the choice of a daily rate plus extra ancillary service charges or the all-inclusive rate. Ninety-two percent of all patients chose the all-inclusive rate. This system was in effect at University Hospitals for close to 50 years.

In this process, I realized that we were taking the cost of all the ancillary services and dividing them among all the persons hospitalized, regardless of the use of these services by the individual patient. Recognizing this, it occurred to me that we could carry this basic idea of cost averaging even further. Instead of just taking the rate and dividing it among people hospitalized, you could average it, or divide it, among all people, whether they were hospitalized or not. This simple notion was and still is the basis of Blue Cross.

Cleveland Blue Cross

With this idea as the base, I attempted to convince the Cleveland hospitals to take some official action with respect to developing a prepayment plan. I was having difficulty making much headway. However, in November 1932, and I think only because I continued to press the issue, the Cleveland Hospital Council, which was the local association of hospitals, now known as the Greater Cleveland Hospital Association, decided to appoint a committee to study the development of a program for the prepayment of hospital care in Cleveland.

As so often happens, and as much as I argued against it, I was appointed chairman. We had a committee of three people. The other members were a Dr. Woods, who was the administrator of St. Luke's Hospital, and a Dr. Rockwood, the administrator of Mt. Sinai Hospital. The three of us worked for more than 18 months, until mid-1934, to establish a hospital care prepayment plan—a Blue Cross plan.

Having helped to establish the plan, I thought my contribution had been made, particularly since I was viewed by some, because of my work in starting the plan, as a "Communist, out to socialize medicine." At the time, I had no intent or interest in becoming connected with Blue Cross as a paid employee. My interest was in hospital management. I thought that was where my future was.

We had the problem therefore of finding an executive for this new organization. With a large number of Americans out of work, there was no scarcity of applicants. My feeling, however, was—because this idea of prepayment was so new—that we should hire somebody who knew not only something about the hospital and health field, but someone who also had promotional ability.

At that time, John McNamara was editor of *Modern Hospital* magazine. I recommended him for the position. He ultimately accepted it, and he was very successful. In a very short time the Cleveland plan became, from an enrollment standpoint, the largest in the country. From 1934 to 1939, because I was chairman of the committee that started the plan, I was called upon by a great many people around the country, mostly hospital people, to help them develop their own Blue Cross plans. For example, I had some part in starting all the Ohio plans: Akron, Youngstown, Toledo, Columbus, and Cincinnati. In every one of these plans, I met with key people at their request.

I also met with people in Rochester [New York], Chicago, Des Moines, and Indianapolis and had some part in the development of those plans. All during this time, I was the associate administrator at University Hospitals of Cleveland. I did all this on a gratis basis and in most cases paid my own expenses.

I ran into many interesting things in those local meetings. It was not unusual to have somebody get up in the audience and ask, "What are you getting out of this?" There was disbelief that someone would be willing to do what I was doing just because he believed in an idea.

Michigan Blue Cross

As noted, Mannix felt that his main career interest was in hospital administration. In fact, as is discussed in later chapters, he was actively involved in the 1930s in reshaping and energizing the AHA. Therefore, it was a surprise to many in the hospital field when it was learned that he had accepted the job of establishing, promoting, and directing a statewide Michigan Blue Cross Plan, with headquarters in Detroit.

MANNIX:[3]
I had been working with some of the hospital administrators in Detroit. They had contacted me sometime in the middle of 1938 because they had formed a committee to study the development of a hospital prepayment plan for Michigan. I met with their committee several times in September and October 1938.

In about November they asked me if I would be interested in becoming the executive of their plan. I said no, that my interest was in hospital administration. They made more attractive offers over the following several months.

I liked the Michigan people. Some of them were important leaders in the hospital field. I was working principally with the administrators of the Harper, Grace, and Ford hospitals. At that time Stewart Hamilton was the head of Harper Hospital; his son, J. Stewart Hamilton, later became the executive of Hartford [Connecticut] Hospital. In 1963, the son served as president of the American Hospital Association.

Warren Babcock was the administrator of Grace Hospital. He was the father of Kenneth Babcock, who was later to become the chief executive of the Joint Commission on Accreditation of Hospitals. Ira Peters was the administrator of Ford Hospital. Henry Ford, Sr., was chairman of the board of the hospital at that time.

The committee persuaded me to take the Michigan position. I was interested for two reasons. First, the Michigan plan would be a statewide program. Second, the state medical society was at the same time also very interested in developing a medical plan. At that time there was only one other medical prepayment plan in operation. California had started one in August 1939, but it was making very little headway. The Michigan State Medical Society was interested, and I was intrigued with the potential for a statewide hospital plan combined with a statewide medical plan.

So I took the job. My idea was that I would stay for two years and then go back to hospital administration.

The Michigan Blue Cross Plan began with only a $10,000 loan, a third of which was contributed by Grace Hospital, a third by Harper Hospital, and a third by Ford Hospital. Edsel Ford gave his personal check for the Ford share. He also gave the odd penny, by the way.

I arrived in Detroit in February of 1939. Almost immediately, the plan had spectacular growth. We enrolled some sizeable organizations in Detroit, including J.L. Hudson, the large department store, and Parke, Davis, the drug house. Ford Motor Company also expressed interest from the very beginning. (As I said, a third of the original financing came from Edsel Ford.) As a result, we enrolled Ford in the latter part of 1939.

There were also at the same time some dark clouds. In 1939, General Motors elected the Metropolitan Life Insurance Company's hospital plan. The General Motors decision made me wonder about the future of Blue Cross plans; here was the largest corporation in the country going with a private insurance company rather than with Blue Cross.

Metropolitan's hospital plan only provided $4 a day toward hospital care and $20 toward all ancillary services. I was convinced that the way to solve the problem of financing hospital care was not through a cash indemnity arrangement. What people needed at the time of hospitalization was service benefits, complete payment—full financial access to services. Blue Cross provided service benefits. We paid for a semiprivate room in full and for ancillary services in full.

I continued to work with General Motors. Two years later, in November 1941, General Motors changed to Blue Cross. This was a great impetus not only to Blue Cross of Michigan, but also to Blue Cross nationally, because we enrolled General Motors nationwide.

There is an interesting story in connection with the General Motors enrollment. To get ready to implement the General Motors contract, we brought together Blue Cross plan executives from all around the country for a meeting. We discussed with them the details of General Motors enrollment.

Following the meeting, one of the Blue Cross executives said to me, "That was a mighty fine thing you did [enrolling General Motors], mighty fine thing for Blue Cross, but I can't take those subscribers."

I laughed and said, "What are you talking about?"

He said, "I can't take those subscribers."

I said, "What in the world are you talking about?"

I am quoting: he said, "I've got 25,000 subscribers in my plan. I don't know what I would do with more subscribers."

There was only one thing that saved me from having a real problem. The General Motors benefit was scheduled to go into effect in Michigan on November 1, 1941. For General Motors employees in all other states, the benefit was not scheduled to go into effect until January 1, 1942. Pearl Harbor occurred in the meantime, and General Motors closed their plant in the state where the plan had said that they could not take any more subscribers. In fact, General Motors did not reopen that plant until some years later. By that time, taking on new subscribers was no problem.

The success of the program with Ford and General Motors resulted, a year or so later, in Chrysler enrolling in Blue Cross.

At the same time that we were making enrollment gains, we also made progress in other areas. For example, at the outset, we had only a hospital plan in Michigan. Ford Motor Company, however, insisted upon having coverage for both hospital care and for surgical care. This resulted in a whole series of meetings with the Wayne County Medical Society, as well as with representatives of the state medical society. In March 1940, about a year after I arrived in Detroit, the state medical society finally agreed to start a companion organization, Michigan Medical Service, to cover surgical care. The Ford Motor Company was the first participant in this joint program.

Michigan Medical Service maintained its own organization for claim payment purposes. A dual arrangement continued for many years; however, within the last few years these two organizations have merged into a single corporation.

Also during the early 1940s, the United Auto Workers developed an interest in the hospital and medical plan. The driving force behind their interest was basically a desire on their part to have a means of protecting their members from the cost of hospital and medical care.

Their position for achieving this goal was not, however, what you might guess. During the early part of the 1940s, the entire cost of hospital and medical benefit coverage was paid by the employees. There was no company contribution. The motor companies simply agreed to deduct the cost of coverage from the employee's paycheck.

Walter Reuther, president of the UAW, seemed comfortable with this approach. In fact, I can remember at one meeting with General Motors officials, the matter of company contributions came up. Reuther made the statement that the company should give the union members the money and let them pay for the care. He actually was opposed to direct company contributions.

The movement toward direct company contributions probably, however, was inevitable. As far as I know, it started developing nationally during World War II. The reasons for this were several. One was the cost-plus basis for paying for war production. Another was the fact that there was a great labor shortage. Employers could not attract workers by raising wages, because wages were frozen by the federal government. Employers could, however, increase fringe benefits. Employers therefore became interested in paying very liberal fringe benefits, one of which was health care benefits. There also developed another situation, which still pertains today: The cost of health care for employees was tax deductible as far as the employer was concerned, and it was tax exempt to the employees.

What really changed the situation on company contributions, however, was the refusal of the steel companies in 1948 to bargain on health benefits with the United Steel Workers union. The steelworkers went into court. The case ultimately went to the United States Supreme Court. The Supreme Court decided that fringe benefits were a bargainable item. After that decision, the spread of company contributions greatly increased. Today it is a rare company of any size that is not paying at least part of the cost of health benefits.

There is an interesting sidelight in this connection. When I first went to the Michigan plan, I took the position that the cost of health care should be paid by the employee rather than the company. I made this position pretty much a rigid rule. Some people in one Michigan area, primarily county employees and school teachers, wanted the county and the school board to pay part of the costs of hospital and medical care. I would not agree to this. The county commissioners went to the state legislature and secured legislation to permit the county to make contributions. This is interesting, because many people believe organized labor took the initiative and forced contributions from employers. Historically, at least in Michigan, this was not true.

Chicago Blue Cross

The statewide Michigan Blue Cross and the payroll medical plan (now called Blue Shield) were precedent-setting organizations. Here also were the beginnings of contracts for national coverage for employees of corporations doing business and maintaining branches throughout the country. After such a sensational start-up, based on original capital of only $10,000, it seemed strange that John Mannix would leave Detroit to become director of the Chicago plan. He explains his reasons for leaving Detroit.

MANNIX:[4]

When I took the position at the Michigan plan, I had no intention, as I said before, of staying on the operational side of Blue Cross for more than a couple of years. Not surprisingly, my plans changed. I guess I should have realized from the outset that it was more likely than not that things would change.

As it turned out, after I had been in Michigan for five years, I was approached by the trustees of the Chicago Blue Cross Plan. They wanted to know if I would be interested in being the chief executive of their plan.

I went to Chicago for several reasons. First, it was the center of health activities in the country. It had the American Medical Association and the American Hospital Association, the national Blue Cross headquarters, and the American College of Surgeons. *Hospitals* magazine was published there; *Modern Hospital* was published there. There were meetings of health groups in Chicago nearly every day in the year. Illinois was also a much more populous state than Michigan; and Chicago was a much more populous city than Detroit.

The Chicago Blue Cross Plan had been started more than two years before the Michigan plan but was only about half the size. Also, I thought it was very important in the city that was the center of health activity to have a strong Blue Cross and Blue Shield Plan. There was no Blue Shield Plan there at all, although at that time the Michigan Blue Shield Plan was five years old. By that time [1944] I had also forgotten about my two-year limit away from hospital administration.

Taken all together, the challenge and opportunity were too attractive to turn away from. So I went to Chicago.

During the 24 months I was chief executive of the Chicago plan, we increased the membership from half-a-million to a million, enrolling as many people in two years as they had in the previous seven, and had the development of the medical [the Blue Shield] plan very much under way.

Prior to Mannix's arrival as director of the Chicago Blue Cross Plan, Robert M. Cunningham, Jr.,[5] worked for the plan. Cunningham later went on to be editor and publisher of *Modern Hospital* and chairman of the editorial board of its successor, *Modern Healthcare.* In his reminiscence about his time with Blue Cross, Cunningham provides an interesting insight into the early operation of a Blue Cross plan.

CUNNINGHAM:[6]

The plan started operations in 1936. I went there full-time in 1938, doing public relations work and being the general errand boy for the plan director. I also got involved in hospital relations activities, such as they were.

We had an obvious interest in hospitals, as we were a major paying agent with maybe 10,000 to 20,000 subscribers in the Chicago metropolitan area. We represented enough revenue that the hospitals were concerned about the rate of payment. We, in turn, were concerned about setting up a sensible accounting base for payment so that it had some relationship to costs and charges.

My recollection is that our payments at that time amounted to about $6.00 per patient day. However, the director of the plan was concerned about the rather casual accounting that he observed in some of the hospitals, so he hired a certified public accountant, who had done some work for some of the hospitals, to put on a series of lectures on cost accounting through the Chicago Hospital Council.

I remember the president of the Chicago Hospital Council, who was the administrator of a respected hospital and who also was a retired clergyman, as many of the administrators were in those days, expressing himself at the end of one of the lectures. He said, "I don't know if we have to go through all these details. You are either going along all right, or you are not going along all right, and that's all there is to it." That always entertained me as an indication of the level of sophistication of accounting in hospitals at the time.

One of the organizers of the Chicago Blue Cross Plan was chairman of the board of trustees of one of the Chicago-area hospitals. He arranged for the director of the plan to come to a meeting of the medical staff of his hospital to explain what the plan was doing and what hospital prepayment was all about. As it turned out, I went along; it was part of my education.

When the director started to explain what we were doing, it began to appear that the doctors didn't want any part of it. During the question and answer period it became clear not only that they didn't want anything to do with it, but that they also thought that Blue Cross was probably Communistic. It was a very awkward situation and an angry crowd. Of course, the chairman of the board, who was there and who had arranged the whole thing, was upset about it. I was upset, but the director of the plan took it all calmly.

When the meeting was finally ended, he said, "Don't worry about that, don't worry about anything. It doesn't make any difference if those fellows don't like it. They will learn to like it. I can foresee a time when there may be as many as a million members in hospital plans like ours all over the country."

I thought he was smoking opium.

*   *   *

Another episode I haven't thought of in many years happened at one of the Catholic hospitals. We had a complicated basis for payment, even in those early times.

We discovered that we had overpaid this particular hospital. As one of my miscellaneous duties, I was sent as an emissary to go out and explain to the Sisters that they had been overpaid and arrange for a settlement of the account.

It turned out that the hospital was run by an order of Eastern European nuns who had come to this country fairly recently and had a little difficulty with the language. The administrator and the business manager were both Sisters. None of us understood what we were doing very well, and also we had a little language problem. Finally, we worked our way through the accounting statement and the Sisters agreed that, yes, indeed, it was four or five hundred dollars that they had been overpaid.

I said, "You can either send us a check or we will take it out of your next payment."

She said, "Oh, no. We owe, we pay."

She dug into her habit and pulled out a roll of bills and counted out $400 or whatever it was and insisted on me taking the money in cash. I have often thought about that. "We owe, we pay" is kind of outdated. Nonetheless, it seems like a fairly sound basis for running a hospital, or any other business.

The John Marshall Insurance Company

Mannix spent two years in Chicago and rapidly expanded the enrollment there, making the plan a successful operation. After two years, he evidently felt there was something missing in the Blue Cross format that could only be corrected by establishing a single organization operating and offering benefits nationwide. The proposed organization apparently seemed beyond the scope of Blue Cross plans. When it was mentioned that his move from Chicago to found a commercial insurance company (the John Marshall Insurance Company) to offer Blue Cross–like service benefits nationwide was surprising, he explained.

MANNIX:[7]

I can't speak to the level of surprise.

Let me, however, tell you a bit about why the John Marshall Insurance

Company was created, how it was to operate, and what happened to it.

In 1939, right after I went to Michigan, I felt that there were too many separate Blue Cross corporations. I felt that there needed to be much more coordination among the plans. For example, because of the lack of coordination or the number of plans, I had encountered great difficulty in working with national employers. This started with the enrollment of Ford Motor Company, which wanted coverage for its employees throughout the country. As I mentioned, we also saw this, and saw it to a much greater degree, when General Motors enrolled.

In view of all the circumstances, I think we did a very good job in working with national employers. There was, however, much difficulty, because hardly any two Blue Cross plans in the country had the same set of benefits.

I first proposed a national organization with the chartering of local units in 1939. The head of one of the larger plans in the country nearly read me out of the Blue Cross movement as a result of this. The plan executives were concerned about their local autonomy.

In 1944, I proposed an American Blue Cross with a national charter similar to the charters of the American Red Cross or the American Legion, with chapters throughout the country. Again, there was little support.

Later, however, the executive of the Blue Cross plan in Huntington, West Virginia, approached me. He was very interested in solving some of the problems of nationwide enrollment and serving national employers. He asked me if I would be willing to consider starting an insurance company that could be licensed in all 48 states and which would then be able to solve some of these problems. I was. The result was the John Marshall Insurance Company.

Even though it was organized as a commercial insurance company, one of the things I insisted on, and had a written agreement on, was that at least 99 percent of the income would be used for hospital and medical care, or for necessary overhead, limiting corporate dividends to 1 percent of gross income. People were willing to finance this and agreeable to the 1 percent limitation on any dividends. Although I had been connected with nonprofit organizations, I felt we could afford 1 percent of the gross income for stockholders if it solved many of the other national problems.

Among other things, I was interested in extending benefits to at least 120 days. At that time, it was difficult to get many Blue Cross plans to provide a benefit period of more than 70 days. It was difficult even though (1) there was a national demand for this kind of benefit on the part of the large employers and (2) it did not cost very much. The greatest cost of hospital care, as you know, is in the earlier days of the patient's stay.

As I said, the ultimate result was the establishment of the John Marshall

Insurance Company. I began the company in July of 1946. We started with $500,000 in capital.

The $500,000 originally seemed like a great deal. It would have been more than enough, except for the fact that hospital costs increased substantially right after the war.

From the outset, I had been concerned about possible inflation and its effects on this venture. I was assured by everyone that after the war we were going to have a major deflationary period. Everybody thought that with the stopping of munitions manufacturing that there was going to be a deflationary period. Well, we were wrong. Exactly the opposite occurred; we had severe inflation.

As a result of inflation, the $500,000 in capital was not enough. We had real financial problems. Finally, we had an opportunity to sell the company to Bankers Life and Casualty, which was owned by John MacArthur. We did.

Just about the time I sold John Marshall Insurance Company to Bankers Life and Casualty, the chief executive of the Cleveland Blue Cross Plan retired. I was contacted by the trustees of the Cleveland plan as to whether I would be willing to come back.

I came back to Cleveland in August 1948 to be the chief executive of the Cleveland plan for the next 17 years. I retired early in 1965.

———

Few people in the Blue Cross movement could understand why Mannix lent his name to the John Marshall Insurance Company. Among his Blue Cross peers it was considered close to immoral to handle hospital care as a commercial venture, to profit on people's illness. The fact that Mannix was trying to solve the national account benefit problem, to provide a service that the confederation of Blue Cross plans could not, was given secondary consideration. Mannix was shunned by his former colleagues. It was only several years after he went back to the Cleveland plan that he was again accepted back into the movement and elected to offices in the Blue Cross Commission.

Minnesota Blue Cross

While Mannix was working on one track, there were a father and son in Minnesota who were also making significant contributions to the growth of the prepaid group hospitalization movement.

The father, Joseph G. Norby, was superintendent of Fairview Hospital in Minneapolis and one of the early leaders of the prepaid group hospitalization movement in the Minneapolis–St. Paul area. (In 1949 Joseph Norby was president of the AHA.)

The son, Maurice J. Norby,[8] was a schoolteacher in Minnesota in the earliest days of the prepaid group hospitalization movement. Norby was a valuable link between the Blue Cross movement and hospitals, working at the Blue Cross Plan Commission with C. Rufus Rorem,[9] developing and operating the Pittsburgh plan after working in the St. Paul plan under E.A. van Steenwyk, and rounding out his career with George Bugbee[10] and Dr. Edwin L. Crosby[11] on the staff of the AHA. His experience and contributions in these three settings proved invaluable.

Norby describes those days and his work with E.A. van Steenwyk.

NORBY:[12]

My awareness of what's come to be known as Blue Cross began in the early 1930s, when my father came back from an AHA convention. At that AHA meeting a paper was given—authored by Justin Ford Kimball—describing the experiment or program he had initiated in group hospitalization. It wasn't Blue Cross in those days, it was called group hospitalization.

My father was intrigued by the idea. Other hospital people also were. Whether the motivation of all these people was altruistic or more financially pragmatic—a way of helping to assure that hospitals would be paid—one can only speculate. Regardless of the motivating force, the results have been beneficial for both patients and hospitals.

My father worked diligently to get hospitals in the Minneapolis and St. Paul area to get behind a group hospitalization program. They were successful, organizing a group hospitalization plan in which the hospitals contracted with each other to provide service. Hospital A contracted with hospital B, and hospital A and hospital B contracted with hospital C. A, B, and C contracted with D. They had interhospital agency contracts. These contracts called for the hospitals collectively to guarantee performance under a prepayment plan for hospital care. In those days they were charging 75¢ a month for an individual.

If those 75¢ payments didn't stretch enough to pay the full bill, then the hospital was required to accept what money the plan had as payment for the services provided to the plan's subscribers. The hospitals in effect provided a guarantee to the subscribers. All the hospitals in Minneapolis and St. Paul were partners in this program.

My father was very influential in getting the Blue Cross plan started. He was one of the key movers in it. He was, I think, one of the first officers.

The plan was run by a man named E.A. van Steenwyk.

Van Steenwyk had gone to the University of Minnesota and gravitated to Chicago somehow. He borrowed money to build houses. He became known in the West Side of Chicago as the Boy Builder.

The way he did it, he told me, was that he would find someone who wanted a house built and who could get money. Van Steenwyk would then dig the basement and charge the would-be owner the amount that it cost to dig the basement plus 10 percent, or some such figure. Then he would frame up the first floor and collect again for work completed to that point—and so on until the house was completed. He had little of his own money involved. In fact, he was operating on a shoestring. He kept on pyramiding until he had a number of houses being built that way.

This was before the depression. Then came the depression. Those folks who had contracted to have their basements dug couldn't make payments, and Van couldn't follow through. He had borrowed money to keep himself liquid, to keep ahead of the game. He had many holes in the ground with foundations in when he had to give up. He didn't go bankrupt, he just quit. He was even when he quit, but he had no money.

He came back to Minneapolis and got a job with a printer. He sorted the type, a menial job. They were printing primarily the *Minnesota Medical Journal* for the medical society. He got interested. He got to know them, and they got him doing some writing for the journal.

Then he heard about this group hospitalization development.

The committee that was organizing the group hospitalization plan also somehow heard about Van and got interested in him. He was a very persuasive fellow and a good thinker and honest. They hired him.

Van, one girl, and one room in the Globe building in St. Paul was how it began.

As this was going on, the public press got interested. There was much publicity about this new way to pay for hospital care. The radio station gave him free time. Van would go to the radio station, which was a block away from his office, and make his pitch to the public. He would then run back to the office to answer any phone calls that might come in. He also made a promotional movie. Even with these efforts, the plan grew fairly slowly.

In the summer of 1936, I was working on my doctorate degree. I had matriculated for summer school. One day that summer I went to the riverbank overlooking the Mississippi River and sat there thinking—I have my master's, my doctorate is practically done (I didn't have my dissertation), and I am being paid $107 a month to teach school. I sat on the riverbank thinking that my situation didn't make sense. I had to be worth more than that $107. I went back to the business office at the university and—I don't know how you would say it—"unmatriculated." I said that I had decided not to go to summer school and wanted my registration money back.

Then I went to see Mr. van Steenwyk. My Dad had told me much about him, but I had never met him. I asked him for a job. He said he was sorry, he would like to give me something to do, but he couldn't put me on the regular payroll, because my father was on the board or president or something. Finally, he did give me a job of selling subscriptions to groups that his regular salesman had said were impossible to enroll.

Van said, "You can take those groups and try to sell them."

Blue Cross in those days was very sticky about not paying sales commissions. They didn't want to support salesmen who forced sales. They wanted low-keyed salesmen, so they paid them salaries. Van broke the rule with me a bit. He said that I could go out and try to sell those dead accounts and that he would pay me in proportion to my success.

So I did that during the summer and made an acceptable amount of money. I was a high-key operation, which Van didn't want. For example, the owner of the Minneapolis ball team, Walter Seeger, had a big manufacturing plant on the border of Minneapolis–St. Paul. He made bodies for refrigerators. They called it Body by Seeger. He was having union trouble. Management had been approached and had not permitted enrollment. The employees wanted it.

So I went to Seeger and said, "If you don't allow these folks to enroll with payroll deductions, I am hiring a calliope and I am going to run it up and down the street here with big banners on the side reading "Walter Seeger is a SOB." With the labor trouble you have now, it's going to make it worse."

I got Walter Seeger enrolled. It was a big feather in my cap. Van's hotshot salesman hadn't been able to do it. It was a group of about 400 people, a great big group. I was OK with Walter Seeger. He gave me season tickets in a box in the ball park—in his own box, I should say.

I went back to teaching school in the fall.

I was teaching in Fergus Falls, which was close to a small, rural town of Wadina, Minnesota (population 3,000–4,000). Van was interested in trying to get rural enrollment. Up to that time everybody had been working in metropolitan areas. Van knew I was near Wadina, so he asked me if I would try to get the people in the town interested in enrolling.

I went to the town and got to the chamber of commerce and got them to agree to promote a big town meeting for a certain night. As I mentioned, Van had made a motion picture called "How Pennies and Seconds Count." It showed an ambulance picking up somebody and rushing them to the hospital and so on. It was a good film. We showed that and then Abbot Fletcher, the treasurer of the plan, made a sales speech. Then I made a speech. I asked employers to take enough enrollment cards to cover their employees—a grocery store, a hardware store, a barber shop where there were two or three employees—and to find out how many of their people would enroll in this program if it was available to them. We said we needed their signatures on the enrollment cards in the event we decided to come in. Whether we could enroll them or not was a question, because we weren't allowed by the Hospital Council of Minneapolis–St. Paul to enroll outside the city boundaries. They said that the plan should be strictly localized to the metropolitan area.

I asked them to sign the cards and told them that I would be back the following week to collect them.

The reason Van wanted to move so fast was that the state hospital association was meeting in Rochester, Minnesota, the following week. He wanted to report on rural enrollment at that meeting. When I picked up the enrollment cards and totaled the numbers who had signed up, we had 90 percent of that town enrolled in one meeting—90 percent of the town! This was really something. This showed that the rural people wanted group hospitalization protection.

I went to the state hospital association meeting in Rochester and was on the program to report our experience in Wadina. I really was enthusiastic. There was a lot of discussion. The net result, however, was that the state hospital association voted *not* to permit group hospitalization outside the city limits of Minneapolis–St. Paul. They were afraid of allowing the Mayos and the hospitals of Rochester into the plan for fear that everyone in the state would run to the Mayos for their hospitalization. So that ended our rural enrollment efforts.

I went to work for Van that next summer again. That was about 1936. Then at Christmas 1937 I got a telephone call from Rufus Rorem in Chicago. Rufus wanted me to come down and see him.

Rufus knew Van. Van had told him about this rural enrollment experience that I'd had.

I went to Chicago to talk with Rufus. He offered me a job at twice what I was making teaching school.

Rufus wanted me to come and set up his office. (He had just left the Rosenwald Fund and had gone over to the AHA with his grant.) He said that it would take about a month. After that, he said, something would turn up. He mentioned van Steenwyk and said that he and Van got along real well.

I said OK.

I worked for Rufus for about three months. I then went back to Minnesota and worked full time for van Steenwyk.

By that time, my father had moved from Fairview Hospital to Columbia Hospital in Milwaukee. So there was no problem in my working for the Minnesota plan.

Pittsburgh Blue Cross

Shortly after I got back to Minnesota, Pennsylvania passed what they called an enabling act to govern the operation of hospital care prepayment plans. There was a fellow in Pittsburgh by the name of Abe Oseroff, administrator of Montefiore Hospital, [13] who was very instrumental in obtaining approval of that legislative act. Prior to this time, most state legislatures had not passed enabling legislation.

The enabling act was passed, and the hospital administrators in Pittsburgh were looking for a developer and administrator for a prepayment plan. They invited van Steenwyk to come. He did not want to move from Minnesota, so he said, "Why don't you look at my man Norby?"

So I went to Pittsburgh and was interviewed by an organizing committee of hospital administrators and trustees.

Abe Oseroff, the promoter of the plan, was part of the committee. There was also the head of the Harbison-Walker Refractories, the president of Gulf Oil, an officer of the Mellon Bank, the president of U.S. Steel, and an officer of the Koppers Company. They were big names. Not only big names, but they had demonstrated their abilities. I was interviewed by them. However, I had the complete advantage, total advantage, because they knew nothing about group hospitalization and they were intrigued with the idea. Anything they got was new information, so they thought I was a fountain of knowledge in this endeavor.

I was still very young in chronological age but old in terms of experience with group hospital plans, because this was a newly developing phenomenon. I started work in Pittsburgh in the fall of 1939.

At the age of 31, I was starting a prepayment plan. I began by working on operational issues and systems. For example, I developed a very simple subscriber's contract. I wrote a contract on one page. In those days, the lawyers got to the early plan directors and put about four pages of whereases and all that kind of legal language into the subscriber contracts.

Well, I put in a simple system of operation. I insisted that all subscriptions be paid by payroll deductions. We sold hard. At the end of the first year we had grown to 100,000 subscribers—the largest first-year growth of any plan.

In 1940, I went to the American Hospital Association meeting in Cleveland. As part of the AHA's overall program there was a sectional meeting for directors of group hospitalization plans. The subject scheduled for the sectional meeting was a proposal to establish a public education program to promote the idea of group hospitalization.

Before the proposal could be debated, word came that the New York group hospitalization plan was broke and that there was big public hue and cry about possible mismanagement. Van Steenwyk recognized the real issue and said, "We don't need a public education program, we need a self-information program. We have got to know what is going on in our own plans and programs."

So they agreed that they would put money into a common fund and hire somebody who could run a program that would analyze their activities and give them facts and figures about how they were doing, statistically and actuarially and financially.

I was ready to go home at the end of the convention. My Dad was there at that meeting. He and I were having breakfast in the hotel coffee shop when Rufus came looking for me.

Rufus said, "Maurice, how would you like to go to work with me again?"

I asked, "What's going on?"

He said, "You were at the meeting. You heard the discussion and approval of the idea that the plans pay into a common fund to finance and distribute statistical information, and financial and operational information—a self-educational program."

Rufus repeated his offer, "How about doing it?"

I said, "Rufus, I don't know. I am happy where I am. Things are going well."

He said, "I have got to get somebody. You think it over. I want you in that job. It would complement my promotional work."

About one week later I got a call from Rufus.

He said, "How about this new job assignment?"

I said, "Rufus, I don't think I can really do it. I have got to keep this Pittsburgh plan going."

He said, "Think it over for another week."

I did that and sort of semi turned it down in my mind.

Then a couple of weeks later, on a Sunday morning, the telephone rang. Here was Rufus again on the phone. "Maurice, I have to know your decision right now," he said, "because the plan directors want their new program to get started. It has been delayed over a month. They want action."

I said, "I know, but how are you going to finance it?"

"They all agreed to make a payment."

"On what basis?"

"Just whatever they think is reasonable."

"How much have you actually got?"

Well, he had a couple of thousand dollars.

I said, "That isn't going to go very far—about a month—by the time I get a girl, furniture, and that stuff."

"Yes," he said, "but they will come through."

I said, "Just a minute and I'll get some advice." So I described the project and asked Judge Wasson, one of my board members who happened to be at my home when Rufus called, what he thought.

He said, "Mr. Norby, why don't you get a leave of absence for a year

from here. Then you will protect yourself and yet you might get into something that is important. A central office program is important in this kind
of growing activity."

So I turned back to the phone and said, "Okay, I'll be there."

"When?" asked Rufus.

Of course he wanted me right away—the next day. I told him I couldn't
come that soon, that I would be there in about two weeks. So I called a
hurried-up meeting of my board. Judge Wasson led the pitch for me to get
a leave of absence.

I went to Chicago.

The Blue Cross Commission

My first job when I got to Chicago was to go to New York and find
out what had happened, why they had gone broke. There was a fellow
named Pyle (I don't remember his first name) who, I think, had been chairman of the board. Van Dyk was the executive director of the plan. Pyle took
over as the chief administrative officer. Van Dyk was still there working on
the program. The main problem turned out to be the result of poor enrollment policy. They had relaxed group requirements and had been enrolling
too many sick people.

Mr. Pyle and Mr. Van Dyk put in corrective measures, and the New
York plan worked out its difficulties.

After the first year of making contributions to a central fund, the plans
set up a permanent system of financing based on the size of the plan, the
number of subscribers. A system for approving plans was also established.
To be approved, a plan had to meet certain specified criteria. It would apply
for approval, submitting data in support of its application, and if it met the
criteria, it would be approved by the AHA. Later, only approved plans could
use the Blue Cross name and the Blue Cross symbol, a blue cross with the
AHA's seal in the center of it. The matter of the symbol, as Norby notes
below, was a sensitive issue.

NORBY:[14]

The plans were meeting in Biloxi, Mississippi. The issue was, shall we
turn the Blue Cross mark or trademark over to the American Hospital Association, shall we turn it over to the Blue Cross Commission, or shall we
keep it ourselves in the individual states? A compromise was finally worked
out whereby the American Hospital Association would allow its seal to be
placed in the center of the blue cross. The Blue Cross plans would transfer

the mark to the AHA as the administrative agency of the mark until such time as three-fourths of the plans voted to take it back again. So the AHA actually was the administrator of the use of the Blue Cross mark and name.

It was a very emotional meeting, because some plans felt the Blue Cross mark was a valuable property. They did not want to give it to AHA. So they didn't give it. They gave the right to administer it. Subsequently, in the early 1970s, the Blue Cross plans withdrew this authority.

In the early 1970s, the AHA and the Blue Cross Association (the successor to the Blue Cross Commission) began a new era of formal organizational relationship. The approval program and the administration of the Blue Cross name and symbol were transferred from the AHA to the Blue Cross Association. Also, the representation on each other's boards was discontinued. In chapter 8, we talk more about the development of the Blue Cross Association and its separation from the AHA.

Early Benefits

Several persons have talked about rates and benefits in the beginning of Blue Cross, but it seems fitting to add a few more comments.

In the early days of Blue Cross, coverage was limited to just the employee, the worker. Later, provision was made to extend benefits to dependents. Also, coverage initially included only hospital care. Norby comments below on the development of benefits.

NORBY:[15]

The emphasis was on the employed person. In Minnesota, the employed person paid 75¢ a month for hospital care. He could enroll his family for another 75¢—all members of the family—but they would get only 50 percent of their hospital bill paid. Gradually, however, coverage of dependents became better. This was good not only for the employee, but for the whole family.

In Pittsburgh, for example, I charged $1.00 for the individual and $2.25 for the individual and the family. It was identical coverage for every person in the family.

Maternity care was not covered by some plans. Some charged an extra 25¢ a month if they included it. Mental health care was never included.

As far as medical care was concerned, there was continuous dispute for the first ten years as to whether or not X-ray, anesthesia, and laboratory should be included in the Blue Cross plan benefits. Local medical societies said that they were medical services and that you could not include medical service in a hospital program.

In Pittsburgh, for example, when I started that plan, we moved so fast that we couldn't talk to the medical society. We said, "We will talk to you a little later." When we got to the end of our first year, we had to talk to them. They were really upset. So we said we would talk with them.

In those days we were paying hospitals $6.00 a day for hospital care. We said we would pay the hospitals $4.00 a day for hospital care and send another check for $2.00 a day for medical care administered through the hospital by whatever device, contract, or commission for the hospital uses. The doctors were happy with that arrangement, because we identified clinical laboratory and anesthesiology as medical services. They wanted them identified as medical services. The fact that we sent two checks, one for the hospital care and one for medical, pleased them in Pittsburgh. Those disputes were satisfied or overcome in many different ways.

In addition to expanding benefits locally, the plans had to find ways of making benefits available nationally. Norby comments on this.

NORBY:[16]

The director of the plan in Chicago would enroll Harvester, because Harvester had its home office there and its biggest manufacturing plants were in Illinois. Also, Harvester had plants out in California and Alabama and so on. The plans there would enroll them. The Chicago plan, the plan where you had the head office, would act as the national account control plan. Through the control plan, they would enroll the employees of the account all over the country under the same contract, a single contract—different from the local plan's contract.

A second issue with respect to national benefits was the question of out-of-area services. For example, if I belonged to the Chicago plan and became ill in San Francisco, what benefits did I get? How could San Francisco give me Chicago benefits? That wasn't what the hospitals had agreed to do. So they formed what they called the Interplan Benefit Bank. It worked like a clearinghouse of a commercial bank.

Through the Interplan Benefit Bank, I got the benefits of the plan of the community in which I was hospitalized. That was just the opposite of the national account enrollment program. In the national account program, all were enrolled under one contract. But in the Interplan Bank, as a member of the Chicago plan, I got a day of care with the benefits of the San Francisco plan if I were hospitalized there. The San Francisco member would come to Chicago, the Chicago plan would give him the Chicago benefits even though the San Francisco benefits might be much greater than those in Chicago. The patient would then have to take the lower benefits he got in Chicago. That was better than none. Prior to Interplan Bank, I got benefits only in the hospitals in my plan's area, not in hospitals in other plans' areas or in other states.

Notes

(Transcripts of the oral histories cited here are housed in the library of the American Hospital Association, 840 North Lake Shore Drive, Chicago, Illinois 60611. The Oral History Collection is a joint project of the Hospital Research and Educational Trust and the AHA.)

1. See Profiles of Participants, in the center of this book, for biographical information.

2. *John R. Mannix, In the First Person: An Oral History.*

3. Ibid.

4. Ibid.

5. See Profiles of Participants for biographical information.

6. *Robert M. Cunningham, Jr., In the First Person: An Oral History.*

7. *Mannix, Oral History.*

8. See Profiles of Participants for biographical information.

9. See Profiles of Participants for biographical information.

10. See Profiles of Participants for biographical information.

11. Crosby was executive director of the American Hospital Association from 1943 to 1972.

12. *Maurice J. Norby, In the First Person: An Oral History.*

13. When Norby moved from Minnesota to Pittsburgh to start a Blue Cross plan there, one of the leaders in the Pittsburgh hospital community was Abe Oseroff. Oseroff was the administrator of Montefiore Hospital. He also was a leading force in setting up the Hospital Council of Western Pennsylvania, under the auspices of the Community Chest, and in establishing the Pittsburgh Blue Cross Plan. The funding of the plan, in fact, came from a foundation grant to the hospital council.

Oseroff later served as director of the Pittsburgh Blue Cross Plan (after Norby left to rejoin Rorem in Chicago). Thus, Oseroff was head of three organizations—the council, the hospital, and the Blue Cross plan—simultaneously. In 1942, he resigned his hospital post, but he continued as head of the hospital council and the Blue Cross plan until he retired in 1955.

14. *Norby, Oral History.*

15. Ibid.

16. Ibid.

8

The National Focus

The Blue Cross Association, which became the national association of Blue Cross plans, had a modest beginning. Originally, a Blue Cross Plan Commission had been developed under the leadership of C. Rufus Rorem to set up guidelines and an approval system for Blue Cross plans. By the late 1940s, the commission was faced with problems of how to handle accounts for firms with employees in more than one Blue Cross territory. In an attempt to solve this problem, an agency, Health Service, Inc., was founded "to operate as a national enrollment office and as an underwriter to fill benefit gaps in national contracts and thus level out the peaks and valleys in benefits among plans."[1]

A corporation was needed to provide stock ownership in Health Service, Inc. A paper, nonprofit corporation was established for that purpose. This was called the Blue Cross Association (BCA) and was separate from the Blue Cross Commission and the AHA. The BCA soon addressed other problems besides those of national accounts: retirement plans for Blue Cross employees, a representation role, need for national advertising, and typical national trade association relations.

While the influence of BCA was growing, the effectiveness of the Blue Cross Commission was declining. By 1960, the Blue Cross Commission had disbanded; BCA became the national organization.

James (Jeb) Stuart,[2] who had acted as president of BCA during the changeover, retired in 1961. In his place the directors chose a young, forceful leader, Walter J. McNerney.[3] McNerney was a graduate of Yale and had a master's degree in hospital administration from the University of Minnesota. He went to BCA from the University of Michigan, where he had been the founding director of the Program and Bureau of Hospital Administration. While at Michigan, McNerney led a research staff in an impressive study of hospital and medical economics. This study came about at the request of the governor of Michigan, who wanted information on which the state could base Blue Cross rates.

Under McNerney, the Blue Cross Association grew from a loose-knit organization into one that spoke with authority and influence.

McNerney describes his coming to BCA as president in 1961.

McNERNEY:[4]

My formal beginning with the Blue Cross Association was in 1961, when I was asked to become its president.

I was in Hawaii with some friends on a Ford Foundation grant. The phone rang. On the other end was Bill McNary, then president of the Michigan Blue Cross Plan. He said, "How would you like to be President of the Blue Cross Association?" I thought about it for about ten seconds. I said, "Yes."

It was interesting because Bill spent another two or three minutes convincing me that it would be a good idea. I said, "Bill, I said yes."

On reflection, either subconsciously or consciously, I still don't know which, I think that the leadership within the Blue Cross movement was preparing for the time that Jeb Stuart would retire as president of BCA and a replacement would need to be found.

Beginning about two years prior to McNary's phone call, I had been getting invitations to appear before Blue Cross plans and some Blue Cross national meetings. I would get up and talk big language and be full of mission, full of zeal. One day, I remember getting up to speak at the Mid-Atlantic Hospital Assembly. There, sitting in the front row, were van Steenwyck,[5] Rorem,[6] and Colman.[7] This was in advance of the telephone call to me in Hawaii by, say, six months. Why would Rorem, van Steenwyck, and Colman be sitting there? I thought it was strange. I was conceited enough by then to think I was such a good speaker that almost anybody would show up and enjoy it. Later, it occurred to me that they may have been tracking me.

Now maybe none of them would admit that's what they were doing. Only Rufus Rorem is still alive. I have the feeling that, in an institutional sense, Blue Cross had a survival instinct.

It showed that the Blue Cross pioneers, and I have just named three of them, had the foresight, the sense of continuity, and the sense of survival to attend to things like that.

At any rate, I said yes and left Ann Arbor with my family and came to Chicago at the age of 36 to assume the presidency of the Blue Cross Association. At that time, BCA's main office was in New York. One of my first decisions was to move the main office to Chicago.

I made the move to Chicago because the leading health and hospital institutions were in Chicago. A lot happens on an informal, everyday basis in most industries. My thought was, why not be part of these informal contacts by being in the same place? At the same time, a national association with members in every state is well located in Chicago for travel and other purposes.

There were some at this point who said we should move to Washington. I resisted it then, and I would still now.

What Washington needs are forces within the private sector that look at the country from a different point of view than that which one gradually assumes when they live in Washington. People who move to Washington, I have observed, become preoccupied with the congressional process, with what Senator X is going to do next. They almost unconsciously seem to mold their lives in reaction to government.

What government needs in the health field, I believe, is a force or forces that have decided what their mission is, where they want to go. These forces must then work with government, not reactively but proactively. So Washington was rejected.

It was interesting that when I got to BCA Jeb Stuart, to his everlasting credit, said, "There's your chair, I'll see you later." He didn't stay around to second-guess me even though I was obviously wet behind the ears. He just said goodbye and good luck.

Jeb did, however, give me some good advice. He told me that there were three people in the Blue Cross field that I should meet with, and meet with fast. He said, "They are tough to begin with and they are not sure where you are coming from. You had better get out to see J. Philo Nelson, Walter R. McBee, and Robert T. Evans." All three were chief executives of major Blue Cross plans: Nelson was in San Francisco, Oakland technically; McBee was in Texas; Evans in Illinois. Jeb told me, "Make your peace with these fellows."

That was it. That was my portfolio. Well, I got to see those three and a lot of others. Then I started the process of helping to move the Blue Cross Association from being essentially a trade association to what it had to become: that is, a combination of a trade association and an operating arm of the total Blue Cross system.

A Changing Role

When I actually got to BCA, I found a staff that was a tenth or less in size of what it is now. The staff had a lot of experience and knowledge.

They were very conversant with Blue Cross and very loyal and dedicated to the idea and ideals of Blue Cross. However, they were a loose organization, held together by individual respect and familiarity with one another. Also, at that point, they were not well tuned to some of the things that were going to lie ahead. So, I had a job to do.

I began by working with that staff to think through how BCA could represent the plans with Washington or industry or labor when there was a national situation; convene meetings to discuss topics of common interest; work with the plans to strengthen them as operational and management entities; and further begin to debate, with a little more forcefulness at the national level, what Blue Cross should be doing and why. More specially, this meant some dialogues about whether Blue Cross simply traded money or whether part of its role was to intervene and help shape the delivery of care.

Through the late sixties and early seventies the Blue Cross Association got itself involved more deeply in plan administrative and operational issues. The means of doing this was the plan performance review program. Through the plan performance review program, we went out into all the Blue Cross plans in the country, on a periodic basis, to examine specific aspects of management and work with them to strengthen their total performance. Where a plan was reluctant to act, the BCA executive committee might talk to the board members of the plan. The plan performance review program provided a discipline. It also gave reality to a striving for excellence.

Other programs were also developed and pursued on a systemwide basis. Cost containment is one example.

I emphasized its importance in the sixties. Fresh out of Ann Arbor, I had a lot of ideas about how to improve the delivery system through the financing process. A fair number of those ideas ended up as polite policy statements, or worse, as exhortations.

In the seventies, however, cost-containment standards were developed which were made a condition of plan membership in BCA. It happened also in Blue Shield. Under the cost-containment program, certain cost-containment activities had to be implemented by the plans. These included utilization review capacity, developing relations with areawide planning, and so forth.

We have also been quite active in urging plans to get into alternative delivery systems, into HMOs. We developed a national network of HMOs.

We grew to a new and different type of maturity.

I want to hasten to add that the end result of all this was not to make Blue Cross monolithic, that is to say, a national underwriting capacity that takes care of all national business and all local business, or some combination of the two. Unquestionably part of Blue Cross' strength is its ability to walk both sides of the street. Blue Cross can be strong nationally when it has to be. Importantly, it has at the same time, through the plans, strong local connections: politically, marketwise, laborwise, and communitywise. It is through this local base that Blue Cross is able to reflect the kaleidoscopic patterns of tradition, income groups, etc. around this country—in effect, to be an integral part of a community.

The question, therefore, becomes: To what degree do you centralize to strengthen the overall Blue Cross system without replacing valuable local capabilities? What emerged was a strategy to centralize or regionalize certain functions like data processing and actuarial work but leave intact provider, professional, and community relations, etc. It's a practical admixture of economies of scale and standards on the one hand and local nuance, political and market relations, and economic attachments on the other.

Nobody that I have discovered yet has a pat answer to the balance required. We are seeking our way in a competitive market, influenced greatly by what it takes to get and keep the business while at the same time do a good job. We are being controlled, in effect, as much by outside practical forces as we are by our own aspirations. If regionalization, a case in point, gets stronger, as it inevitably will, it will be because we will have to drive our retentions down, our administrative costs down, to stay in the market.

I don't mean to drain out of our history the desire to do a good job and to serve the community better. I do, however, want to underscore the fact that we are continually shaping and reshaping ourselves in a pluralistic, competitive market. Simultaneously, we are trying to achieve self-stated objectives. We are not yet institutionalized to the point where we are not plastic and experimenting.

National Association: Merger

Through the 1960s and 1970s the Blue Cross Association developed programs to represent plans as well as to assist them in their operations. The Blue Shield Association (previously, the National Association of Blue Shield Plans) was undertaking many of the same kinds of activities for its member medical plans. In some parts of the country Blue Cross and Blue Shield plans competed with each other; in other areas the two were a single corporate entity. At the national level, however, they were separate and autonomous, each with its own staff and board. In the late 1970s the two associations merged.

McNerney:[8]

There came a point in the relationship between Blue Cross and Blue Shield when certain things became an issue. The two organizations at both the national and local levels typically always worked closely together. This basic generalization, however, has to be qualified. In a few sections of the country Blue Cross and Blue Shield plans competed. In some sections of the country the two were allied but not well coordinated. In some sections of the country they were organized as one corporation.

This type of variation was sustainable when life was a little less complicated and markets were less competitive.

In the 1970s, however, the environment shifted. Consumers became more informed and had more opinions about how care should be rendered. Also, they were more critical of the performance of health benefit carriers.

Accounts [purchasers] got more articulate and experienced. The economy moved from a supply economy to a demand economy. The federal government was faced with health care cost problems and started to grapple with them. The number of competitors to Blue Cross and Blue Shield grew. You found a more businesslike environment, one which was much more demanding, much more critical, and much more highly penalizing of weakness.

Then not only did Blue Cross have to start to examine concepts of centralization and regionalization, to make better use of limited resources, but also it had to ask the question: What about the relations between Cross and Shield? Were there redundancies and overlaps that were hurting the total system of plans?

When a few of the plan presidents looked at the national associations, they found redundancies. Not only were there people in the Blue Cross Association and the National Association of Blue Shield Plans doing similar things, overlapping, but the national voices were not always synonymous. We weren't always saying the same things in Washington.

Initially some plan presidents got together informally to talk about combining the two associations. Rump meetings were held, I would be invited, and in those days Ned Parrish [president of the National Association of Blue Shield Plans] would also be invited.

I think it is fair to say that from the very beginning the Blue Cross Association thought that combining the two associations was a sound idea. There was a need to bring the two together. But the Blue Shield Association, as it is now called, with equal enthusiasm at first thought it should not be done.

There was a fear on the part of the Blue Shield Association that in any consolidation they might not come out equal. Some physicians feared that through such a consolidation the physician might be subordinated to the Blue Cross idea, which is a combination community idea and hospital idea.

The rump meetings started to formalize. I won't take you through it all other than to say the issue did not die. It went from semiformal meetings to formal meetings then to the members discussing it openly. It involved the appointment of committees, the conduct of formal surveys, the formulation of formal recommendations, and finally a vote on the issue.

During that time, I was encouraged to keep a low profile because I was potentially part of the problem. What would happen to Blue Shield if McNerney were to become the chief executive officer? If I were to have gotten too assertive at that point, it could have prejudiced the question. So, for a while I played a less visible role. I offered my opinion when asked, and I was asked.

Considering market forces, the need to have a more collectively organized posture toward the government, the outright need to save dues money by cutting out redundancies, and the fact that the public viewed the two associations as the same anyway, it was time that the two became the same. The evidence became overwhelming, and the consolidation was voted.

Following the merger, a chief executive officer had to be found to direct the new consolidated organization. After much speculation, McNerney was selected to be the first chief executive officer of the combined associations.

McNERNEY:[9]

Maybe I shouldn't be this personal, but it has been reported that, when the search committee asked a lot of people about the new position, they were told by both the hospital and the doctor representatives, as well as by various consumer and public representatives, that they should move in my direction. That sounds bumptious, and certainly opposition was expressed within and without the system, but I want to make the point that by then the American Medical Association had changed.

Several years earlier [the mid-1960s] I had been cited for malfeasance by the AMA house of delegates (it had to do with the development of HMOs). There were memories about that, but a lot of water had gone under the bridge since. When the chips fell, the AMA and some of the speciality societies were more concerned about having a reasonably articulate spokesman representing the private sector than they were about some past differences of opinion.

They asked me to take the job. I did.

A Different Point of View

An interested observer of the development and progress of Blue Cross was Daniel Pettengill. Pettengill joined the Aetna Life and Casualty Company in 1937. His connection with Aetna's health insurance business began in 1946, and he was a vice president of the company from 1964 to 1978. During the 1960s and 1970s, Pettengill was a major spokesman for the commercial insurance industry on health matters. His observations on the development of health insurance in the United States and the problems and progress of Blue Cross provide an interesting counterpoint to the comments in the previous chapters and to McNerney's views.

***

PETTENGILL:[10]

In 1937, which is the year that I first went to work for the Aetna, the Aetna wrote its first group hospital expense benefit policy for an employer. It provided a $3.00 daily room and board benefit and a $15.00 benefit as the maximum allowance for ancillary services. Interestingly enough, that was very adequate for the day.

My point is simply that it was a relatively easy matter in those early days to design a hospital benefit that was adequate and yet had a modest, finite dollar limit.

Shortly after I came, Aetna introduced the medical expense benefit which paid for physician office and home visits, as well as in-hospital visits. It's important to point out that this benefit was for the services of attending physicians in nonsurgical cases. Later, we also introduced coverage for diagnostic X-ray and laboratory examinations.

The primary competition, in terms of physician service benefits, were the Blue Shield plans. Blue Shield, however, did not expand its benefits beyond inpatient services for quite some time. As a result, because Blue Shield was better known and more familiar, many physicians did not realize that under many insurance company group policies the patient might have available benefits for home and office calls—and more importantly, diagnostic X-ray and laboratory examinations. Not surprisingly, physicians would admit Aetna-covered patients to the hospital, thinking they had to admit them in order to get the diagnostic examination paid for. They assumed that Aetna had the same coverage as Blue Shield, and they knew that they had to do that under their Blue Shield plan.

This was an unfortunate situation, and for many years we were unable to correct this false impression.

In terms of the development of health benefits, one of the most important innovations was created in 1948. In that year, the executives of the General Electric Corporation [sic] became concerned about the "high cost of health care," particularly with respect to serious illnesses and accidents. They were able to persuade the Liberty Mutual Insurance Company, which is a casualty company headquartered in Boston, to write, on an experimental basis, a catastrophe benefit, which was called major medical. Actually, the group that it was written for was known as the Elfund Club. The Elfund

Club was a club to which the General Electric executives belonged. Actually, they took the coverage out as one of the fringe benefits of belonging to the club.

This experiment immediately created tremendous public interest. The typical health benefit policy in the late 1940s, while adequate for an acute, short-term episode, didn't really provide enough help if you got into a real serious or drawn-out medical problem. So there was real pressure on the insurance industry to move ahead with this kind of product. And we did.

Aetna and other major group underwriters went to work; we studied the limited experience that the General Electric executives had, and we came up with major medical coverage in the beginning of the 1950s. I think the Aetna wrote its first policy in 1951.

Major medical benefits became the most rapidly growing form of benefit coverage. This was simply because people who had basic hospital-surgical benefits wanted to add, to superimpose major medical on top of their basic program in order to reduce their potential risk.

The next question for insurers was, why do you have a set of basic hospital, surgical, medical, and diagnostic benefits and then superimpose a major medical benefit? It makes for a very complicated plan to describe to employees and an expensive one to administer with all the separate benefits to calculate and pay. In 1953 the United States Fidelity and Guaranty Company in Baltimore, Maryland, decided to purchase a single-benefit, comprehensive plan for their employees. All medical expenses incurred in a given year were to be combined, the employee was to pay a front-end deductible (I believe it was $50), and then the plan would pay 80 percent of the excess up to a $10,000 maximum lifetime. This comprehensive approach, though logical, is not as popular as first-dollar basic hospital-surgical benefits plus supplementary major medical.

The Blues at first were reluctant to write the supplementary major medical benefits. Their reluctance I believe was due to the fact that major medical didn't fit nicely into their respective areas of operation. The Blue Cross plans had their contractual arrangements with hospitals, and the Blue Shield plans had their arrangements with physicians. So the major medical concept of lumping together all medical expenses in a given period (usually a year), applying a deductible of, say, $100, and then paying 75 percent or 80 percent of the excess up to some specified maximum dollar amount just didn't fit conveniently into their method of operation. The Blues countered with richer hospital-surgical benefits. Ultimately, they were forced to write major medical benefits. They did so by establishing a couple of captive insurance companies which wrote the major medical benefit when the Blues needed it to compete with insurance companies.

In addition to what might be called philosophical differences, there are business practice distinctions between commercial insurance companies and Blue Cross and Blue Shield plans. These differences shape the competitive position of each and influence their ultimate success in the marketplace.

PETTENGILL:[11]

The effect of some of these differences, as contrasted with the example of major medical, are in favor of the Blues. I think you can see this in the experience we all had with the Federal Employees' Health Benefits Program [FEP].

The FEP is also in and of itself an important event in the history of both the commercial insurers and the Blues.

In terms of business practices, it should be appreciated that, in general, insurance companies did not permit employee-pay-all plans, because they didn't get satisfactory participation and the experience was generally poor. The Blue Cross and Blue Shield plans, on the other hand, did. Also they were a bit more aggressive in this regard. They would usually make arrangements with one or more of the employer's employees to act as their agent and go around on payday and collect the employee contributions. As a result, I would estimate that, in the case of federal employees, about half of those employees had local Blue Cross and Blue Shield coverage on an employee-pay-all basis at the time Congress was considering a uniform health insurance plan for federal employees. The Blues, of course, were pushing that their plan be the federal plan.

Henry S. Beers, who was then the vice president in charge of the Aetna group division and who subsequently became president of the company, felt very strongly that coverage of the federal employees by only the Blues would adversely affect insurance company business. So he went to work and lobbied Congress that the federal employees program ought to be either just an insurance company plan or a choice between a Blue plan and an insurance company plan. As I'm sure you can imagine, it was that choice situation which appealed to Congress, because no congressman wants to offend any constituent. By giving the employees the right to choose between a Blue plan and an insurance company plan, a congressman could say, I gave you a choice, I didn't pick for you.

Because Congress did decide that there was to be a choice between the Blues and the insurance companies, both types of insurers have survived. The Blues did gain an advantage, because they kept—that is, they enrolled—most of the 50 percent of the federal employees that they presumably already had covered on an employee-pay-all basis and then gained some of the remaining 50 percent. And the insurance companies got about half of the remaining 50 percent.

Thus, the Blues ended up with 54.4 percent of the enrollees, the commercial insurance companies with 26.7 percent, and employee unions with the remainder. I don't believe the numbers reflected a true preference for the Blues. Rather, I think they reflect the fact that the Blues had federal employees working as agents, something Aetna was not allowed to do.

Another point to keep in mind about the federal employees program is the fact that the various local Blue plans did not initially have a good record of continuing benefits for retired employees. This was due in part to the differences in benefits of the local Blue plans and the fact that many retirees moved to an area served by a different Blue Cross plan. This problem should not have been a factor for federal employees, because the high and low options of the Government-Wide Services Benefit Plan were to be uniform regardless of where an employee worked. But the fear remained. As a consequence, many federal employees, when they reached retirement, switched from the Blue plan to the indemnity plan which the Aetna administered.

While the total number of persons enrolled in the indemnity benefit plan remained relatively constant, this influx of the retirees from the Blues meant that there were fewer and fewer new active employees. This was a great disadvantage in the sense that the retiree has a higher claim cost than the active employee.

In a fundamental sense, I think the FEP saved the Blues, because it gave them the ability to offer a uniform plan nationwide for the first time—an ability the insurance companies had always had and had used effectively. Furthermore, it united them at a time when their prestige in the group health insurance field was slipping.

———

Pettengill then spoke of what a great boon it was for Blue Cross Association to become the fiscal intermediary for Medicare. Blue Cross was particularly well suited for the work because of its claims experience and mechanisms, and Medicare business became a major portion of the Blue Cross workload.

———

PETTENGILL: [12]

Medicare was an even greater savior, because it lowered the high expense rates of the smaller Blue plans. Remember, the Blues are an aggregation of a lot of local plans, frequently one per state, but, in some states, several per state. In 1965, many of these plans were sufficiently small that they had very high expense rates and could not compete with the bigger insurance companies. Getting the contract to administer Medicare in its area gave the small Blue Cross plan a much, much larger base over which to spread its fixed expenses. This was a salvation for them. If they had not gotten that, a number of them would have simply folded their tents and gone away.

Walter McNerney achieved for the Blues a major success, for which they should be eternally grateful.

The Blue Cross–hospital relationship was also noted by Pettengill as a business practice that worked to the advantage of Blue Cross.

PETTENGILL:[13]

Probably the most important relationship between Blue Cross plans in particular and the hospitals is their payment arrangement. Traditionally, Blue Cross plans paid hospitals on either a cost basis or a discounted charge basis. In either event, Blue Cross paid a differential price which was less than the hospital's listed full charges—the price charged to commercial insurance company beneficiaries.

I know of situations where the hospital charge differential (the Blues' discount) had become so great that an employer could not afford to insure his group plan with an insurance company. From a purely economic perspective his only choice was to go with Blue Cross. In that kind of situation the hospital becomes trapped, for it has essentially nowhere to go to recover its deficits.

The ultimate answer to this kind of situation has to be reasonable equality of charges for all types of carriers. But equality doesn't exist today, although the insurance companies have tried their darndest to secure it.

The problem started way back in the Great Depression, when several hospitals asked insurance companies to write hospital expense insurance and we, properly, said it's not insurable. So the hospitals formed their own entities to write the coverage, and these eventually became the Blue Cross plans. Because, relatively speaking, both the benefits sold and the amounts of service provided by hospitals were modest, Blue Cross succeeded in those early days. Insurance companies, seeing the market, responded by writing health coverages in order to compete.

But neither type of carrier, Blue Cross nor insurance company, was insuring in the normal sense. They were and still are providing an annual budgeting mechanism. At the end of each year, the insurer reassesses and says, "Next year the budget's got to be bigger. So if you want the same benefits, Mr. Employer or Mr. Union, you have to pay more." Essentially, that's been the story ever since about 1961. We're kidding ourselves when we say we insure it. We insure it for the year, and if you are able to change carriers at the end of the year and leave the carrier with a loss, yes, you've had insurance.

Insurance companies tried to eliminate these differentials on the basis that they constituted a restraint of trade. The Travelers actually brought an antitrust suit against the Western Pennsylvania Blue Cross Plan, only to have the Pennsylvania Supreme Court say, yes, this is discrimination but the state may do so if it chooses. The state licenses the Blue Cross plan. If it chooses to discriminate, the state has the power to discriminate. So, it has been established that there is discrimination, but, unfortunately, there is not a thing insurance companies can do about it.

There was one other advantage that some Blue Cross plans had initially, but I think it's pretty well gone now. Michigan was a classic example. Namely, the hospitals actually reinsured the Blues. Thus, if, at the end of any year, Blue Cross had suffered a financial loss, the member hospitals had to pay a special assessment to bail out the plan. Such reinsurance, however, has pretty well disappeared.

But the fact that the hospital will sell service to the Blues at cost or less, then charge the public rates for those same services which are higher than costs has been the Blues' greatest advantage. For example, in the Federal Employees' Health Benefits Program, I estimated, and the Civil Service Commission never denied it, that Blue Cross enjoyed at least the equivalent of a 10 percent discount. It wasn't an actual discount per se, but the amounts that Blue Cross plans were paying the hospitals were at least 10 percent below the charges that commercial companies were having to pay under the indemnity benefit plan.

Medicare eased the discount problem initially. But the present situation, where a state merely holds down the rates that Medicaid, and in some cases Blue Cross, will pay but not what the hospitals can charge the rest of the people, has made it worse than ever.

Nevertheless, hospitals should set charges at amounts reasonably related to their costs. Those charges should then be the basis of payment for everybody, whether it is a Blue Cross plan under an agreement whereby it pays the hospital directly or whether it's an insurance company which, because it sells such modest benefits, the hospital wouldn't touch with a ten-foot pole. The point is that everybody should pay the same fair charge for a given service at a given hospital.

Has the competition between the Blue Cross plans and the commercial insurance companies been good for the country?

PETTENGILL:[14]

Ever since the 1944 Southeastern Underwriters decision [which prohibited collective actions among insurance companies], insurance companies have not been able to do anything in concert without specific legislative authorization. I know it shocks people, but prior to that time there was a small committee, composed of the heads of the group divisions of various insurance companies. This committee would meet every other month for lunch in New York City and would discuss group insurance problems. Group insurance in those days was as nice a controlled commodity as you would hope to see. There was a lot of competition in the individual insurance business, but the group side was remarkably controlled.

Now, in one sense I don't think this control actually hurt the American people, because you've got to remember the insurance companies were competing against Blue Cross and Blue Shield, so there was competition. And many of the decisions the committee made dealt with how to compete with the Blues. Furthermore, in the early days of group health insurance, this competition was vital. Because if the nation had only had the Blues, it would not have had the development of new coverages anywhere near as rapidly as they actually occurred. The insurance companies were constantly trying to find ways to compete against the Blues' discount, their preferred tax status, etc.

                    *   *   *

Both the Blues and the insurance companies have lost a substantial portion of the group health care insurance market. It has been lost to self-insurance. The loss has been the result partly because of the premium tax and partly because of claim reserves.

In virtually all states, if an employer self-insures his group plan, he is not subject to premium taxes. Let's face it, for a large employer, the premium tax was frequently 40 percent to 50 percent of the total administrative cost of the benefit. Forgetting the claims, say the insurer's actual expense rate was 3 percent and the premium tax was 2 percent, so a large employer would have to pay an insurance company a total of 5 percent over claims. Whereas, if the employer self-insured, he could save the 2 percent premium tax or 40 percent of the total expense. This assumes he could administer the plan as cheaply as the insurance company, which is questionable, but large employers often feel they can.

The other problem was the claim reserve, and this applied to both the Blues and insurance companies. An insurance company, and in most states the Blues as well, is obligated to set up a reserve for claims which have been incurred but haven't yet been paid. Such claims range all the way from the accident that just happened but which the insurer does not yet know a thing about, to the claim that has been reviewed and approved but the check has not yet been mailed to the claimant. The claim reserve is the actuary's best estimate of the aggregate of all these claims that are in process.

The claim reserve depends on the type of coverage, but the reserve for a typical health insurance plan would amount to anywhere from two to three months of premium. That can be a substantial amount of money. If an employer is paying you, for example, a million dollars a year, and you've got to set up three months' premium as the claim reserve, that's $250,000.

So large employers argue, if we self-insure, we won't have to pay premium taxes, which will save us anywhere from 2 percent to 3 percent, depending on the state, and we won't have to set up claim reserves.

Thus, employers started to self-insure. They found, however, that the job of claims administration was not simple. As a result, there was pressure on the insurance company to sell its claim administration services. In other words, the employer self-insured but then hired the insurance company to settle the claims. Most insurance companies refused to write such administrative services contracts for a long, long time.

Unfortunately, or fortunately, depending on which side of the fence you sit on, independent agencies started to say, "We'll be very happy to settle the claims for you." And then one insurance company after another weakened and agreed to sell their claim service.

* * *

Self-insurance has had the same effect as far as the Blues are concerned. Indeed, I suspect an administrative service contract is more difficult for Blue Cross plans because they are used to paying costs to hospitals rather than charges.

I think that's the thing that is hurting the Blues.

* * *

I think the American Hospital Association finally came to realize that the long-term solution that's viable, from the hospital's point of view, is to set charges so that they are reasonably related to the cost of the service provided, but with a little margin. After all, you've got to set your charges today and your costs don't get incurred until tomorrow. It's humanly impossible to set your charges precisely equal to your costs. You've got to have a little margin in there for breakage.

The following observations by Robert Sigmond expand on Mc-Nerney's comments about performance discipline and striving for excellence.

SIGMOND:[15]

Maintaining performance levels is a very complicated process. Let me see if I can discuss it in terms of different levels. But, let me talk about Blue Cross.

First and most formally, the plans must conform to the approval standards which were originally developed by Rufus Rorem and have been amended from time to time. The plans are required each year to complete certain forms which signify that they think they're in conformance with the approval standards, along with supplemental information. There's an entire staff that reviews that material and takes appropriate action.

What does appropriate action mean? In theory, it means that a plan could lose the Blue Cross symbol by action of the board on recommendation of the approval committee. In practice that has not happened in over 20 years and it's not likely ever to happen again.

At least once every three or five years there's a full-fledged site visit [plan performance review visit]. This visit has to do with fiscal stability, with management, with relationships, with hospitals—the whole approval standards. It is very much like a Joint Commission on Accreditation [of Hospitals] visit or an AAMC [Association of American Medical Colleges] visit for accreditation of a medical school. The visits always result in assessments, in which areas of performance weakness and strength are pointed out.

This is all done in a relatively confidential manner, with nothing said to the public, etc. But, of course, the reports of this activity go to the board of directors of the BCA, which is made up of plan executives. As a result, any plan executive who gets a critical letter tends to respond. If his response is inadequate, that fact will be reported to the board. There are different kinds of actions that are taken. Really, the most extreme action that I can think of that's been taken in the last few years was when, following a number of intermediate steps, the BCA executive committee requested the chief executive officer of a plan to arrange a meeting with his board. The meeting took place and had considerable effect. So that kind of thing goes on.

Action moves from an exchange of letters through to a delegation of plan executives that meet with the plan CEO, and so on. I don't want to mislead you: I cannot imagine a situation where BCA would actually take the symbol away any more, but that doesn't mean that it is a totally powerless process. It is a very powerful process.

Second, BCA is the prime contractor for Medicare. The plans subcontract with BCA. Nationally, as a group, the plans handle more Medicare money than subscriber money, especially in the smaller plans. If these plans didn't have Medicare, they'd be dead.

BCA has the power—obviously through the board structure—to say that this plan isn't measuring up and it's threatening the prime contract with Medicare, which means it's threatening the stability of every Blue Cross plan. So, Blue Cross might have to take Medicare away from the Oklahoma plan and give the work to the Texas plan. That sort of thing has been done.

Point three is national accounts. A national account is an employer who has employees in various plan areas but whose health benefits are uniform and centrally administered through common policies.

National accounts are not handled by the national association. They are typically handled by a syndicate of plans. Plans participating in the syndicate are those in which that national account has a specified minimum number of subscribers in the plan's area. The plan in the corporate home office town is the head of the syndicate—the control plan. So, the Michigan plan obviously is the control plan for all the Detroit auto companies, and the Pittsburgh plan for the steel companies. The Allentown Plan—Allentown, Pennsylvania—probably wouldn't exist if Bethlehem Steel went to commercial health insurance. It's there because Bethlehem Steel wanted to have its own Blue Cross plan.

Now again, the national association has the power, by the agreement of the plans, that, if a national account control plan is doing an unsatisfactory job, after going through an appropriate process, to take its role as head of the syndicate away. To say, for example, "Sorry Michigan, the Illinois plan is going to handle General Motors."

Well, aside from the financial implications of that, there would be a lot of embarrassment. The national association doesn't do something like this very often, but it has been done.

Finally, when a plan gets into real trouble, it doesn't get into trouble with the national association, it gets into real trouble with the state insurance commissioner.

One of the things Rufus did early on was sponsor model legislation—enabling acts for establishing local Blue Cross plans. The enabling acts almost all provide for the insurance commissioner to supervise the plan.

Now, we get calls in Chicago. There have been two of them since I've been there in five years, two that I know about. An insurance commissioner calls McNerney, "I'm in trouble." He doesn't say to McNerney, "You're in trouble," he says, "I'm in trouble."

McNerney says, "What are you in trouble about?"

"I'm going to have to declare plan X bankrupt. I can't afford to do that politically. You've got to help me."

I'm fantasizing that conversation, but in effect an insurance commissioner with a problem Blue Cross plan has got a problem on his hands. He doesn't have that many people to turn to, and BCA is there. He invites in the national association—and BCA has every reason to call the plan and say, "Hey, we'd better come in."

They usually say yes.

In the two situations I know about, the national association representatives sat down with the plan's board and urged that they get new management. The insurance commissioner is usually scared to death and accepts that course of action. BCA doesn't take over the management, but they do make specific recommendations to the plan board. Also, in one of the two cases they did, for the first time and I hope the only time, lend the plan some money, which they are now paying back.

So BCA has all those kinds of powers. Now that adds up to a lot of power.

Notes

(Transcripts of the oral histories cited here are housed in the library of the American Hospital Association, 840 North Lake Shore Drive, Chicago, Illinois 60611. The Oral History Collection is a joint project of the Hospital Research and Educational Trust and the AHA.)

1. Odin W. Anderson, *Blue Cross Since 1929* (Cambridge, Mass.: Ballinger, 1975), pp. 59–60.

2. Stuart was interim president of the Blue Cross Association from 1959 to 1961. Formerly he had directed the Cincinnati Blue Cross Plan.

3. See Profiles of Participants, in the center of this book, for biographical information.

4. *Walter J. McNerney, In the First Person: An Oral History.*

5. E. A. van Steenwyk was chief executive officer of the Philadelphia Blue Cross Plan.

6. C. Rufus Rorem. See Profiles of Participants for biographical information.

7. J. Douglas Colman was chief executive officer of the New York City Blue Cross Plan.

8. *McNerney, Oral History.*

9. Ibid.

10. *Daniel Pettengill, In the First Person: An Oral History.* See Profiles of Participants for biographical information.

11. Ibid.

12. Ibid.

13. Ibid.

14. Ibid.

15. *Robert M. Sigmond, In the First Person: An Oral History.* See Profiles of Participants for biographical information.

PART III

The Emergence of a Profession

9

The American Hospital Association

In this chapter, we look at the creation and evolution of the American Hospital Association. We focus on its development from almost a small "chowder and marching society" to an organization of institutions committed to helping hospitals realize their potential as community resources.

The organization that became the AHA was created in 1899, when a group of hospital superintendents got together at the Colonial Hotel in Cleveland, Ohio, organized, and called themselves the National Hospital Superintendents' Association. It was a personal membership group, with affiliation limited to only what today would be called hospital chief executive officers. Eligibility was later enlarged to include assistant superintendents.

At the outset, the organization was essentially a correspondence club that met once a year. The results of the annual meeting were published verbatim as proceedings.

A few years after its founding, the group changed its name to the American Hospital Association. More important, in 1917 it changed from a personal membership society to an organization of institutions. At about the same time, the AHA hired its first paid chief executive and established hospital sections, subgroups of hospitals, within the national association.

Dr. William Walsh was the first paid secretary (chief executive) of the AHA. He served in this capacity on a part-time basis from 1916 to 1918, when he went into active military service and was granted a leave of absence. M. Howell Wright was appointed secretary during Walsh's absence. In 1919,

Dr. A.R. Warner was elected permanent secretary and served until his death in 1926. Walsh resumed the position of secretary and served until 1928, when he resigned. He was replaced by Dr. Bert W. Caldwell.

Ohio was the first state to be recognized as a section of the AHA. Wisconsin was second, and Michigan was third. Interestingly, a group of Protestant hospitals, the American Protestant Hospital Association, asked to be recognized as a section. The leadership of the AHA rejected its request, feeling that AHA sections should not be based just on religious affiliation.

By the time Caldwell became chief executive, the association had a headquarters building in Chicago (at 18 East Division Street), a small full-time staff, and an annual convention.

Gerhard Hartman was the executive secretary of the American College of Hospital Administrators from 1937 to 1942.[1] During this time, the ACHA had its offices in the AHA building, and Hartman knew and worked with Caldwell.

_____

HARTMAN:[2]

I would describe Bert Caldwell as a well-dressed, powerfully competent, singularly devoted, operative executive.

Intellectually he was a profound adversary. He didn't cater to Michael Davis,[3] because he felt Michael was too much to the left with national health insurance. Even though Bert was a physician of the old school, and I mean the Latin-type old school, he would not buy Morris Fishbein's[4] diatribes and Fishbein's resistance to prepayment.

I have a story which I think shows Bert at his best. He was a very cavalier gentleman. He had absolute self-control of his person and how he wanted to present his person. There was to be an AHA convention at the Royal York Hotel in Toronto. It also was to be my second ACHA convocation.

Bert said, "Gerry, how about getting on the train with me; we'll go up together. I would like to show you how I put the convention together."

We went up about a week before. He took a suite. I took a room. About ten in the morning the next day we had breakfast in Bert's suite.

He picked up the phone and said to the operator, "I want to see Mr. Sweet, the hotel manager."

The manager came up and said, "Yes, Dr. Caldwell, what can I do for you?"

Bert was in an elegant silk robe, and silk pajamas, and satin slippers.

Bert asked, "What have you to offer this time around?"

Poor Ray Sweet said, "Well, we'll have to come to that."

Bert said, "Fine, come back when you are ready to come to it."

That went on for about three days. Bert kept him on the prod. When

Bert finished (I may be exaggerating, but my recollection is quite vivid), I think he ended up with 24 or 26 complimentary suites for the use of the AHA's officers and board. He also knocked down the price of the banquet, and he got the complete ACHA convocation taken care of, just to be nice to me.

Well, when the convention was over, he called Mr. Sweet again.

Caldwell said, "Were you pleased?"

Sweet said, "The attendance was excellent and we made out very well."

Bert said, "I know you did."

Bert had his faults: he was a bit pompous; he was a bully if he could get away with it. But I also have to say that he was intellectually honest.

During the 1930s the AHA was a modest organization. Caldwell kept it small, with limited new activities. The annual convention was its major function until the mid-1930s, when it also began to publish a journal.

By the mid-1930s, however, people like John Mannix were beginning to press the AHA to change, to restructure its governance so that it would be more representative of the country's hospitals, and to provide more services for its membership.

Restructuring the AHA

MANNIX:[5]

As secretary of the Ohio Hospital Association from 1927 to 1933, I had the opportunity to observe the activities of the AHA on a first-hand basis. I also had the opportunity to make various program activity suggestions. I always felt that my suggestions received a lot of attention. Not much, however, was actually done, though. I was actually told the association did not have the money to finance the implementation of whatever it was that I was suggesting.

I felt that the American Hospital Association should be well supported, that it should have the funds to enable it to carry out the many projects that were needed—projects that could not be performed by a state or a metropolitan area association.

In 1932 the president of the AHA was Paul Fesler, who was the administrator of the University of Minnesota Hospitals. Paul showed some real interest in not only the need for what I called the reorganization of the AHA but also the financing of it.

With this encouragement, I continued to press for some kind of action. Dr. Nathaniel W. Faxon [president of the AHA in 1934], who was administrator of Strong Memorial Hospital in Rochester, New York, and later administrator of Massachusetts General Hospital, became very interested in what I was proposing. I think he was influenced by my previous conversations with Fesler.

Dr. Faxon agreed to appoint a committee on membership structure to study the American Hospital Association. I was appointed chairman. He inquired who I wanted on the committee, and I proposed three trustees of the AHA and three members representing state hospital associations.

The original group of AHA trustees were Dr. Robin C. Buerki, from Henry Ford Hospital in Detroit; Asa Bacon, who was at Presbyterian Hospital in Chicago and who also was the treasurer of the AHA; and G. Harvey Agnew, who was with the Canadian Hospital Association. The three people representing state associations were James A. Hamilton of New England; Graham Davis, who was with the Carolina-Virginia association and was in charge of hospital activities of the Duke Endowment and later the executive for health activities of the W.K. Kellogg Foundation; and John Hatfield, who was secretary of the Pennsylvania Hospital Association.

It was an excellent committee. Asa Bacon had been president of the AHA, and Agnew, Buerki, Hamilton, Davis, and Hatfield later became presidents of the association.[6]

That committee met from 1934 to 1937. Prior to the AHA's annual meeting in 1935, we developed a report with certain recommendations. The bylaws of the AHA at that time provided that any change in the constitution and bylaws had to be cleared through the constitution and bylaws committee.

In many ways the old leaders of the hospital field were satisfied with the way the AHA was operating and what it was doing. They did not want to change. As a result, our committee's attempts to contact the chairman of the constitution and bylaws committee were not successful. He did not answer our correspondence in advance of the meeting. At the meeting itself, he was completely unavailable. He would not answer our calls at his hotel room, although we knew he was in town. We spent from Monday until Thursday trying to reach him to arrange the required meeting of the constitution and bylaws committee. A meeting never came about, so there was no action. Our committee, however, was reappointed.

In view of later history, it might be just as well that those early recommendations were not acted on, although the final recommendations were not particularly different. The delay provided us with the opportunity to become a little more adept at association politics.

At the 1936 meeting, we had a report, but we insisted that it be a progress report. We argued that we needed another year to acquaint the membership with what we were proposing. We presented the progress report, and some of the then leaders of the AHA insisted on calling for a vote. We stated there was nothing to vote on, that this was just a progress report and we were not making any recommendations. The chairman of the meeting finally ruled there was nothing to vote on. Actually, they wanted to vote it down. We knew this. Moreover, we knew that they probably had the votes to do it.

The committee continued to meet and to improve its recommendations. There must have been 15 or 20 full-day and two-day meetings over a period of three years.

By 1937 whatever opposition might have initially existed had now vanished. By that time, we had met with a great many of the state associations and we had contacted a lot of key people in the field. So in 1937 the AHA board approved the report and decided that the committee's recommendations should be implemented.

The recommendations included the establishment of a house of delegates of 100 people, with representation from all the states, with the larger states having greater representation. We recommended setting up what we called councils. Prior to this time it was customary for the president of the AHA to appoint committees each year. A president generally would have some special interest and appoint a committee for that purpose. There was no sunset law. Thus, once a committee was appointed, it could continue ad infinitum. This resulted in a lot of overlapping of committee functions and duplicate effort.

We recommended six councils in what we considered six principal areas of association activity and provided that all committees in the future should report to one of the six councils. The councils were to coordinate committee activities. In addition, we recommended a coordinating council which consisted of the chairmen of the six councils.

We also recommended quadrupling the association's dues.

Dr. Caldwell was very concerned about the dues increase. He felt that as a result of the dues increase the association might wind up with only 20 percent of the hospitals remaining as members. Thus, even though the dues would be four times as much, the total income of the AHA would be less. In actuality, the hospitals not only paid the increased dues, but the association had an increase in membership.

For the first time the AHA had the money to do the things that we had been talking about for years. In my opinion, the work of that committee gave the AHA, for the first time, the kind of financing required to do the national job which the hospital field needed.

The restructuring of the AHA was a major accomplishment. As reflected in the comments below by Kenneth Williamson, former director of the AHA's Washington Service Bureau, it provided the basis for a stronger organization. Williamson also notes that later changes may have had an opposite effect.

The committee's plan, however, was not enough. To achieve results, the organizational architecture had to be implemented and pursued with commitment. Comments by James Hague, former editor-in-chief, associate director, and secretary of the AHA, address the problem of moving from a plan to practice. Williamson's comments are presented first, followed by Hague's.

WILLIAMSON:[7]

The AHA structure can be described as consisting of councils, a coordinating council, the board, and the house of delegates. The house is an open forum for debate and discussion of issues. The board's policy recommendations have to be debated and approved in the house.

The AHA leadership was smarter in this regard than the American Medical Association, in that the AHA bylaws provided that the house of delegates could argue about an issue and then turn it back, but it had to come back to the board. The AHA house could not initiate an independent action different than the board's. This has been one of the problems of AMA: they would think on the floor and take actions that would refute the thoughtful recommendations of their committees.

The AHA membership had a voice, a strong voice, and at every meeting you had to think of who the people were in the hospital field who might raise questions and argue. You had to be ready for it, which was good and healthy. It strengthened the association.

Later, to streamline things, the AHA also established regional advisory boards [RABs]. There are nine of them.

The idea underlying the RABs was the desire to provide a means for placing the board's recommendations on the major issues in front of the field. The chairman of each RAB is automatically a member of the board. The regional groups would discuss the issues and argue about them, and then their recommendations would come back to the board.

That brought a lot of input and had many values. It had value for the people in the field, but it also lost something. You can organize to the point where you ruin dissent and you ruin individuality. I think that's what happened to the AHA. The process is now so neat, so slick, and so organized that things get so talked out, that by the time they come to the house of delegates, there is often little interest in the matter.

Caldwell's reaction to the agreed-upon changes in the organization of the AHA was seemingly less than enthusiastic. James Hague comments on this.

HAGUE:[8]

I was told by someone who really should know that Dr. Caldwell was satisfied with the way things were. He didn't want to spend the money made available to him. He was apparently frightened of guys like Mannix and Jim Hamilton.

I am told that what he [Caldwell] would do every year was say, "I think I am going to retire." This kind of comment had the effect of quieting down the efforts to oust him. Then another year would come, a new set of officers would come in, and he would say the same thing.

The officers would say, "Let's not do anything. Bert has been around for a long time. He is a very nice guy. He knows all the right restaurants. Things are going along nicely. We have big crowds at the convention. It's good."

Then a new face came along. It was Jim Hamilton. Hamilton's arrival in the elected leadership positions changed things. Hamilton got great support from guys like Mannix, but it was Hamilton who did what had to be done.

As I understand it, it began with his going to the nominating committee and saying, "Look, I am going to be president of the AHA some day, I'd like to get it behind me, so I want you to nominate me."

I think Harvey Agnew was chairman of the nominating committee. According to Jim Hamilton, Agnew said, "You are going to be president, but it's not your turn yet."

Hamilton said, "I don't care whether it's my turn. I want to be nominated. If you don't nominate me, I will have the votes anyway."

He was nominated, and, of course, he was elected president of the AHA [in 1943]. He made it his business to make the necessary changes. He had to do a fairly dirty job.

There was a lot of pressure on the board not to fire Caldwell. Hamilton said, "At the first meeting of the board at which I preside, he's going to go. Period."

The board was meeting at the Drake Hotel. Hamilton recalls that he was in his room when John Mannix called him from the lobby. Mannix said, "Jim, I am here with Monsignor Griffin.[9] Come on down, will you please? We would like to talk with you."

Hamilton said, "Look, I just got to bed. It's been a tough day."

John said, "We have lived together for a long time. Come on down."

So Hamilton went down. As he tells it, the conversation was nothing but a straight-out appeal for a delay in dealing with the Caldwell situation. Caldwell apparently aroused a great deal of sympathy among Catholic hospitals and among the Catholic hierarchy.

Hamilton said, "Now look, I have to do it." He said, "I am up to here with the pressure from the church on this. Now I am going to tell you what I am prepared to do, then I am going to leave. If Caldwell resigns, I will see to it that he is taken care of (a pension or something). If I don't have his resignation by tomorrow morning, he will be fired and that will be the end of it. I have the votes and I am going to do it."

He went out of the room and the next morning he had the resignation. That was the end of that.

___

Hamilton's own recollections of the events add detail and a first-person perspective.

___

HAMILTON:[10]

Finally I said to Caldwell, "I'm going to become president." (I was only president-elect at that time.) You have to decide whether you are going to be editor of the AHA magazine, *Hospitals,* or the executive secretary (chief executive) of the hospital association."

He wouldn't choose.

So finally I said, "All right, Bert, that's the answer. I am going before the association and have you fired."

"They won't do that," he said. He thought that they wouldn't fire him. He was relying on Monsignor Griffin, who was the power behind the throne.

I said, "Don't count on that, Bert."

I sat down with John Mannix and with Monsignor Griffin, whom I knew and whom John also knew very well.

I said to Monsignor Griffin, "Tomorrow morning I am going into the board meeting and I am going to suggest that you be kicked off the board and somebody take your place. Also, I am going to say that Caldwell must be fired."

We argued about it until I said, "I don't want to argue about it any more. What you have done is wrong. You have made this a religious issue. You have stirred up bishops all around the country, and, the first thing you know, I've got Wilinsky[11] of Boston getting in touch with me saying, 'What the hell are you doing with the bishops? The bishops are coming around and telling me that Hamilton's doing terrible things at the hospital association and that he is going to do something horrible.' So that's what has made it religious."

So I said, "The best thing I know to do is get Caldwell out, let's give him a pension or something. We owe him something for all those years of service. Let's get that office going with somebody in charge that can really do it. Then ask the members again to put up more money to do it. We can't run the association on chicken feed. Compare our dues with that of other associations and it doesn't amount to a row of pins."

The next morning I met with Monsignor Griffin and Dr. Caldwell.

Griffin said to Caldwell, "I guess the jig is up. I can't hold it any longer. Hamilton says he is going to the board and you are going to be kicked out. But Hamilton says if you will resign, he'll fight like hell for a pension for you and a few things like that."

Caldwell resigned and we set him up with a pension.

After Caldwell resigned, we had to look for somebody to replace him as executive secretary. That wasn't easy.

It finally got down to three people: John Mannix, O.G. Pratt,[12] and George Bugbee.[13]

I said to all of them, "George says he would like the job. George is just the kind of guy that will do the job well. He has an understanding of human relations and is able to quietly get things done. The three of us must support him."

They agreed, and we did.

After deliberation, the board chose Bugbee.

Building the Organization

In addition to engineering the change in leadership, Hamilton obtained a fourfold increase in the association's dues. With George Bugbee as chief executive and with adequate revenues, the AHA was now ready to meet the growing needs of the nation's hospitals. James Hague comments on how Bugbee built the organization and set out a clear direction for it to take.

HAGUE:[14]

George went to work. Using the additional dues money, he began to hire a good staff.

He got good people and he set the association on the right track.

The key staff—C.J. Foley, of the AHA editorial staff; Dr. Hullerman, secretary of the council on professional practice; Maurice Norby; Kenny Williamson; and Bugbee—met in what Bugbee called a "retreat." They came up with a clear statement of what the association should be.

First was representation. You think of representation in more recent years with an emphasis on Washington. Actually there was and is far more to it than just that. Representation meant the AMA, the pathologists, the radiologists, the anesthesiologists, and so forth.

The second had a double name, research and standardization. The AHA was influential in the study of the anesthetic gases.

The third one was education—publications, conventions. George thought of the commercial aspect of conventions as a necessary evil. He wouldn't give the exhibitors the time of day if they interfered with the educational program. He would take their money, but that's it. He ran good conventions, so they came.

Those three—basically three, because research and standardization could be considered one—dominated the AHA's work. The council chairmen were given these three goals, and then George asked them what these councils should be doing and thinking about to further AHA activities toward these goals. They came up with some very exciting things.

———

Maurice Norby was one of the staff persons who participated in the direction-setting retreat. He came to the association from the Blue Cross Plan Commission, where he had worked directly with Rufus Rorem[15] and the chief executives of the various Blue Cross plans.

———

NORBY:[16]

I liked George. I liked what I saw in him and in the association. It was growing. It was growing without the problems of youthful growth and ego ambition that the Blue Cross Commission had. I thought that maybe the AHA would benefit if it better understood what Blue Cross' problems were. I thought that I could serve both Blue Cross and hospitals best if I was on the hospital platform.

George offered me the secretaryship of the committee on Blue Cross and prepayment plans. From this position, I was an officer of the American Hospital Association. At the same time, I could continue to deal with my peers on the Blue Cross Commission. I thought I could do the commission a better service if I was on the inside of hospital circles than I could if I was back in the commission family. Also, I liked George's method of operation. He was direct, and he was not personally ambitious. He was, however, ambitious for the association.

Shortly after I came to work at the AHA, George called for a "think meeting" with Kenny Williamson, Foley, myself, and Dr. Hullerman. We went to a hotel and locked ourselves in a room. It was what George called a retreat, and its purpose was to decide what the association should be doing.

We decided that the work programs of the association should include education, representation, research, and standardization. All the programs of the association should have some phase of those activities intertwined in their work.

George then brought the proposed work program guidelines to the board. They agreed with it. So, for example, the council on administrative practice had more education in it. Standardization was emphasized by the council on professional practice. I can remember hospitals were using about 70 kinds of suture needles. They got them standardized down to 20 or a number like that. They got everyone to agree to the standards.

This was the kind of thing that George did. His emphasis was on how to do it, how to improve hospital administration, how to help hospitals and hospital administrators, how to assure better care for all the people.

We also produced manuals. For example, they got out a laundry manual. They had a committee with a couple of administrators and three or four good laundry managers. The secretary of the council on administrative practice was present to assist the committee. They would first agree on what the table of contents should be and then assign people to write chapters. Then they would criticize the chapters and edit them and so on.

They were how-to-do-it manuals. They had quite a number of them, each on a different hospital department. There was no hospital literature at that time, so we gave every hospital a free copy of each manual.

Kenneth Williamson was another of the participants in the Bugbee retreat. Williamson came to the AHA from the California Hospital Association and the Association of Western Hospitals. His comments, while similar to the foregoing, also show another aspect of the direction the association was taking.

WILLIAMSON:[17]

Jim Hamilton convinced George Bugbee to leave City Hospital in Cleveland and take the AHA's chief executive position. George, though he came from a hospital and knew hospital operations, didn't know the field. Therefore, he wanted someone who knew the hospital field. I went to Chicago to interview for the job. It sounded interesting. I liked him, and he liked me; so I joined AHA. The staff at that time consisted of 13 people.

When George came to the AHA, there was really not much there. There was no organized hospital field. There were a few spots of organization. Generally, however, the field was unorganized and disconnected. The association had no platform, it had no program, it didn't know where it was going. There was nothing. The association was essentially just a group of people with lots of goodwill.

With George, we used to go and sit together, about three or four of us, and think and talk. Even with the dues increase there were still limited funds. The management task was to spend the funds, spend them in a way that would accomplish the most good.

One of the things that came out of the talking, thinking, and our own experience was a recognition of a need to organize the field. That meant developing state hospital associations all over the country. That was one of my first jobs. I think there were 36 or 38 state hospital associations I had a hand in organizing. I met with their committees, wrote their bylaws with them, met with the hospital leaders, sold them on doing this and that, and so on. It was a lot of fun, but I was away traveling much of the time. After the state associations came the local or metropolitan hospital councils. We also had a hand in helping some of them get started.

We also developed a series of manuals or textbooks, or perhaps more precisely primers on how to operate every aspect of a hospital. We got the best laundry people together, for example, to learn every phase of how you operate a laundry, and then wrote a text on operating a hospital laundry. We also wrote a textbook, a manual, on hospital housekeeping. That housekeeping manual was interesting, because we got a fellow from the Fleischman Yeast Company to come and talk to us about sterility. He went around and looked in some hospital operating rooms. He said that, if the areas where they made yeast were as dirty as those operating rooms, they would be in trouble.

I also got the chief housekeeper of Marshall Field's, the Chicago department store, to talk with us. If you ever want an interesting experience, go into Marshall Field's when they open in the morning. It is something to behold. The floors shine, and there isn't a fingerprint on any of the glass cases. As I said, it is something to behold. I got this man to go into some hospitals. He said, "If Marshall Field's was as dirty as some of those hospitals, they wouldn't have any customers."

We wrote manuals on all aspects of hospital operations. This was very important, for it affected the economy of the hospital. For instance, the purchasing manual written by purchasing agents who really knew their business led to standardization of supplies for hospitals. We went about the standardization process with a set of objectives that weren't there before. Fortunately, this standardization helped us keep up as medical care changed and evolved. I think it was very fortunate for the public that hospitals were somewhat ready for those changes.

George Bugbee himself describes the organizational context he was moving into and the goals he was trying to achieve.

BUGBEE: [18]
Jim Hamilton resigned from Cleveland City Hospital to go to the University Hospital in New Haven. A search committee was set up to find a new superintendent for City Hospital. I ended up with that appointment.

Hamilton, by that time, had become very active in the American Hospital Association. As a result, he drew me into various activities, including, eventually, appointment as chairman of the association's council on hospital planning—or construction—perhaps hospital planning and construction.

That job, with Jim at the helm as president of AHA [1943], precipitated an evaluation of the staff of the association.

Dr. Bert Caldwell had been the executive secretary of the association for a number of years. He had set up an operation where he did most of the work, with some clerical help. As World War II continued, hospitals needed representation in Washington. Also, they needed many other services. Dr. Caldwell, however, was reluctant to increase his staff or change his style of operations. As you can guess, the situation came to a head, and the board ultimately asked Dr. Caldwell to retire. Then there was a search for an executive to replace him. I was eventually the selection of the board. I took office in May of 1943.

I think it's important to appreciate that Bert Caldwell's conservatism was understandable, even if no longer pertinent. The association just prior to the depression had purchased what had been the Boys' Latin School building at 18 East Division. The association did not have reserve funds, and the purchase required that it take out a substantial mortgage. With the depression, the association's income decreased, and at one point it was thought that it would be impossible to meet the payments on the mortgage. The situation was saved by the sale of bonds to AHA members. Undoubtedly, the danger of losing the building and of the collapse of the association was very much on Bert Caldwell's mind and supported his objection to all the new plans of the so-called Young Turks.

Prior to my being in office, Jim Hamilton, with a committee on association resources, had gone to the board and recommended that the dues of the association be quadrupled. The amount would be rather inconsequential compared to present dues, but the size of the increase was startling in the field. The board recommended it to the house of delegates.

The house of delegates approved the dues increase. In anticipation of their approval, and because there had been a great deal of interest in expanding the role of the association, I was asked to begin planning what the association's program should be. This was pretty short notice, since I hadn't had any association management experience. However, there was a core of people, led by Jim Hamilton, to advise me. Included in this group was John Mannix, who had been instrumental in the reorganization of the association a few years earlier, and O.G. Pratt, who was at that time in Massachusetts administering a hospital, I think in Salem. Bob Buerki and Dr. Robert Bishop[19] were also involved. I won't go into all the locations these men were in, but they were all in key positions. Importantly, they had ideas about what the association should be doing.

The first thing, of course, in support of the dues increase, was money for a Washington office. It would need almost as much money as the total association had been spending up to that time.

It was also decided that the councils of the association, other than the council on government relations, which was in charge of the Washington office, should be staffed and have funds for travel. This may sound inconsequential, but the councils weren't meeting, because there wasn't any money to pay the travel expenses of the council members. Also, there hadn't been money to provide staff support to the various councils. So this was the second item, travel expenses and staff support to the councils, for which the dues increase was used.

The accomplishments of the councils can easily be evaluated by looking at the annual convention transactions published by the association. These were a verbatim transcript of everything said at the annual convention, both the papers delivered and the proceedings of the business meetings. The transactions were discontinued a few years after I was appointed, because both the number of program sessions and the detail of the reports to the house of delegates became so lengthy that they could not all be published in one volume.

Another priority for the new dues money was a public relations program. Jim Hamilton and I arranged an appointment with a vice president of American Bell Telephone to see what his advice would be. Our thinking in seeking them out for advice was based on the fact that the telephone company had done an unusually good job of communicating with the public.

We made the appointment and saw him in New York City. He was very kind and visited with us for a while and asked us how much money we had. I don't recall exactly, but it was around $150,000. He tried not to laugh, but we got the idea. He said that $150,000 would buy just about one page in the *Saturday Evening Post,* which was then, probably, as good a medium for reaching the public as any.

We finally ended up hiring a public relations director and working with internal staff to furnish materials to member hospitals. They, in turn, could use these materials for local public relations. I think this met with some success for the hospitals that wanted to do it.

There was also need to employ a staff. I think Kenny Williamson was the first. At the time we hired him, he was secretary of the California Hospital Association and the director of the Association of Western Hospitals. He was experienced. He had worked for Blue Cross also. He was a good addition to the staff.

I also became editor of *Hospitals.* When I took the job as executive secretary, I insisted on not having a separate editor, calling whoever ran the magazine managing editor. The model I wanted to avoid was the Dr. Olin

West and Dr. Morris Fishbein situation at the AMA, where the editor of the American Medical Association journal, Dr. Fishbein, was more powerful than the chief executive, Dr. West. It wasn't a matter of a power play, I just didn't care to have a division of accountability. I also insisted that the director of the Washington Service Bureau, as we called the Washington office, report to me rather than to the council on goverment relations. If I were going to run the association, I was going to try to do it.

I didn't do as well in staffing the journal. I got a very honest, able fellow named John Storm. John, however, was not a flashy publisher.

Dr. Otho Ball, who was then the owner and editor of *Modern Hospital,* had recommended that I hire someone else. I probably should have followed Ball's advice, but I didn't want him to feel that he had control of the association. You have to remember that at one time the association had been only a desk in the *Modern Hospital* office. Otho Ball was a powerful man, and I wanted to avoid having him think that he was going to continue to play any dominant role. So I got John Storm and then built up the journal's staff.

Up to that time Bert Caldwell had been the editor of *Hospitals.* Really, all he did was publish convention papers. It was hardly, as the library would show, a sparkling journal. I think we did improve it. However, I never thought that we were able to catch up with *Modern Hospital.* That was always a matter of personal frustration with me.

After a few staff members were recruited and on duty, we began to think about the future of the association, whether the budget that was formulated a few months after I got there was a sensible one. I recall we had what was somewhat pretentiously called a retreat, where staff talked over what the functions of the AHA should be.

Of the functions of the association, one was education—running all the way from institutes to the convention and including the journal.

A second function, little understood, I think, by many people, was research moving toward standardization. Its focus was on helping the field develop "best" practice. We spent a great deal of effort bringing in the most knowledgeable people on a given subject, asking them to formulate what might be a manual or a discussion of a procedure, and getting this information out to the field.

The third major function was representation. The obvious level of representation, of course, is with government—all levels of government. However, representation was needed also with the professional associations which affected hospitals. There were many of these, all the way from the American Medical Association to the National Fire Protection Association. If AHA didn't work closely with these groups, they would proceed with their own interests without any attention to what their actions might do to hospitals or hospital care.

Having formulated those three functions, we structured the staff organization to accomplish them and moved ahead to do them.

I stayed at the association until 1954, when I left to become president of the Health Information Foundation. HIF was an organization committed to doing research and public relations, particularly in regard to the advances in medicine that had been useful to people. They also tried to focus on research in areas where research might be helpful in finding the solutions to real problems. HIF's financing came from the pharmaceutical industry, primarily the ethical and proprietary drug companies.

The reasons one voluntarily changes jobs are always complex and perhaps in part just rationalizations. The HIF job was interesting. It also paid a great deal of money. Additionally, it would let me spend more time with my family.

I had another reason, but I think it was part rationalization. When I was hired for the American Hospital Association job, Jim Hamilton told me about one of the engineering associations which had hired an executive for a ten-year term with the promise that they would get him a job at the end of ten years. Their theory was that ten years was about as long as an executive was productive. That might be true.

The other reason for leaving was more pertinent. I never could find a way to run the association easily. It seemed to me that I almost had to be the center of contact between the membership, the councils, the committees, the board, and the house of delegates. I don't mean decide everything, but communication was very important if you weren't going to have a revolt of one sort or another. It got to the point where really every waking hour was occupied, and too much from the standpoint of my family. It would have continued, because it was the only way I could see to do the job properly. I told Ed Crosby[20] that when he succeeded me, but he said, "I am not going to work so hard." Of course he did. He did things differently, but he worked equally hard.

A Washington Presence

Under George Bugbee's leadership the AHA came of age, achieving national stature and respect. The strategy that Bugbee employed to accomplish this was twofold. One part focused on membership services: technical support and education. The other concentrated on representation. The following comments by James Hamilton and Kenneth Williamson address representation in Washington, D.C. Hamilton speaks to the needs during the war years. Williamson, who headed the AHA's Washington Service Bureau from 1954 to 1972, follows, taking a longer perspective.

HAMILTON:[21]

When I was at Yale [1938–1946] I was appointed by the secretary of war to be on the National Commission of War. The secretary of war happened to be a Yale graduate.

I also knew the secretary of the treasury. I'd known him for years through Rotary activities. I went to see him and began to talk about the things that were affecting hospitals. About that time, they were shutting down hospitals because of the war effort. There was nobody in Washington telling the government what harm they were doing to the nation's hospitals in the name of war economies.

So I would go to Washington to tell the hospital side of the story. I was going around Washington doing this on my own, feeling that hospitals didn't have anyone in Washington to represent them. Bert Caldwell, who was the executive secretary of the AHA, wasn't focused on Washington.

In those days, the head of each of the major hospital associations (the AHA, the Catholic Hospital Association, etc.) would periodically get together and talk about how the hospital field could or should be represented in Washington. The Catholic Hospital Association fellows would say, "We've got a guy in Washington. We should let him represent the field."

Finally, when I became president of AHA (1943), I said that it was inappropriate to have the Catholic Hospital Association try to represent the whole field. I felt that representation of the entire hospital field should be the job of the AHA. So I established the AHA's wartime service bureau in Washington.

I was asked, "How are we going to finance it?"

I said, "By assessment."

The Catholic hospitals said, "We have a representative in Washington; we won't pay any assessment."

I said, "Fine, we won't represent you."

Well, they came back into the fold. They really had no choice; they were part of the hospital field.

So the AHA started its wartime service bureau in Washington with one guy.

His job was simply to go around and represent hospitals, to bring the hospital point of view to those in government who were making decisions. They (the people in government) were begging for it. The people I found down the line, under secretaries and assistant secretaries, would ask where they could go to get information on hospitals. So we provided it. From that small beginning quite a lot has developed.

WILLIAMSON:[22]

You can plot several distinct phases of the hospital field's relationship with government. The first was a time of total voluntary involvement. The federal government really had very little to do with hospitals. Perhaps the exception to this was during World War II, when there was a more formal relationship through the Emergency Maternal and Infant Care program. The EMIC was a program run by the government to take care of the wives and children of the men who were serving overseas. Government assured these men that their families would get care so they would not have to worry about them while they were away.

Then Hill-Burton came along. It also was voluntary. You didn't have to ask for money if you didn't want to. There were other things that the hospital could choose to do or not to do.

A second phase is represented by direct interaction with government. It started where we began to get exemptions for hospitals from such things as unemployment compensation, the minimum wage law, the National Labor Relations Board, and the Taft-Hartley Act. The AHA worked to get exemptions for the hospital field from the effects of participating under those laws.

Later, hospitals began to lose their exemptions under those laws, and the government began to be a party to the operations of hospitals in a big way. Hospitals came under the kind of rules and regulations that commercial firms were used to. So the ability of hospitals to decide whether or not to relate to government went out the window. They had to relate to government. This had-to-relate phase grew as government programs and government money grew.

At the Washington Service Bureau we got involved with trying to prevent the passage of a lot of bills and propositions that were aimed at controlling the hospital field. Sometimes we were the sole voice, sometimes we were a party with others. Part of our work was in helping to organize the hospital field for political action. This was done through the state hospital association executives. Some of them did it pretty well, some of them very poorly.

In the early years, an annual effort for the AHA was to get adequate funding passed for the Hill-Burton program. The program was no good without money. That took a lot of work and a lot of support. Incidentally, it was interesting how, by and large, the support came from hospitals who hoped to get money from Hill-Burton—some support from those and less support from those who had no interest in it. It was quite a problem.

We also worked on medical education financing. Here, we succeeded in including in the financing program hospitals that weren't owned and operated by universities. If they were recognized medical teaching facilities, even if they were not owned and operated by medical schools, they could get some of the money. In fact, these hospitals got a lot of it.

The AHA really instituted the federal government's role in participating in the cost of nursing education. This was helpful to the hospitals because they needed nurses and many nursing students didn't have money to pay for tuition. So it was self-interest and public interest at the same time. Organized nursing had less of a role in that than did the AHA. They supported it, but we instigated the legislation and followed it through with their help.

Later, we also instituted our annual meeting in Washington. The notion was that we would have a national meeting in Washington to foster the political side of things, to get people into contact with their elected officials so that they could talk to them about issues. We would have a meeting, then turn the people loose on their congressmen.

A great deal has come from the Washington meeting. A lot of things happened. The hospital people now know the legislators in a way they never did. It has stimulated a lot of contact, not just here in Washington but there has been follow-up. It goes on all the time. I think a lot of definite good comes from it. The hospital field, without a doubt, is now a lot better known.

━━━━━━

Representation had another aspect to it, one involving other organizations in the health field. George Bugbee's experience with the AMA, the American College of Surgeons, the American College of Physicians, and what ultimately became the Joint Commission on Accreditation of Hospitals provides not only an example of this aspect of representation, but also an interesting story. The episode is told by Maurice Norby and Bugbee himself.

By way of background: the American College of Surgeons had established a standardization program for hospitals in 1916. It established such a program because it needed a means of assuring that it admitted to membership only surgeons of proven ability. Deciding just who these surgeons were was very difficult. To help in this process, the college decided that it needed accurate medical records of surgery performed. Most hospital records were not very good at that time. The American College of Surgeons therefore set up a voluntary hospital accreditation program requiring complete medical records and review of quality of care and plant operation.

The college provided the financial support for the program until the late 1940s, at which time it requested the AHA to assume the operation and financing of the standardization program. Not surprisingly, there were objections to this from the AMA and the American College of Physicians.

━━━━━━

NORBY:[23]
Dr. MacEachern was the director of the American College of Surgeons [ACS]. He was responsible for the hospital standardization program conducted by the college and was a frequent speaker at hospital association meetings. He also had served on many important committees of the AHA.

So when ACS decided they didn't have the money to continue to support the standardization program, MacEachern suggested that the logical organization to do hospital accreditation was the American Hospital Association.

So, the American College of Surgeons actually approached George Bugbee and asked him to approach the AHA board and determine whether the AHA would like to take on that work and expense. George presented it to the board and recommended acceptance of the transfer of the program to AHA.

Admittedly, there was not a lot of love lost between the American College of Surgeons and the American Medical Association. That, however, wasn't the reason why the ACS came to the AHA. They approached the AHA because it was the logical move.

When the AHA accepted the ACS's invitation to assume the accreditation program, the AMA formally disapproved the transfer. They asked that it be transferred to them, so that it would remain within the medical framework, within medicine's control. There was a little jockeying, then they said, "Let's have a meeting and see how we can do this, maybe jointly."

For that joint meeting, it was decided that the American College of Surgeons should be represented, the American College of Physicians, the AMA, and the AHA—just those four. Each organization was represented by its president and, I think, the president-elect or the past president, one or the other, plus their executive secretaries (chief executives). How I was selected to be recording secretary I do not know, but I was.

At the first meeting, the doctors sat on one side of the table, except the college of surgeons representatives—they sat on the other side of the table with the American Hospital Association group. Both sides seemed to be glaring at each other. I have never been in such an uncomfortable position. Dr. Gundersen from LaCrosse, Wisconsin, who was representing the AMA, was elected chairman.

The objective was to write up a program of accreditation of hospitals. They wrote their objectives, which really would be the preamble to bylaws. They did this at the first meeting and seemed to get along pretty well with it. They knew they would have to have bylaws and would begin drafting them at the next meeting.

Someone said, "Mr. Norby, would you please bring in some 'boiler-plate,' some things you think ought to be in the bylaws? We can then go from there."

This I did. I went to the bylaws of various medical groups and selected sections within the objectives which the organizing committee had stated. I brought this material to the committee, and they started working it over at the next meeting. As they worked, they began to feel more comfortable. We had frequent meetings. They would take a section that I brought in and go through it. I would note their objections and make changes. We would bring that in to the next meeting and then work on a new section. Finally everybody was happy. Then the Canadian Medical Association said they would like to be in the program; so the committee expanded the bylaws to include them.

Then, they needed to find a director, and they were searching around. At one meeting I said, "How about Dr. Crosby[24] at Hopkins?" They said that we couldn't possibly get him. I knew a very good friend of his, Dr. Russell Nelson,[25] so I said, "I think we may be able to get him." I said, "Dr. Gundersen, if you wait, I'll make some inquiries around, and then I'll let you know. Don't invite Crosby before he is softened up a bit."

So I got Nelson to approach Crosby. To Crosby, it was unthinkable at first. Then Gundersen formally invited him, and, to everyone's surprise and delight, he accepted.

Then we were going to have the formal organizing meeting at the Drake Hotel[26] on a Sunday morning. (The doctors almost always met on Sundays; they didn't want to interfere with their practice on weekdays.) I knew the people at the Drake very well, all the kitchen people, the waiters, and all their work force. I arranged the meeting and the breakfast. That Sunday morning, we sat down for breakfast. It was a good breakfast. However, as soon as the meal was over and the plates had been cleared, in walked the waiters carrying trays with stemmed glassware, goblets with bubbles coming up through the amber liquid.

Gundersen, who was still chairman, said, "No, no. Stay away. We are here to do business; we don't want any drinks."

I had told the waiters to bring in the glasses and set one down in front of each person, no matter what the chairman said. So the waiters did as I had requested.

One of the other physicians, a fellow from the Napa Valley in California looked at what was going on and said, "It looks like good California champagne. As long as it is here, let's all stand up and toast to the success of the joint commission."

We all stood up, put our lips to the glass, then, with funny looks on their faces, the committee members began to sit down.

Bugbee said in a loud voice, "Maurice, you are up to your old tricks again, aren't you!"

They saw the bubbles coming up through the amber liquid and thought it was champagne. It was beer.

They then elected officers. It was hard for the chairman to get that meeting adjourned. They were complimenting each other, saying great things. Everyone had to make a speech complimenting the other people. They were so happy and so pleased. I never have seen such a change in a group. The animosity was completely gone. They were ready to go to work and do a good job. Crosby had accepted. He was there.

================

BUGBEE:[27]

The college of surgeons reluctantly decided for economic reasons that they were going to get out of the accreditation program. Then the question was, what's going to happen to it? I knew one thing, if the accreditation program were going to go on, the hospitals had better jump in and be in favor of it and keep it alive. So I proposed to the AHA board that we get in.

The AHA board decided to do it. The AMA got wind of it and showed up in an uproar to tell the AHA that they had no right to be involved. The AMA had pretty good support, particularly from the general practitioners, who had always been seemingly threatened by the accreditation program.

The criticism of the AMA didn't bother me. I thought it added stature to the association. I think I have to admit, however, that we were wrong. The resolution of the argument, and there was plenty of argument, was better than if the AHA had taken it over alone.

The board of trustees of the AHA and the board of trustees of the AMA met together and then appointed a committee, which met repeatedly. The president of AHA at the time [1951] was Dr. Charles Wilinsky of Boston, a wonderful man who had been president of the American Public Health Association and most everything else. He was deaf, but he heard enough so he did better than most who heard everything. He also was unusually adept with the physicians.

The argument, of course, was over how much medicine and how much hospital should be on the commission [Joint Commission on Accreditation of Hospitals]. The AHA by that time, with people like Wilinsky, were not worried about doctors per se. They were worried, however, about the AMA and the attitude of the general practitioner either emasculating the program or killing it. They thought it was a program primarily approved by specialists rather than generalists. So AHA insisted that there be representation from the American College of Surgeons and the balance from the American College of Physicians. It ended up with six AHA commissioners, six AMA commissioners, and three commissioners from each of the colleges. Then somebody said, What about Canada? The Canadian Medical Association was given one, and, since there wasn't a Canadian national hospital association at the time, the AHA was given a seventh commissioner. That was the early texture of the joint commission.

================

Maturity

Bugbee left the AHA to become president of the Health Information

Foundation. He was succeeded by Dr. Edwin L. Crosby. Crosby went to the AHA from the Joint Commission on Accreditation of Hospitals. He died in 1972 at the relatively young age of 64, while still serving as the AHA's chief executive.

The maturing of the AHA under Crosby's leadership is described by James Hague and Maurice Norby, two of the association's senior staff at that time, and Robert M. Cunningham, Jr., the former editor of *Modern Hospital*.

HAGUE:[28]

Ed Crosby was not a medical scholar. In fact, he never saw himself as a practicing physician at all. He said he wouldn't treat someone's cat.

He brought to the AHA his belief in doing good for as many people as possible. In the field of health, except for the classical public health things like sanitation and immunization, the hospital was the major agency for doing good for people. The hospital had, indeed, supplanted the family physician. It was in the hospital that care was given, and it was in the hospitals that the care givers were trained. Therefore, it was natural for someone who was dedicated to doing good for a lot of people, if they were in the health field, to be working in and for hospitals.

I think he believed that. He had an amazing personality. He knew everyone, and everyone liked him. He was trusted by them, and he could get things done.

He was a Salvation Army child. He married a Salvation Army woman. He quickly went into public health in New York State. The New York State Department of Health had a habit of choosing its brightest people and sending them on to Johns Hopkins for further training in public health. He did his work for his master's and his doctorate in public health at Hopkins, where he came under the strong influence of a man named Lowell Reed.

Reed was an outstanding man, eventually becoming the president of Johns Hopkins. Lowell Reed was not an M.D.-type doctor. He was a Ph.D., a biostatistician. At one time, every chair of biostatistics in the country was held by a graduate of his.

The School of Hygiene and Public Health at Hopkins is right across the street from the hospital. Until recently, the Johns Hopkins Hospital had no formal relationship with the university. The only thing that held them together was one sentence in a letter from Johns Hopkins to both the university and the hospital saying that he wanted them to work together. That's all, and, by God, they did.

Crosby was sent over to the hospital to work in the vital statistics area. Unlike most institutions, Johns Hopkins Hospital placed great reliance on statistical reporting to judge the quality of its care. Its annual reports were full of statistics from the hospital. Not enough attention is paid to that these days.

From this beginning, Crosby moved into the broader field of hospital administration and became Dr. Winford Smith's [the hospital director] chief assistant. Subsequently, he became the hospital director.

Later he took over the Joint Commission on Accreditation of Hospitals. Then he came here to the AHA. He built the AHA into what it is today, or just about what it is today, on the foundation that Bugbee had left him.

NORBY:[29]

Crosby was decisive and would make decisions fast—and I think he got more than his share of correct ones. For example, building the building at 840 North Lake Shore Drive. The board had agreed that they were not going to buy a used facility. He was the one who talked with Northwestern University about getting the land, convincing them that we could rent it. He decided that we should dig the foundation immediately, because prices were only going to go up. The excavation was there for a whole year, sitting full of water. He acted decisively and speedily.

CUNNINGHAM:[30]

As editor of *Modern Hospital,* I did notice a difference right away when Bugbee moved to the Health Information Foundation and Dr. Crosby came to AHA. They continued to be our competitors, but in a different way. Ed Crosby's basic position was, "You are in the same field as we are, providing information for this professional society, and if we can be of help to you in any way, let us know."

The advertising salesmen continued to cut each other's throats on the street, but we had a different relationship. I expect Crosby may have known what he was doing, because inevitably we were not as critical as we had been in the past.

I had known Ed Crosby when he was at Johns Hopkins. This was even before he was director of Johns Hopkins Hospital, when Winford Smith was the senior director and Ed was his assistant. Then Crosby came to the Joint Commission on Accreditation of Hospitals as its first director. He was in Chicago and I knew him better. Then, of course, when he moved to AHA, it was a different kind of relationship.

I think that Ed Crosby's contribution was very significant. George Bugbee took the association from a one-man organization that lived in the shadow of the AMA and made it into a real trade association with useful programs in all of a hospital's major fields of interest and responsibility. I think Crosby moved it into a new and still larger sphere by adding services; getting the AHA building built; and creating a continuing relationship with the medical profession.

Retrospective

John Mannix, who was one of the forces for change in the 1930s and who has watched and helped the AHA grow and develop since then, provides an interesting closing perspective. His observations help to bring into focus the process as well as the progress.

MANNIX:[31]

I think you can say that all the men who have held the position of chief executive of the AHA have done a very good job. It is not easy to keep 6,000 member hospitals happy. In many ways, Caldwell, Bugbee, and Crosby had very similar personalities. All were very good executives, all personable, all well-liked by the field, and all meeting a need of the field which differed with the specific times.

There is no question in my mind that the AHA has gained greatly in national stature. It is an effective national organization today, well-recognized by the medical profession and other organizations in the health field. A large part of this is unquestionably due to these top executives.

Notes

(Transcripts of the oral histories cited here are housed in the library of the American Hospital Association, 840 North Lake Shore Drive, Chicago, Illinois 60611. The Oral History Collection is a joint project of the Hospital Research and Educational Trust and the AHA.)

1. See Profiles of Participants, in the center of this book, for biographical information.

2. *Gerhard Hartman, In the First Person: An Oral History.*

3. Davis was a director of the medical economics division of the Julius Rosenwald Fund and founder of the University of Chicago Program in Hospital Administration.

4. Fishbein was for many years editor of the *Journal of the American Medical Association.*

5. *John R. Mannix, In the First Person: An Oral History.* See Profiles of Participants for biographical information.

6. Robin Buerki was president of the AHA in 1936; Asa S. Bacon in 1923; G. Harvey Agnew in 1939; James A. Hamilton in 1943; Graham L. Davis in 1948; and John H. Hatfield in 1950.

7. *Kenneth Williamson, In the First Person: An Oral History.* See Profiles of Participants for biographical information.

8. *James Hague, In the First Person: An Oral History.* See Profiles of Participants for biographical information.

9. Monsignor Maurice Griffin was a priest in Youngstown, Ohio, in a parish which included St. Elizabeth's Hospital. During World War I, he was pastor of a church and also the Catholic chaplain for St. Elizabeth's. He became interested in the hospital field and was very active in the Ohio Hospital Association. For many years he was a trustee of the Ohio Hospital Association, and at one point he was president of it. He later became a trustee of the AHA, which he served for more than 25 years. He was also at one time president of the Catholic Hospital Association. He and Caldwell worked very closely together. Besides being professional friends, they were close personal friends. They were about the same age, and both were extremely well-traveled individuals, having been around the world several times.

10. *James A. Hamilton, In the First Person: An Oral History.* See Profiles of Participants for biographical information.

11. Dr. Charles F. Wilinsky was president of the American Hospital Association in 1951.

12. Pratt became administrator of the Rhode Island Hospital in 1946. He was a close personal friend of Hamilton.

13. At this time, Bugbee was superintendent of the Cleveland City Hospital, where he had succeeded Hamilton.

14. *Hague, Oral History.*

15. See Profiles of Participants for biographical information.

16. *Maurice J. Norby, In the First Person: An Oral History.* See Profiles of Participants for biographical information.

17. *Williamson, Oral History.*

18. *George Bugbee, In the First Person: An Oral History.* See Profiles of Participants for biographical information.

19. Bishop was administrator of University Hospitals of Cleveland.

20. Dr. Edwin L. Crosby was executive director of the AHA from 1954 to 1972.

21. *Hamilton, Oral History.*

22. *Williamson, Oral History.*

23. *Norby, Oral History.*

24. Crosby was then executive director of the Johns Hopkins Hospital.

25. Nelson succeeded Crosby as executive director of the Johns Hopkins Hospital.

26. Drake Hotel, Chicago.

27. *Bugbee, Oral History.*

28. *Hague, Oral History.*

29. *Norby, Oral History.*

30. *Robert M. Cunningham, Jr., In the First Person: An Oral History.* See Profiles of Participants for biographical information.

31. *Mannix, Oral History.*

10

Educating for a Profession

Education in hospital administration has followed a pattern prevalent in many, if not most, other professions. In the early stages there is a period of apprenticeship or learning on the job, then advancement to college-level training, and finally possible licensing.

The physician of three or more generations ago was likely to have learned his skills at the side of an older, practicing physician. He learned to set bones and bleed his patient. He learned to use some of the "heroic" drugs to dose and purge his patients. He had only a few useful drugs, including so-called specifics: quinine for malaria, digitalis for the heart muscle, and ipecac as an emetic. If he were lucky, he might have had some chloroform to use as an anesthetic when he attempted surgery. Lacking chloroform, there was always whiskey.

The learning process for physicians changed somewhat for some of them. These physicians sought better ways of treating patients than the bleeding, purging regimen. Some began to think of treatment in terms of rest, heat treatments, and water cures, or hydrotherapy. But, for all its change, medicine in the nineteenth century was a far cry from medicine in the 1980s.

An alternative mode of medical education in the 1870s was the medical school of the day. For example, Dr. John Harvey Kellogg, the famous medical director of the Battle Creek Sanitarium for over 60 years, received his formal medical education in several places. Kellogg spent 20 weeks at Dr. Russell Trall's Hygieo-Therapeutic College in Florence Heights, New Jersey. Richard W. Schwarz has described the school: "Instruction at the Hygieo-

Therapeutic College emphasized the curative powers of the internal and external use of water, a simple diet, proper exercise, and fresh air."[1] The school placed little reliance on drugs of any kind. Kellogg, however, was not satisfied with his medical competence, so he enrolled at the University of Michigan Medical School for two sets of lectures of 24 weeks each. This would earn him an M.D. degree. A short time before the end of the university lecture course, he became disillusioned because of what today we would call a lack of clinical experience. He left the University of Michigan and enrolled at the Bellevue Hospital and Medical College in New York City, where he got experience in taking care of patients, in addition to classroom lectures.

On his graduation from Bellevue after one year, in 1875, Kellogg received his M.D. degree and joined the medical staff of the Western Health Reform Institute in Battle Creek, Michigan, his hometown.[2] A short time later, he became medical director of the institute and convinced its board that Battle Creek Sanitarium was a better name for the institution.

The medical treatment that Kellogg supervised at the Battle Creek Sanitarium was quite different from that prescribed by most other physicians of the time. He used very few drugs, depending instead on diet, hydrotherapy where indicated, exercise, fresh air, rest, and heat treatments. The diet was principally vegetables, fruits, and nuts. He had his patients abstain from alcohol, tobacco, tea, coffee, and meat. He attempted very little surgery because of lack of training and his preference for what he called "biologic living."

Medical education in America was sketchy, at the very best, until after the reforms that followed the publication of the Flexner report in 1910.[3] It was generally believed, among persons who were interested, that to get a really good medical education one had to study in one of the great medical centers of Europe, for example in Vienna, Edinburgh, or Paris. Kellogg also believed that one must go to the fountainhead in order to get the best possible medical education. Consequently, he made several extended visits to Europe over the years in order to observe noted doctors in practice.

Education in nursing developed somewhat differently. In its earliest stages, nursing was done by those most able to care for the sick because of their experience in the work. Later, nurses generally were trained in hospital schools of nursing, where students learned through practice and instruction by senior nurses. This course of instruction gave way to two-year curriculums connected with colleges and offering an associate degree in nursing and to four-year courses offering a bachelor's degree. The baccalaureate training is preferred by educators, but it is not yet clear whether there will be a sufficient number of candidates to produce the number of nurses needed by the field.

Another health profession that has changed in respect to educational standards over the years has been pharmacy. For example, after the Civil War a person could become a pharmacist by merely opening a drugstore for business. This was the case in Michigan. As late as 1928 in Michigan, a person could take the state pharmacy licensing examination with only a high school diploma and one year's apprenticeship; grandfather clauses granted a license to any applicant who could show 20 years' or more experience working in a drugstore. Today the qualifications needed for taking the Michigan state examination are graduation from a five-year college of pharmacy course and an apprenticeship. Other states have done the same thing.

The same general pattern developed in hospital administration. In the early days, hospital managers, with no special administrative training, often learned by trial and error. Physicians became administrators because they owned their own little hospitals, or they came into the field because management seemed more attractive than medical practice. Nurses became hospital administrators because the institution was small or because there was no other health professional to take on the responsibility. Church-connected hospitals were likely to have a nun or a minister in charge, not so much because of any administrative training, but because of their religious role.

In time, hospitals grew larger and more complex. Finances, personnel, community and government relations, advancing technology, and medical staff privileges and relations became programs that required professional management skills. As with other professions, the trial and error method had to give way first to on-the-job training and then to formal college training in management.

John Mannix is an outstanding result of apprenticeship, or on-the-job training. He himself would respond, modestly, that his teacher and mentor, Frank Chapman of Cleveland, was responsible.

―――――――

MANNIX:[4]

I was born in Cleveland on June 4, 1902. When I finished high school, I took a position at Mt. Sinai Hospital in Cleveland. Frank E. Chapman was the hospital administrator there at that time. He took me under his wing. He was one of the few business-oriented people serving as a hospital executive, although I was not at all aware of this at the time.

In the 1920s, the larger hospitals of 300 beds or more were generally administered by physicians who, for one reason or another, had given up the practice of medicine. Many of the medium-sized hospitals of 100 to 300 beds were religious hospitals. If they were Catholic hospitals, they were administered by Catholic Sisters. The Protestant hospitals were often administered by ministers. The smaller hospitals of 100 beds or less were, for the most part, administered by nurses. I am generalizing, but it is surprising, in looking back on it later, how true that was.

I worked at Mt. Sinai for a couple months during the summer and then told Mr. Chapman that I was going to go back to school. He said, "I want to talk to you about that."

He was a very persuasive man. He called me into his office and talked to me about a career in hospital administration. As far as I was concerned, hospitals were operated by doctors, Sisters, ministers, and nurses—and he was a very, very rare exception. I felt the future of hospital administration was in the hands of physicians. I felt that anyone other than a physician would not have much success in the long run in hospital administration. This situation, in my opinion, changed only after World War II.

Several forces brought about the shift in responsibility for hospital management to trained, professional hospital administrators: the increase in the number of hospitals in the late 1940s and 1950, the need for physicians, and the experiences of World War II. The W.K. Kellogg Foundation also played a major role in this movement. In particular, it was instrumental in promoting the development of the graduate education programs needed to train hospital managers. Andrew Pattullo,[5] who over his career became synonymous with the foundation's interest in health services management, talked of the foundation's pioneering initiative.

PATTULLO:[6]

In the early 1940s the W.K. Kellogg Foundation was an "operating" foundation. That is, it ran things or had a major part in making things happen. In the post–World War II era, it was committed to changing its character. It became a national and, in fact, an international kind of operation focused on grant-making activities.

Pattullo became a Kellogg Fellow in 1943 after receiving his master's degree in hospital administration from the University of Chicago. He worked out of the Battle Creek office of the foundation under the direction of Graham Davis, who headed the foundation's hospital program.

PATTULLO:[7]

In 1944 my fellowship year with the foundation ended. I was asked, however, to stay on and help plan for the postwar era. I was named associate director of the division of hospitals. Graham Davis[8] was the director.

I guess you could say that the Kellogg Foundation's romance with health administration education began at about this time. Part of our strategy was to bring together advisory committees.

The first hospital advisory committee was appointed in 1944. Its membership consisted of people such as Jim Hamilton,[9] who was a past president of the American Hospital Association and had really turned that organization around. John Mannix, a pioneer in the prepayment movement,[10] was another committee member, as was Robin Buerki,[11] a physician and very prominent hospital administrator. Dr. Buerki had been the director of a national study on graduate medical education in the early 1940s. He went on to become the chief executive of Henry Ford Hospital in Detroit. Dr. Harvey Agnew,[12] who was regarded as the patron saint of hospitals in Canada, was on the committee, as was Dr. Basil MacLean,[13] another great hospital administration figure of that time.

Over the subsequent years, our hospital advisory committee changed in composition but continued to contribute a great deal to our program concept and work in the hospital field. Such individuals as George Bugbee,[14] Ed Crosby,[15] Jim Dixon,[16] Ray Brown,[17] Art Bachmeyer,[18] Walter McNerney,[19] Jack Haldeman,[20] George Cartmill,[21] and Mat McNulty[22] were later members. In the mid-1960s we dropped the standing committee format, going to ad hoc groups which focused on a single problem. This latter approach has also served us well.

As to the original group, we brought them together and asked their advice about what the foundation could do in terms of improving hospital services, quality, etc. It was unanimously agreed that education for hospital administration was a project that had tremendous promise and should be our highest priority.

So, we did two things. First, we decided to create a commission on education for hospital administration. The commission wasn't under our direct sponsorship. Rather, we went to the AHA and to the American College of Hospital Administrators and asked them to take the lead. They agreed and became the cosponsors for what was called a "joint commission" because of the two organizations.

The commission was formed, and Robert Bishop, a prominent Cleveland physician-administrator,[23] was selected as chairman. The commission was politically very sound, with good people on it. The study director was Charles E. Prall, who had been the dean of education at Pittsburgh. They embarked on a two-year study to determine what a model curriculum might be like and then some strategies for developing specific programs.

Charlie Prall did a very neat thing. He decided to go out into the field and poll not only administrators themselves, but trustees, department heads, physicians, and so forth as to what they thought the responsibilities and the problems of a hospital, not the administrator, might be. He made that analysis, and then from that the commission tried to derive a curriculum. There were two publications that came out of this: one concerning the problems of hospital administration, and a second focused on curriculum.

By 1945, the Northwestern University Program in Hospital Administration had come into being; it was the second program to be viable—the University of Chicago Program in Hospital Administration started in 1934, and then Northwestern began in 1943. So in 1945 there were two graduate-level degree-granting programs, probably with a combined annual output of 25 to 30 graduates.

Given the limited number of existing training programs, we then, as the second part of our effort, went to a number of universities that we thought might be interested, if we provided initial support, in starting a program in hospital administration. The hospital advisory committee had a great deal to do with the selection of those original universities.

There was a very definite orientation towards schools of public health as a site for these initial programs. In good part this was due to the influence of Dr. Basil MacLean. Dr. MacLean, a past president of the AHA, was the director of Strong Memorial Hospital in Rochester. He had a strong feeling about the need for administrators to have, in addition to management capabilities, an appreciation for community health concerns. He felt that this latter understanding could best be conveyed in schools of public health. That was the bias, and we followed it.

With the exception of Washington University in St. Louis, every program that we helped to initiate at that time was located in a school of public health. There were six, one in Toronto and then, in this country, Yale, Columbia, Johns Hopkins, Minnesota, and Washington University in St. Louis (situated in the medical school). Of those initial programs, all survived except Hopkins, where there was a hiatus for many years and then later a reincarnation.

Our interest in the mid-1940s was also in attracting to hospital administration the many people returning from World War II who had served in the Medical Administrative Corps (MAC). These people were presumed to be a potential pool of students.

My recollection is that ACHA, in cooperation with the army's surgeon general, developed a questionnaire which was distributed to MAC personnel, inquiring as to their interest upon discharge etc., in a civilian hospital administration career. The response was very positive. Consequently, when the new hospital administration programs came into place, beginning in January 1946 (I think Columbia started at that time), there was a pool of students and a ready acceptance. Well, following that (the development of a number of new programs) we have been involved, I guess one could say, with education for health administration ever since, supporting one dimension or one phase or another.

———

In addition to the formal academic programs at the University of Chicago and Northwestern University, Duke University had a hospital administration training program. The Duke program was essentially a controlled on-the-job learning experience, culminating in a Certificate of Hospital Administration as opposed to a master's degree. Richard Stull, a graduate of the Duke program, talks about it.

_____

STULL:[24]

My career in hospital administration probably started by a coincidence.

I was hospitalized at the Duke University Medical Center for an extended period. During that time I became acquainted with my nurse. She was a friend of Ross Porter, the assistant superintendent of the hospital. Following my return to school, and through social relations with these individuals, I found out that Porter, along with Harold Mickey, the other assistant superintendent, and Vernon Altwater, superintendent of the hospital, with support from the dean of the School of Medicine, Wilbur C. Davison, were involved in a program for training in hospital administration. I began to explore the program.

After conversation with Mickey, Porter, and Altwater on what the program offered, I applied. I was accepted in September of 1940.

The Duke program at that time was in the form of what they called a "residency type" or "preceptor type" program, which took the individual into the hospital setting. It started out with a rotation, with your working in every area of the hospital. In addition to working in the various divisions and departments of the hospital, you were allowed to take some courses on campus, but that was purely by your own personal election. Periodically, at least once a week, the superintendent and the assistant superintendents would lecture, or they would bring in people from the outside to talk to the students about things that related to hospital care.

Also as part of the preceptor program, if they had a particular problem area in the hospital, they would give a student an assignment in that area. At the time of my experience, they were having difficulties in two areas of the outpatient department. One was handling and scheduling appointments, the other was in financing. I was given the assignment to try to do something about the outpatient department. I concentrated my efforts on that department for a while. I am happy to say we turned it around by improving the scheduling of the clinic appointments and in establishing arrangements for financial screening. After a period of time the department was in the black.

What I am trying to point out is that in the environment of Duke Medical Center you were given every opportunity to be intimately involved, to play a role in and participate in the operations of the institution. Therefore, you became knowledgeable about the purposes and functions of each department, about their interrelationships, and a great deal about the people relationships in a complex environment of that kind. So, despite the fact there wasn't the emphasis on the basic management skills which currently is the point of focus in graduate education, you learned a lot about the environment in which you were going to apply the skills. This was an essential thing.

_____

Another person who entered the health field without formal hospital administration education and rose to be a leader of national prominence was Kenneth Williamson. He described his training.

_____

WILLIAMSON:[25]

When I was about 17, I worked Saturdays and after school in the pharmacy of a hospital, the Methodist Hospital of Southern California in Los Angeles. I got really interested in hospitals. I began to think about it as a career at a time when it was not visualized as a career to manage a hospital. People, through a series of circumstances, fell into it. Physicians became administrators, ministers became attached to hospitals and became administrators. Hospitals turned to somebody they thought had a social conscience, you know. Many, many nurses moved from supervisor to superintendent of nursing then into hospital administration.

I thought it would be a smart thing to write to the leaders in the field whose names I had read in the journals at the time. I wrote, as I remember, to five of them: Dr. Benjamin Black, in Alameda County, California, who probably was considered *the* leader in the United States in hospital administration; Harvey Agnew in Canada, a physician; Malcolm MacEachern;[26] and a couple of others I can't remember right now. The letters I got back from each of them indicated they couldn't suggest a formal approach for becoming an administrator. Moreover it seemed that they didn't think there was such a thing.

The only one I got an answer from which had any vision of the future was Malcolm MacEachern's reply. He said there weren't any formal courses yet. He said, "I suggest you take these courses in school." He laid out a course: some hygiene, some physics, some economics, administration, some of the health sciences, and so on. So I set out to try to get a handle on some of these subjects.

Also, it seemed obvious, if I could talk the hospital into allowing me to move around in various capacities, i.e., various jobs in the hospital, that I might learn something. So I did. I went from pharmacy to working in the operating room for a period, then working as an assistant to the purchasing agent, working in medical records for a while, then into administration. I started into school, and I worked nights. I was in charge of admitting. Going to school in the daytime and working at night, I became the night admitting officer and handled accounts receivable. From this experience I learned a lot about hospitals—not from the textbooks, but from a very practical standpoint. I think anyone would be fortunate to have that opportunity today.

After the W.K. Kellogg Foundation showed its interest in formal, graduate training in hospital administration, some innovative programs were developed.

The Minnesota Program

The Minnesota program was one of those programs. Under the direction of James Hamilton, it established a new model for training hospital managers. Below, Hamilton describes how the program was established and the philosophy it embodied. Two of the graduates of the Minnesota program, Gary Filerman and Edward Connors, also describe it, giving, after some years in the field, a perspective on their education.

HAMILTON:[27]

I was one of the people who served on the W.K. Kellogg Foundation hospital advisory committee.

Graham Davis, assisted by Andy Pattullo, and the hospital advisory committee would meet, I would say, about every three months. On the first hospital advisory committee were Basil MacLean, Bob Buerki, Harvey Agnew, John Mannix, and myself.

Supposedly Graham had chosen us as leaders of the hospital field or various aspects of the hospital field. We didn't always see eye to eye. The other members besides John Mannix and I were medical men.

It was at that committee that we would advise Kellogg where they ought to be putting some of their money. That was the idea of the committee. We had no authority except to advise. Then Kellogg would decide what they wanted to do.

I was responsible on that committee for recommending that graduate schools be established for training hospital administrators. Two of the medical men, I remember, pooh-poohed the idea in no uncertain terms—the idea that you could train an administrator. This seemed to them a strange approach, because they believed very strongly that the only good administrators were medical ones. As a result, and I think it was startling to many, Kellogg came out and decided to establish graduate hospital administration programs.

Nearly all the early hospital administration graduate programs were started with money put in them by the Kellogg Foundation. The University of Minnesota was one of the schools which approached the foundation and which was given money.

A fellow by the name of Gaylord Anderson and a fellow by the name of Ray Amberg[28] had gone to the Kellogg Foundation, on behalf of the university, to request money to establish a program in hospital administration. The practice of Kellogg was to give a grantee $20,000, provided they also got $20,000 from the university.

They said, "Now we have got to start looking for a director."

Graham Davis said, "How about Hamilton?"

Ray Amberg, who was running the hospital up there, said, "We can't get Hamilton. We can't afford him."

Graham said, "Well, you might try."

Gaylord Anderson, who was the dean of the school of public health, said, "I only know one Hamilton, a guy by the name of Jim Hamilton."

As it happens, Gaylord was a classmate of mine at Dartmouth College. His father had taught there. We didn't know each other very well, but we knew of each other.

While I was still in New Haven, at the New Haven Hospital, I had given some thought to what would be necessary for a strong program in hospital administration. I had done this mostly because I was on the Kellogg advisory committee and I wanted to serve them intelligently. In the process of thinking it through, I became convinced, at least for myself, that, if I was going to run a hospital administration graduate degree program, it would have to be from a position which had some degree of independence. If it didn't have independence, then the program would be forced to follow the lead and meet the requirements of other programs at the university which *did* have the independence to determine their own curriculum and graduation requirements.

For example, at Yale a hospital administration student had to take all the requirements for a master's degree in public health and then add to that some hospital administration courses. I didn't want that. I didn't want hospital administration students to take a graduate degree in some other field and then fill in with hospital administration subjects. I wanted a degree in hospital administration.

I finally got the independence which I thought was needed at Minnesota. So I went there. I said what the requirements were going to be. Although I was located for administrative reasons in the school of public health, I had complete authority. I was able to run it without having requirements to meet for some other kind of degree. I ran it in such a way that the students were taught what they ought to be taught—what I thought they ought to be taught, let's put it that way.

It has been said that I tried to make the program in hospital administration at Minnesota different from other programs. Well, you see, that was the point, the goal. Each of those other programs was put in a school and had to meet the requirements of a degree in that school. Then they tacked on a little hospital administration. So it would vary in whatever school we were talking about as to how much hospital administration the student really got.

I had come up fundamentally as a teacher, therefore I insisted that we take the field of hospital administration and break it down into subject areas that would teach that field. For example, there are courses in organization and so forth that you take in a business school and which are taught by the business faculty. So if you went to Columbia, for example, for hospital administration, you went into the business school and learned hospital administration by business methods. Then you had to translate it back into hospitals. I didn't. I taught organization and used hospitals all along the way. I taught hospital organization. I taught the fundamental principles of organization, but I taught hospital organization. I applied those principles immediately to hospitals. The fellow who was teaching at Columbia had to keep changing his illustrations because he had mixed classes—some hospital administration students and some business students.

As a result of this, my program was unique. There was no course in the country at that time which was built that way. There have been some since then.

―――――

Gary L. Filerman, a former student of Hamilton's and president and chief developer of the Association of University Programs in Health Administration (AUPHA), comments on his experience at Minnesota with unusual insight.

―――――

FILERMAN:[29]

There is no question that Hamilton accomplished an immense amount of education with that program. Hamilton was an extraordinary educator.

There was something about the group process in that program which was very intimidating and at the same time motivating. That's exactly what he wanted to accomplish. He was like a staff sergeant. Hamilton was convinced, and I think he was right, that successful administrators first of all had to have style. You had to believe it to do it. To believe it, you had to learn how to act in certain ways—carry yourself in a certain way, to express yourself a certain way. He convinced us that we were decision makers, and there is a style to decisiveness.

The idea was if there was anything that a Minnesota graduate knew how to do, it was to make a decision, live with it, and go on from there.

Now, there's no question that I benefited greatly from the experience. If nothing else, the elitism of the Minnesota program was a great asset, and has continued to be a great asset. For a young profession making its way, it was one of the fundamental building blocks. It was an effective instrument toward achieving a broader objective.

━━━━━

Edward J. Connors, president of the Sisters of Mercy Health Corporation, Farmington Hills, Michigan, looks back after years of experience in the health field to his days as a student under James A. Hamilton at Minnesota.

━━━━━

CONNORS:[30]

I found the academic experience under Jim Hamilton's leadership to be perhaps not very technically helpful, but enormously helpful in terms of attitude, point of view, concern, understanding, and values. I kind of chuckle occasionally when current persons in academic hospital administration sort of disdain or look down on or criticize or say, "Well, we used to teach a lot about the laundry and so on." Well, that opinion is just nonsense and not accurate.

I don't think such persons knew what Jim Hamilton was like in the classroom. Jim Hamilton was a man of tremendous capacity and ability. He had the day-to-day ability to really challenge students, to stretch them, to make them think. He did it with a lot of tough techniques of teaching. He was a first-class actor. I told him later, after I got to know him a bit better, that he really belonged in the theater. He was a dramatic teacher, but he had a way of making us very, very excited about the career that we had chosen. Realistic, but excited.

Jim Hamilton, I think, made us think very deeply about what is the purpose and role of the hospital. Why does the hospital exist in the first place? What is its basic mission? Why is it there? I think that was so important in the formulation of attitudes and opinions that I am everlastingly grateful to him.

━━━━━

The Michigan Program

In the mid-1950s the University of Michigan established a program in hospital administration. The Michigan program not only built on the Minnesota model, but also went a step further, emphasizing research and community service. Walter McNerney, the first director of the Michigan program, describes what he was trying to create.

━━━━━

MCNERNEY:[31]

Michigan was my first real opportunity to stand back and develop a hospital administration program totally in my own style. At the University of Pittsburgh (prior to going to Michigan) I had been trying to balance several jobs at once.[32] Also, the fact that the program at Pittsburgh was tightly contained within the department of public health practice gave it less elbow room. Under those circumstances, I followed more orthodox program lines and simply capitalized on the assets of the school, of the university, and of the medical center to the extent that I could. On the whole, I think the Pittsburgh program was good. It had to start quickly in 1950, but the resources were rich.

So when I went to Michigan I had some experience behind me. Also, being program director was to be my full-time job. I was going to be able to devote the time to it that it needed.

The Michigan program was to be located in the School of Business [Administration] because politically that was how it fit best at that point. The tension between the university hospital and the School of Public Health, and between public health and the Medical School was such that locating the program in the School of Public Health would not have been a smart choice at that point. Since you can compensate for site very easily, why wrestle with it? I said it was fine, let's set it up in the school of business.

I also asked for, and got, an advisory committee comprised of the dean of the school of medicine, the dean of the School of Public Health, the director of the university hospital, and the vice president of the university for academic affairs. That committee met routinely. I reviewed curriculum with them; I reviewed appointments with them; etc. This was a very powerful step, because I was able in good conscience to represent the program as having a firm connection with the Medical School and the School of Public Health, as well as with the business school. It also provided a pipeline to the hospital. It was an important step.

The next thing I did was lay very heavy emphasis on the fact that any program in health administration, then called hospital administration, should operate on three mutually reinforcing planes: education, research, and community service.

The focus on education was apparent. Education alone was not enough. I felt that research was absolutely necessary, because both the teaching programs and the hospital administration field in general needed a firmer factual base, a firmer conceptual underpinning. The field was growing in complexity. If it were to be managed, it needed more facts and more concepts.

Michigan was an innovator in health administration research. All the hospital administration programs tipped their hats to research. They would write papers and so forth. I think our degree of formality of research, for which I took a chiding from a lot of the practitioners who led programs, was special. It was dedicated, it was identified. It stood the scrutiny of the university community as being valid and good research.

The third critical element was community service. I felt that the faculty, particularly in administration, needed to get its feet wet in community and institutional life. This was necessary both to enhance the teaching and also to raise the questions that should be researched. So we developed an active community service program. Of course, that had the added benefit of getting us into Michigan communities, Upper Peninsula, Lower Peninsula, Detroit area, etc.

When the university would go to Lansing[33] in regard to the budget, one of the things they heard from the legislators was, "I understand you are helping the hospital in Charlevoix," or such and such. Understandably, this would please the administration of the university.

In addition to positioning the program at Michigan to draw widely on a variety of resources in the university, and to develop mutually reinforcing tracks of teaching, research, and community service, I felt at that time that two other things were very important. One was that the orientation of the program should be health administration rather than hospital administration.

I gave a speech on this idea at the University of Chicago and later published a paper on it. I forget what group it was, but I remember that Bugbee and Hamilton and others were there. The point of view I had, and I guess this was about 1958, was that the more challenging academic problems, as opposed to operational problems, involved the total community. One had to understand the environment of health (the problems of industry, of water pollution, of the family, of disease, etc.) before one could develop intelligent goals. Intelligent goals were absolutely indispensable if one were to conceptualize institutions correctly and manage them correctly. Towards that end, I was very careful that the students in the Michigan program got exposed to public health ideas as well as to business school and public administration ideas.

The other thing that I thought was important was that the head of a health administration program should be a full-time director. The early programs in health administration were started by prominent people who in themselves had a lot to offer. Actually there was no one else around, they had to do it. I admired them for it. However, often the program was ancillary to a lot of other interests. Also, due to the fact that the director was not on the grounds all the time, there was a temptation to use a long list of visiting lecturers to pick up the slack. Some of them were good, some of them were dreary. The connections were not always that good among them. That kind of program had a vocationalism about it that reflected the experience of the individual and the fact that there wasn't time to work on the curriculum with the intensity it deserved.

All in all, Michigan was absolutely superb as a site for a program in hospital-health administration. The university was outstanding. It had a wide variety of forces, and they were put at the disposal of the program. The Blue

Cross–Blue Shield Plan there was outstanding and cooperative. There were talented people in management and labor that thought a lot about health. I exchanged classes with Wilbur Cohen[34] and with Bill Haber. Bill Haber was one of the early architects of social legislation; subsequently he became a vice president of the university [actually, "adviser to the executive officers"]. Wilbur Cohen later became secretary of HEW. These were the men who helped me out, taught in my classes, and there was a certain limited amount of reciprocity. That gives you an idea of what there was to offer there.

Edward J. Connors was the first faculty member hired by Walter McNerney for the new University of Michigan program in hospital administration. He talks about this teaching experience.

CONNORS:[35]
I left the Rhode Island Hospital a few months after my administrative residency to join Walt McNerney at the University of Michigan. There was only the two of us at first. The university took us under its wing and helped us enormously.

In those days we were in the business school, plus we were a part of a very excellent university that was committed to quality education. The business school, the Medical School, the university hospital, and the School of Public Health made good their commitment that they would do what it took to develop quality graduate education in hospital administration.

There was quite a debate before Michigan decided to get into the hospital administration field. After the war, when some of the first programs in hospital administration sprung up, Michigan did not develop a program. One of the reasons why they stayed out of it until the mid-1950s, as I understand it, was because there was an understandable rivalry between the School of Public Health, the graduate school of business, and the Medical School as to who should own the turf that health administration represented. There was an impasse for several years. I suppose like most things, given that kind of infighting, university officials decided it wasn't worth a faculty fight as to whether the Medical School, public health school, business school, or university hospital should win.

The decision at Michigan was helped through by the Olsen report.[36] The Olsen report was the result of a study financed by the Kellogg Foundation in the early 1950s as to the content of and the responsibility for graduate education in health administration. One of the conclusions of the report, at least the way the report was interpreted, included the idea that it really didn't make any difference whether a program in hospital administration was in the medical school, business school, or graduate school or whatever. It did make a difference, though, that all the relevant disciplines were brought to bear upon this emerging field. I think Michigan picked up that cue and developed a multidisciplinary approach.

Residency

One of the hallmarks of the early years of graduate hospital administration education was the requirement that students complete a one-year residency. The residency experience was the second year of the two-year graduate program. Like the Duke University training program, it was a controlled work experience in which the student was exposed, under the supervision of a senior administrator, to the operations of the hospital.

The Minnesota residency is described below, first by James Hamilton and then by Gary Filerman and Edward Connors.

HAMILTON:[37]

I have had very strong feelings about the master's degree program and the residency, or internship, none of which were universally accepted. My thesis was that you could not teach a graduate course like hospital administration and then have the graduates immediately begin to do work of any stature without a practice period. How long should that practice period be? There was a great debate. I said a year.

I began to use the residency system, and I began to impress upon the guys I was using as preceptors of the residents that preceptors were members of the faculty. I had them all voted members of the faculty. The University of Minnesota put them on the faculty as clinical preceptors. This was not any hogwash. It was real. Then, I made the preceptors come back to campus every year for a faculty meeting.

I picked the leading people in the field, from all around the country as preceptors.

We used people like Frank Groner[38] and Boone Powell.[39] We picked them from different parts of the country. Then I would say to them, "You have got to come back to campus and learn how to be a preceptor. Don't talk to me and tell me how you are going to take this student and put him to work. That's just part of his exposure. You have got to be sure he is being taught this and this and this."

So I brought them back to Minnesota, had faculty meetings, and had them put down on paper what a preceptor should be doing. Then it was all mimeographed in different forms for them to use.

I did this to make them honest-to-God members of the faculty. This lasted for about six or seven years, then the older preceptors began to delegate the job to graduates that they had hired from the program.

The residency was a serious business. We didn't do it lightly. I finally dwindled the number of preceptors down to a few. They had to take a resident every year. They didn't choose him, I did.

I said, "You don't ask a teacher of algebra to choose his students. The dean of the school sends the teacher a student, and he has to teach him. You are going to have to do the same thing."

Other hospital administration courses in other schools had been working it in a different manner than this, so I was running into all kinds of comments and criticism. People wanted to know, why didn't I do it like Columbia, which sends its residents to hospitals right close by? Even Kellogg had an idea at one time that they ought to be located in a certain geographic area around each school.

I said, "I think that's a lot of hogwash. What you should do is pick a faculty member and an atmosphere where the student will learn what he needs to learn, what he doesn't know now, or what he needs to know in whatever he is headed for."

I made the residency matching a major process. I would ask the students in November to put down on paper the three places they would like to go. I would then take that information and begin to study that individual. I would not let it be known until April where he was going. In the meantime, I had been studying where to put him.

I would study the appointment and the student very carefully as to the personalities, what the student needed, what the environment was apt to give him—as much as I knew how. Of course, I thought I knew how, without any question. I really did try to match the appointment to the student's wishes wherever possible. If it were going to be different from what he had on his list, I would call him in and discuss that with him. Sometimes I would change my mind after he talked with me—usually against my better judgment.

In other words, I thought I had given enough personal thought to it that I knew more about what a student ought to have than he did. That was an assumption on my part, but it seemed to work pretty well. A lot of students, who at first hated to go where I sent them, told me later how glad they were that I sent them.

———

FILERMAN:[40]

As one began to look ahead, the critical decision was where to take a residency. I believe that two of my choices were Johns Hopkins and Strong Memorial, so I was definitely interested in a university hospital setting. Hopkins was somewhat selective, in spite of their institutional arrangements with Minnesota, in which Minnesota virtually picked the resident. Hopkins retained a veto, and you had to go there for an interview. If they decided you didn't have two heads, you were accepted.

My motivating factor in picking Hopkins was the prestige of the name. I didn't know anything about the residency. The director of the hospital, Dr. Russell Nelson, was at that point a major figure in the field, and that added to the stature of going there.

If I had known what kind of a residency it was, I might not have gone there. Maybe I would have anyway, however, because of the prestige of it.

I thought later, as I was in the residency, and I still believe, that the residency experience I had demonstrates some of the fallacies of the residency process. An experience like mine shows some of the traps that the field had fallen into, such as confusing the prestige of the institution with the quality of the residency, or the stature of the administrator with the quality of the preceptorship.

Obviously what I'm saying is that, for many reasons, mine was not a very good residency. Part of the problem was that it was a delegated residency. The hospital's director was not readily accessible to the residents. He had limited knowledge of the program. Beyond that, he wasn't interested and, in fact, didn't really believe in the residency. He really didn't think that it was part of the way by which you learned hospital administration. So he delegated it to an assistant. Russ Nelson believed that the way you learned to run the Johns Hopkins Hospital, and this is a direct quote, was, "You start in the storeroom killing cockroaches and work your way up, or you started on a clinical service as a physician."

Somehow those were not equal. It was not a good residency, because Nelson believed in the separation of the administrative side of the house from the medical side and that the only people who bridged that gap were the medical administrators, the physician administrators. So the residency would by definition be limited to the administrative side of the house. It was also limited in a hierarchical sense, because you were delegated to an assistant administrator. I suppose that I had five hours with Nelson that year and only because I fought for it.

In fact, I had a good residency, but it was in spite of the residency program.

━━━━━

CONNORS:[41]

I went to the Rhode Island Hospital in my administrative residency. I found out that the transition from the classroom to the practical world was difficult and that the real problems were tough. The power struggles, the competing points of view were real.

Mr. Oliver G. Pratt was administrator at that time and was very influential in my life and my development. He prided himself and his organization on the fact that he took young men from the University of Minnesota—he and Mr. Hamilton were close friends.

I was fortunate enough to be asked to stay on at the Rhode Island Hospital as an administrative assistant.

The Ph.D.

As the hospital management field matured, interest in Ph.D.-level education increased. The pressures for offering a Ph.D. were several, but, as the following comments by Hamilton reflect, the need for such training was not initially accepted by everyone. Hamilton's comments are followed by those of Gary Filerman, who received a Ph.D. from Minnesota.

HAMILTON:[42]

One of the more controversial subjects was the Ph.D. course in hospital administration.

For a long time I was firmly convinced that a Ph.D. in hospital administration meant nothing. I said I was not going to offer a Ph.D. because I don't think a person just because he had a Ph.D. would be a better administrator. Also, I felt that the student who wanted a Ph.D. just for the degree's sake ought not to be an administrator to begin with.

Finally, however, we began to offer a Ph.D. I was being pushed by Kellogg, mostly, to turn out some teachers. The field was beginning to expand. Where do you get the teachers? You try to get the average hospital administrator to go in and teach in a graduate school, and you find out that he hasn't any teaching background. He can't teach, really. Oh, he can convey some information and get across a certain amount of this and that, but he doesn't use or know the fundamentals of teaching.

Kellogg put some money in three places. They put some in the University of Iowa, where Gerry Hartman[43] was trying to turn out a Ph.D. in one year. (I don't think that can be done, by the way. No Ph.D. can be turned out in that time. He discovered later he couldn't. He had to keep them four or five years to train them.) Also, Columbia was trying to teach them in a regular length of time but didn't have enough institutions to work through.

So we started one at Minnesota. Our strategy was that we'll turn out teachers and scholars provided we don't take more than three a year. We'll select them from that point of view. We don't want them to be administrators. We are only training people who were hopefully going to be good teachers. We are only training people who could be scholars and who could do some research in the field—research in administration, not in medicine.

So we began to turn out three at a time. We had, if I remember right, only two classes before I left.

I think they have continued the Ph.D. program at Minnesota, but I don't think they have very many in it.

I thought a Ph.D. was useless if a person was going to be an administrator. It didn't make any sense to me. If he was going to be a scholar or a teacher, that was different. The fellows I trained almost invariably were in demand before I finished training them. So when the time came around for them to write their thesis, I had to let them take a job and write their thesis at the same time. This extended the period a little bit. It was the pressure of need in the field. The five or six I trained all turned out to be good and to do very well.

_____

FILERMAN:[44]

The doctoral program at Minnesota, on balance, I think, knowing what I do today about doctoral programs, was a pretty good one.

From the standpoint of education in terms of what you were exposed to in breadth and depth, it represented a very good education in a very good university. On the other hand, in terms of education from the standpoint of self-definition, making the optimum use of the resources of the university from the perspective of the individual and his growing understanding of his needs and interests, it was quite limited. You didn't have much flexibility. A good part of the judgment as to what was appropriate for you to study and what wasn't resided with Jim Hamilton. So that if I went to Hamilton and said, "I've decided I want to take a three-course sequence in the philosophy of science or in art history," whether or not I was able to do it depended on whether he thought it made sense. That, in turn, depended to a great extent on how it fit with his idea of what you needed.

The doctoral program at Minnesota was really a very difficult experience for everybody concerned. I was in the second cohort; the first cohort was still there. The third cohort was arriving or had arrived, and so the program had thrust upon it a group of pretty bright, motivated people who came with a different set of expectations and experiences than did the master's students. I don't think that Jim Hamilton was prepared for that difference. The question of style wasn't so important to us.

When Hamilton said, "This is the way it is," we said, "Why? or "I don't think so," or, even worse, "Where is your data?"

That led to a great deal of tension, which was not the same kind of tension as we had experienced as master's students. When we were master's students we were totally encapsulated in that program—its faculty, its traditions, its whole milieu. As doctoral students we were out across the campus and having experiences with many different faculty members and other doctoral students. So you came back to the program with something to compare it to. For me, at least, it was not always a pleasant comparison. Hamilton and I were at odds a good part of the time. A number of the students were at odds with him over the same issues.

I believe that Hamilton made a number of really quite remarkable and pivotal contributions, e.g., creating the master's program, setting up the decision-making model and carrying it through so well and convincing a lot of people that they were part of the self-fulfilling prophecy of leadership. He also contributed a great deal by creating the doctoral program and by the vision of what a doctoral program could do for the field. Where he reached his limits was in attempting to put himself academically into the doctoral program. In later life I have learned to appreciate, if not to genuinely admire, a number of individuals in the field who have recognized and dealt with that in themselves.

The following reminiscences by Andrew Pattullo and George Bugbee illustrate the W.K. Kellogg Foundation's continuing interest in health administration education, and particularly in the Association of University Programs in Hospital (later Health) Administration. Pattullo's comments are presented first. Bugbee's observations, which focus on the AUPHA, follow.

PATTULLO:[45]

The foundation's support to the Association of University Programs in Hospital Administration is another example of its continuing involvement with health administration education. I think their first meeting—an informal grouping—was in 1948 during the AHA annual convention.

Later, in the early 1950s, we helped bring AUPHA together with some other interested parties for a conference in Battle Creek to attempt to identify some of the needs at that time in the field, which was very much in its infancy.

In the early 1950s I expect there must have been only a dozen or so programs, and that conference resulted in a number of suggestions which we followed through on: the need for more research orientation in the field and for more faculty being very prominent. At any rate, we did provide support to a few universities in an effort to strengthen what might be described as the field's "intellectual muscle."

Later on, we funded a second study commission, headed by Jim Hamilton as chairman with Herluf Olsen as director. This commission's report came out in the mid-1950s. The report had a very divisive effect in the field, creating quite a schism between programs in schools of public health and other settings. We tried to mend that rift by bringing the differing factions together through several conferences that tried to concentrate on the positive aspects of the Olsen report. This strategy succeeded, I think, to a reasonable extent.

We were also supporting AUPHA in various ways. At that time, AUPHA had a part-time secretariat that was based at the University of Chicago program. George Bugbee had only recently arrived at the University of Chicago as director of the Center for Health Administration Studies and became interested in AUPHA and its purposes and needs. One evening we had a discussion about AUPHA with Chuck Goulet (who was AUPHA's part-time secretary). I recollect a suggestion was made that the foundation would not be averse to considering support for a reasonable period of time for some kind of full-time secretariat if there was also an agenda toward some objectives. From that conversation they did make such a proposal, and the first secretariat was hired. I think this proved to be a sound investment on our part and a wise decision by AUPHA, allowing it to become a viable organization.

━━━━━━

BUGBEE:[46]

As the director of the Program in Hospital Administration at the University of Chicago, I was drawn into the Association of University Programs in Hospital Administration, as it was then called.

Charles Goulet was superintendent of University of Chicago Hospitals and Clinics, and he was secretary and treasurer of AUPHA. One night Chuck and I had dinner with Andy Pattullo. In the course of the dinner Andy talked about AUPHA. We, Chuck and I, were visualizing the program that AUPHA could have, but Andy was indicating that nothing would ever come of it without more full-time leadership and direction.

Chuck had driven us up from the University of Chicago campus to meet Andy. It was about ten miles. On the way back I said, "Chuck, you know what we were being told? For goodness sake, to do something. Stop talking and do something. I think if we submitted a project that made some sense to Andy, the foundation might approve it."

Chuck had a dictating machine at home. He went home and that night dictated a draft application. We put money figures in to provide for five years of funding. We got the grant and looked for an executive secretary.

Well, who could we hire for the executive secretary of AUPHA? It was a hard thing to know. The grant was there, but it wasn't that much money either, you know. We couldn't hire the most expensive fellow in the field. Chuck Goulet was secretary, and he sat in the executive committee, which was small.

Finally Chuck said, "I had a resident at Johns Hopkins Hospital when I was administrator who did his Ph.D. work with Jim Hamilton. He's smart." That was Gary Filerman. We hired him.

Hiring Filerman set the stage for the resurgence of AUPHA, largely through his hard work and talents, and by establishing an accreditation program.

Since the founding of the Program in Hospital Administration at the University of Chicago[47] in the mid-1930s, the field has grown in graduate and undergraduate programs. Today there are over 50 graduate programs in health administration. There are thousands of students each year taking health administration courses at either the graduate or undergraduate level.

One extension of health administration education that should not be overlooked is the excellent program of postgraduate and continuing education developed by the ACHA for practicing administrators and other members of the college. The program has had a great effect on the maturing process whereby an occupation became truly a profession with dignity and status.

Thus education in health administration has evolved from apprenticeship and on-the-job training to graduate and postgraduate education of growing sophistication. No one has more aptly expressed what education in the health field could mean than John S. Millis, an eminent authority in professional education.

MILLIS:[48]

The image I use in trying to explain my thinking is that, in an apprenticeship, the responsibility of a master is to bring the apprentice to his level. The responsibility of the true teacher is to bring the student to his shoulder so he may stand thereon and go beyond. The difference between training and education is the capacity to go beyond.

Notes

(Transcripts of the oral histories cited here are housed in the library of the American Hospital Association, 840 North Lake Shore Drive, Chicago, Illinois 60611. The Oral History Collection is a joint project of the Hospital Research and Educational Trust and the AHA.)

1. Richard W. Schwarz, *John Harvey Kellogg, M.D.* (Nashville: Southern Publishing Association, 1970), p. 28.

2. The Western Health Reform Institute was opened in Battle Creek, Michigan, by Seventh-Day Adventists on September 5, 1866, to treat the sick with water cure rather than drugs. The institute was patterned somewhat after James Caleb Jackson's Our Home on the Hillside, a water cure retreat in Dansville, New York. The establishment of the institute was a "fulfillment of one of the fondest hopes" of Ellen G. White, the Adventist "prophetess of health reform."

3. See chapter 2 for additional comment on the Flexner Report.

4. *John R. Mannix, In the First Person: An Oral History.* See Profiles of Participants, in the center of this book, for biographical information.

5. See Profiles of Participants for biographical information.

6. *Andrew Pattullo, In the First Person: An Oral History.*

7. Ibid.

8. Davis went to the Kellogg Foundation from the Duke Endowment; he was president of the AHA in 1948.

9. See Profiles of Participants for biographical information.

10. *Mannix, Oral History.*

11. Buerki was president of the AHA in 1936.

12. Agnew was president of the AHA in 1939.

13. MacLean was president of the AHA in 1942.

14. See Profiles of Participants for biographical information.

15. Crosby was president of the AHA in 1953 and executive secretary from 1954 to 1972.

16. Dixon is a graduate of the Columbia University course in hospital administration. He was a Kellogg Fellow, a public health officer, a president of Antioch College, and is now a faculty member at the University of North Carolina, Chapel Hill.

17. Brown held various professional positions, among them: director of the University of Chicago Hospitals and Clinics; director of the University of Chicago Program in Hospital Administration; vice president of the University of Chicago; director of the Duke University Program in Hospital Administration; and executive director of a consortium of New England hospitals.

18. Bachmeyer was director of the University of Chicago Hospitals and Clinics and director of the University of Chicago Program in Hospital Administration. He was also director of the Commission on Hospital Care. Bachmeyer was later director of the Commission on Financing of Hospital Care, where he served until his death in 1953.

19. See Profiles of Participants for biographical information.

20. Haldeman was a public health officer who became director of the Hill-Burton program. At the time of his retirement, he was assistant surgeon general of the Public Health Service.

21. Cartmill is the chief executive officer of Harper-Grace Hospitals in Detroit. He was president of the AHA in 1967.

22. McNulty is chancellor of the Georgetown University Medical Center.

23. Bishop was director of the University Hospitals of Cleveland.

24. *Richard Stull, In the First Person: An Oral History.* See Profiles of Participants for biographical information.

25. *Kenneth Williamson, In the First Person: An Oral History.* See Profiles of Participants for biographical information.

26. MacEachern was director of hospital activities of the American College of Surgeons and author of one of the first textbooks in the field.

27. *James A. Hamilton, In the First Person: An Oral History.*

28. Amberg was president of the AHA in 1959.

29. *Gary L. Filerman, In the First Person: An Oral History.* See Profiles of Participants for biographical information.

30. *Edward J. Connors, In the First Person: An Oral History.* See Profiles of Participants for biographical information.

31. *Walter J. McNerney, In the First Person: An Oral History.*

32. McNerney wore three hats at the University of Pittsburgh: assistant to the coordinator of hospitals and clinics and medical centers; administrator of one of the medical center hospitals; and assistant professor in the Program in Hospital Administration.

33. The state capital of Michigan.

34. See Profiles of Participants for biographical information.

35. *Connors, Oral History.*

36. The Olsen report was from one of the three commissions funded by the W.K. Kellogg Foundation to examine hospital and health services education needs. The first commission was set up in the 1940s under the direction of Charles Prall; it produced the Prall report. The second was set up in the 1950s; it was chaired by James A. Hamilton and directed by Herluf Olsen of Dartmouth College. The third, set up in the 1970s, was chaired by James Dixon; Charles Austin was the study director, and Janet Strauss was assistant director. The report was published in three volumes under the general title *Education in Health Administration* by the Health Administration Press in Ann Arbor. It is often referred to as the Dixon report.

37. *Hamilton, Oral History.*

38. Groner was president of the Baptist Memorial Hospital, Memphis.

39. Powell was president of the Baylor University Medical Center, Dallas.

40. *Filerman, Oral History.*

41. *Connors, Oral History.*

42. *Hamilton, Oral History.*

43. See Profiles of Participants for biographical information.

44. *Filerman, Oral History.*

45. *Pattullo, Oral History.*

46. *George Bugbee, In the First Person: An Oral History.*

47. The Program in Hospital Administration at the University of Chicago was founded by Michael Davis in 1934, with start-up money from the Julius Rosenwald Fund.

48. *John S. Millis, In the First Person: An Oral History.* See Profiles of Participants for biographical information.

PART IV

A Look Backward

11

Five Decades of Change: A Summary

The last five decades have seen a rapid evolution of American health care and political philosophy. This period stretched from the depths of the Great Depression to the nuclear age, from an era in which the federal government exercised little control over health care to one in which it is deeply involved in health care.

The movement that resulted in a long list of health legislation seems to have been an outgrowth of an effort to enact workmen's compensation laws in a majority of states. The American Association for Labor Legislation, organized in 1906 under the direction of John Andrews, worked for the passage of such laws. The AALL wrote a standard, or model, bill that would establish nonprofit organizations to administer state-collected "sickness insurance" funds from employees and employers—health and disability insurance. The standard bill created much interest between 1915 and 1919, but the promoters of the idea, although they were successful in introducing the bill in several state legislatures, were unable to enact it into law. One notable example was in New York State: there the bill had the support of Governor Al Smith, but it still did not pass.

The influence of one man is evident in the efforts of the AALL and other social activist groups during this period. John R. Commons, professor of economics at the University of Wisconsin, was the mentor of many of the persons who were advocating social legislation then as well as later, in the New Deal days. Besides John and Irene Andrews, other members of the Wisconsin group who came to prominence later on were Arthur J. Altmeyer[1] and Edwin E. Witte[2] of the Social Security movement, and Wilbur J. Cohen,[3] secretary of HEW during the Johnson administration.

Workmen's compensation, unemployment insurance, old age pensions, and other aspects of social security naturally led men and women to try to design some kind of health insurance program.

Early Efforts in Health and Hospitalization Insurance

During the years 1915 to 1919, some states considered compulsory state health insurance. Several states set up commissions to consider health and health care. The Metropolitan Life Insurance Co. did a home interview study to determine the extent of illness and loss of days of work. The U.S. Public Health Service collected statistics on sickness among wage earners and concluded that a system of health insurance could be adapted to American conditions. The U.S. Commission on Industrial Relations recommended in 1915 that compulsory health insurance be instituted for all employees in interstate commerce. In 1916 the National Association of Manufacturers viewed health insurance as an extension of medical care under workmen's compensation and favored a compulsory system with free competition among carriers and insurance companies.

The AMA established a committee on social insurance, which met between 1915 and 1919 under the chairmanship of Dr. Alexander Lambert of New York City. Lambert was Theodore Roosevelt's physician, and a few years later was president of the AMA. The committee concluded that compulsory state health insurance was needed.

A few years later, however, the state medical societies and the grass roots general practitioners turned the AMA's position about; the association publicly opposed government at any level impinging in any way on the practice of medicine.

During this same period, the American Federation of Labor was suspicious of government insurance and its effect on labor unions. Prudential Insurance Company spoke out against compulsory health insurance,[4] and several of the states that had seemed favorably inclined toward the standard bill backed away.

In 1920 the AMA's house of delegates stated its position against "any plan embodying the system of compulsory contributory insurance against illness."

Little social legislation was enacted in the period between 1920 and

1932. The Sheppard-Towner Act, benefiting mothers and children, was passed in 1921. It was short-lived, but it did act as a benchmark for that type of legislation later on. There was also some movement for state pension legislation urged by the Association of Old Age Security under the leadership of Abraham Epstein.

At a time when there was disagreement over the state and federal government's role in providing means for compulsory health insurance, prepaid group hospitalization insurance was developing and being financed independent of government.

The year 1929 is often cited as the apex of the prosperity of the 1920s, from which the rapid slide began down to the mass unemployment, hunger, deprivation, and despair of the 1930s. The year 1929 is also the date often given as the beginning of prepaid group hospitalization—and, by extension, of the Blue Cross movement. Actually 1931 is more important in this context, because it was at the AHA's annual meeting in 1931 that a paper written by Justin Ford Kimball was read by Asa S. Bacon.[5]

As discussed in part II, the paper described an experiment in prepaid group hospitalization developed by Kimball at the Baylor University Hospital in Dallas. Kimball, who had been superintendent of schools in Dallas, enrolled over 1,000 teachers in his plan. Later he extended it to employees of the *Dallas News*. This early prepayment plan was limited to services in one hospital, not to others in the community or elsewhere.

The importance of the paper lay in the fact that it was a public announcement of a new idea. Several of the people who attended that AHA meeting went home and tried to start prepaid group hospitalization plans in their own cities. Maurice Norby, for example, spoke of the effect the paper had on his father, Joseph Norby, who went home to Minneapolis–St. Paul recommending that a plan be started there (see chapter 7).

It is difficult to determine whether prepaid group hospitalization plans were started to help patients pay their hospital bills or to help hospitals collect their charges. Whatever the reason, medicine was showing advances in the training of physicians, in standards of practice, and in technology. Also, prepaid group hospitalization was an idea whose time had come.

The economic conditions of the 1920s were misleading as far as general prosperity was concerned. Productivity in manufacturing and other businesses increased tremendously during World War I and on into the 1920s. Unfortunately, this rise in productivity was not paralleled by a similar increase in wages. Buying demand was satisfied by a tremendous increase in consumer credit. As might be expected, prices rose faster than wages, so prepaid group hospitalization was a natural answer for both patients and hospitals.

Committee on the Costs
of Medical Care

Concurrent with the modest beginnings of prepaid group hospitalization was the work of the Committee on the Costs of Medical Care. The committee was composed of a group of concerned health professionals and educators, as well as representatives of the general public, who set about to study the state of medical care in the United States. The group received financial help from foundations and worked under the leadership of Dr. Ray Lyman Wilbur, former president of the AMA, president of Stanford University, and secretary of the Department of the Interior under President Herbert Hoover. The CCMC worked from 1927 until January 1933 trying to get a wide view of a complex and dynamic situation. (I.S. Falk and C. Rufus Rorem relate their roles in the research undertaken by the committee in chapter 2.)

The 28-volume report of the CCMC, issued at the end of 1932 and delivered in January 1933, was almost precognitive. The committee was able to project emerging ideas such as group practice, health insurance, and the government's role in health care matters so accurately that its predictions or recommendations are still relevant and developing after five decades.

The *Journal of the American Medical Association* opposed—adamantly opposed—the CCMC report even before it was officially made public. The editor labeled it as Communistic and liable to incite to revolution. The AMA's stance was that, any time a layman passed judgment on the medical profession or suggested changes in the delivery or financing of health care, it was heresy, an unjust interference in the practice of medicine. Why physicians felt threatened by honest suggestions for change is difficult to understand.

During this time C. Rufus Rorem wrote one of the first books on group practice, while working between the Julius Rosenwald Fund and the CCMC.

Prepaid group hospitalization was emerging simultaneously in several parts of the country. While the growth of the movement cannot be directly attributed to the publication of the CCMC report, it was certainly fortified by the report.

The CCMC report also stressed the need to strengthen medical education. Although there had been improvement in medical education after the Flexner report in 1910, there was still a call for better postgraduate training, for more structured intern and resident training, for better education in public health, and for cognizance of the social aspects of medicine.

Besides its principal report, the CCMC issued the Minority Report Number One, which warrants notice. The signers of the minority report clearly stated their attitude toward government's role in medicine. They recommended that "government competition in medicine be discontinued." They were quite willing, however, to allow government to be responsible for public health, for the medical care of U.S. Army, Navy, and Geodetic Survey personnel, and for "veterans suffering from *bona fide* service-connected disabilities and diseases. . . ."

The minority report "vigorously opposed corporate practice of medicine through intermediary agencies" as being "economically wasteful and inimical to a continued and sustained high quality of medical care."[6]

Roosevelt and Health Care

The year 1933, the year the CCMC report was published, was also a turning point in the role and operation of American government. Because of the Great Depression, government became a part of every citizen's life. Unemployment, hunger, the need for financial and moral support turned citizens toward the government for help in a way never experienced before in this country. The federal government in the following few years spent billions protecting people by providing food, shelter, clothing, and makework. The government was the rock of assurance, protection against want and against the rise of an American dictator.

However, it wasn't long before a natural question was asked: If the government can help with food, shelter, and jobs, why can't it help with health care?

President Roosevelt was not able to answer that question directly, although he showed his interest in some sort of national health insurance plan several times. During his first term in office, 1933–1937, he set up various agencies to combat the economic depression and to provide social security. Although the Social Security Act covered old age pensions, unemployment insurance, and maternal and child health care, as well as increasing the scope of the Public Health Service, it did not include health insurance.

In 1934 Roosevelt saw the need for social insurance in addition to the direct aid the government was furnishing. Some individuals attribute this to the growing pressure of groups demanding old age pensions and other benefits. In the forefront was a group in California led by Dr. Francis E. Townsend. Townsend clubs were formed across the country to promote a plan that would give every citizen of the United States 60 years of age or older $200 a month. The money for Townsend's revolving pension plan would be raised by a 2 percent sales tax. Recipients would have to spend all of one month's benefits before receiving another check. A bill was introduced in

Congress for the Townsend plan even before the Social Security Act was passed.

There was also a threat from Huey Long of Louisiana, who had some indefinite plan of sharing the wealth and making "Every Man a King."[7] The danger was not so much from Long's plan as from the possibility that he might run for the presidency in 1935 as an independent and take enough Democratic votes away from Roosevelt to elect a Republican.

The Committee on Economic Security

The Committee on Economic Security was created in June 1934 by President Roosevelt to "study the problems relating to economic security and to make recommendations for a program of legislation."[8]

In discussions with members of the Committee on Economic Security, the president talked of every child's being issued an insurance policy on the day he was born, a policy that would protect him against any major economic misfortunes that might befall him in his lifetime. This was Roosevelt's "cradle to the grave" idea.

The Committee on Economic Security was a cabinet-level committee headed by Frances Perkins, secretary of labor. Other members were the secretaries of the treasury and agriculture, and the attorney general. Harry Hopkins, administrator and director of FERA, was also a member.

Edwin Witte, from the department of economics at the University of Wisconsin, was named executive director of the committee. Arthur J. Altmeyer was appointed to head a technical committee charged with carrying on studies and collecting information. The technical committee was composed of federal employees expert in the areas to be studied. There was also an advisory council of 23 members. Five of the members were from labor, five from business, and the remainder were individuals interested in social welfare. The advisory council was expected to inform the committee of the views of persons and groups outside the government. It was not expected to submit a report.

The Committee for Economic Security worked expeditiously and had a report ready for the president by the last week in December 1934. A bill was drafted. Although the technical committee had considered the need for health insurance, this item was not included in the bill presented to Congress. One reason given was that the inclusion of a health insurance provision might endanger the passage of the entire Social Security bill. Another reason given was that the committee had not had enough time to study the health insurance situation sufficiently to offer a bill at that time.

On August 14, 1935, the Social Security Act, without health insurance, became law. The voting followed party lines: the Democrats generally supported it, and the Republicans generally opposed it.

The Interdepartmental Committee

The possibility of a health plan's passing Congress was not abandoned just because it was not included in the Social Security Act. The same month that Social Security became law, the president appointed an Interdepartmental Committee to Coordinate Health and Welfare Activities. This committee was composed of the assistant secretaries of the cabinet departments involved: Josephine Roche of treasury, chairman (the Public Health Service was under her jurisdiction); Oscar Chapman of interior; M.L. Wilson of agriculture; and Arthur Altmeyer of labor.

For a year and a half the interdepartmental committee coordinated existing government health activities. In 1937 it began a comprehensive survey of the health needs of the country and the development of a national health program to meet those needs. The interdepartmental committee appointed a Technical Committee on Medical Care to make the survey and submit recommendations.

The technical committee reported in February 1938 and recommended the following:

1. An expansion of public health and maternal and child health services under existing titles of the Social Security Act
2. Federal grants-in-aid to the states for the construction of hospitals and for defraying operating costs during the first three years
3. Federal grants-in-aid to the states toward the costs of a medical care program for medically needy people
4. Federal grants-in-aid to the states toward the costs of a general medical care program
5. Federal action to develop a program of compensation for wages lost due to temporary and permanent disability

President Roosevelt was pleased with the work of the interdepartmental committee and suggested that the health items be made public. He also said there should be a National Health Conference called, with representatives of the health professions and of the public, so that the report could be discussed. The president said, "I hope that at the National Health Conference a chart for continuing concerted action will begin to take form."[9]

About 175 delegates attended the conference, which was held in July 1938. There was generally enthusiastic support for the recommendations of the interdepartmental committee. The AMA offered to support points 1, 2, 3, and 5 if point 4 were abandoned. The members of the committee would not agree to that proposal, so the AMA house of delegates in a special session voted to formally approve the interdepartmental committee report with the exception of point 4.

After the National Health Conference in 1938, there was a growing constituency for some sort of national health program. Some of this positive attitude came from labor unions and Farm Bureau groups. Even the Social Security Board in its 1938 suggestions for changes in the Social Security system endorsed the plan recommended by the interdepartmental committee. Harry Hopkins, then administrator of the Works Progress Administration (WPA), recommended that the WPA build hospitals across the country.

Although some of the leading physicians in the country favored a national health program, the bulk of the doctors represented by the AMA stated their opposition in unmistakable terms.

As a propaganda medium against compulsory health insurance, the AMA created in 1939 the National Physicians' Committee for the Extension of Medical Service (NPC). The purpose of the committee was to oppose any federal health program. The trustees were former AMA and state medical society officers. Financial support for NPC came mainly from drug companies. Over the ten years or so of its existence, NPC printed and distributed millions of pamphlets opposing federal participation in health care. Its lobbying efforts went full force until it sent out a letter that was interpreted as being anti-Semitic. The backfire was so great that the NPC was disbanded in 1949.

The National Health Bill

The next step in the legislative path for a national health services financing plan was the national health bill introduced in Congress by Senator Robert Wagner (D–N.Y.) in 1939. Basically, the bill called for federal aid to state plans of medical care. Five areas for support were identified:

1. Child and maternal health care
2. State public health services
3. State systems of insurance for temporary disability
4. Construction of hospitals and health centers
5. State-sponsored general programs of medical care[10]

Hearings were held before the Senate Committee on Education and Labor to consider the bill. "Liberal labor" spokesmen were in favor of the bill, as was a group of physicians and medical educators called the Committee of Physicians for the Improvement of Medical Care. (This Committee said it had declared itself independent of the AMA in 1937.)

The AMA, as usual, was opposed. The house of delegates voted unanimously in March 1939 to oppose the bill on 22 counts. Officials of the AMA appeared before the Senate to testify in opposition to the bill. The chairman of the AMA board of trustees, Dr. Arthur W. Booth, presented the testimony and revealed in the course of his comments that he had not read the bill. However, the statement that capped the AMA opposition was made by Dr. Morris Fishbein, who said, "A little sickness is not too great a price to pay for maintaining democracy in times like these."[11]

The bill did not pass in 1939; Wagner was hopeful for 1940. Roosevelt, however, slowed any momentum the bill might have had by saying that, for 1940, he favored an experiment with one phase of the bill: the federal construction of hospitals. Wagner therefore introduced a bill for construction of hospitals. The hospital construction bill passed in the Senate, but it lay dormant in the House through the rest of the session.

Problems During World War II

When World War II broke out in Europe in 1939, the United States became involved as the "arsenal of democracy." Every effort went into supplying war material to Britain and Russia and to building our own defense. After Pearl Harbor in December 1941, we were not just a supplier, we were a principal.

There was a great shift in population from the farms to the industrial cities of the Northeast, the Midwest, and California. Supplies for civilian use became scarce. Housing and health care became national problems. The building of hospitals for domestic use practically stopped, because supplies and equipment were in extremely short supply.

Kaiser Industries is an example of a war plant that felt the lack of medical care for its workers. Kaiser shipyards on the West Coast were attempting to build new ships fast enough to replace the ones that were being destroyed with alarming regularity. Kaiser, like other war industries, had to depend for workers on women and 4Fs, men classified as unfit for military service and thus likely to have illnesses and disabilities needing medical attention.

The high incidence of need for medical care and the scarcity of physicians became such a problem that Henry Kaiser had to use his personal influence in Washington to get the release of enough doctors from the draft to take care of the shipbuilders. The doctors were found, the ships were built, and the war was eventually won.

During the war years, when Americans on the home front were tightening their belts and adjusting to ration books, a revolution was taking place in clinical medical care.

Postwar Planning

While the capacity and capability of clinical medicine advanced, the capacity and capability of the domestic hospital system languished. This situation made many thoughtful persons realize that, once the war was won, the nation would have to take stock of itself and bring some kind of order to the industrial and economic confusion that was likely to result during the initial postwar period.

George Bugbee was one of those thoughtful persons. In 1943, he became the executive director of the American Hospital Association. The AHA was in the midst of great organizational change and on its way to assuming a national role in health care. Bugbee believed the war would be over in a year or two and that the country would face great readjustments, particularly in the health field.

Actually, little detail was known about the health care situation in the United States then. The CCMC study, completed in 1932, had been the last major, definitive study. Something more, therefore, was needed to update its work. Dr. Thomas Parran, surgeon general of the U.S. Public Health Service, was of the same mind as George Bugbee: a study should be done, and plans should be laid for the postwar years.

Commission on Hospital Care

The Commission on Hospital Care was born of this need to know and plan. It was founded with the support and help of the AHA, however it was not a part of the AHA. Foundation financial support was found, and a staff and study effort was formed under the leadership of Dr. Arthur Bachmeyer of the University of Chicago. Bachmeyer was assisted by Maurice Norby, who was on leave from the AHA.

Bugbee, Norby, and Pattullo relate in chapter 3 how the commission prepared a voluminous questionnaire designed to gather as much information as possible about hospitals and other health care institutions. The Public Health Service participated unofficially in the study, arranging for the collation of the data obtained through the commission's questionnaire. In turn, the information was immediately made available to the Public Health Service for its use in planning for the postwar years.

Wagner-Murray-Dingell Bill

It was in 1943 that George Bugbee and others began thinking of plans for the postwar years. It was also the year Senator Robert Wagner introduced his second health bill. This bill was usually referred to as the Wagner-Murray-Dingell bill. Senator James Murray (D–Mont.) and Representative John Dingell (D–Mich.) were cosponsors. The bill was a voluminous one, calling for many social measures, including:

1. Compulsory national health insurance
2. Revamping of all programs of grants-in-aid to states for public assistance

3. Nationalizing the U.S. employment service

4. Nationalizing and extending the unemployment insurance system

5. Expanding the coverage and benefits under old age insurance

6. Establishing a national system of temporary and total disability benefits

7. Paid-up benefit rights under Social Security for veterans' time spent in military service

8. Special reemployment benefits for veterans during readjustment to civilian life

The bill was drafted by Senator Wagner's legislative aides under his close supervision and with the advice of many groups, including the AF of L, the CIO, the Committee of Physicians for Improving Medical Care, and the American Association of the Blind. Extensive help was also given by experts from federal agencies with related interests.

The bill was introduced in Congress in June 1943. President Roosevelt gave it his best wishes but little direct support. It was supported by the liberal press and other liberal interests, but it lay in Congress for two years without coming to a vote.

In the meantime, Congress passed in 1944 what is commonly called the GI Bill of Rights. This bill encompassed the veterans' items included in the 1943 Wagner-Murray-Dingell bill.

The 1943 Wagner-Murray-Dingell bill was the first major legislative proposal in which there was a decided shift from state action to federal action in the health field. Up to this point, most federal legislation called for grants-in-aid to states to carry out health programs, even compulsory health insurance. With the Wagner-Murray-Dingell bill, the emphasis was on federally administered programs, many of them to be carried out by the Social Security program.

The historic fourth-term victory for Roosevelt came in November 1944. By December of that year he seemed at last ready to make an all-out drive for a national health program. Harry Hopkins (a confidant and personal assistant to the president) telephoned Michael M. Davis in New York and asked him to come to Washington and work with Judge Samuel Rosenman[12] on a message to Congress. The president planned to deliver the health message in the spring of 1945.[13] The message was expected to present a national health program, including national health insurance. By January 1945, Davis had an initial sketch ready for Rosenman. Unfortunately, the President died in April 1945, before the speech could be completed and delivered.

Truman and Health Care

President Harry S. Truman, on assuming office after the death of Franklin Roosevelt, carried out some of the tasks on FDR's agenda. The health program proposal, which Michael Davis and Samuel Rosenman were working on at the time of Roosevelt's death, was useful in the writing of Truman's message to Congress on health, delivered November 19, 1945.

Many of the recommendations in this presidential message on health—the first to be delivered on this topic—were similar to those of the Wagner bills (of 1943 and 1945), the items stressed by the technical committee of the interdepartmental committee, and other study groups.

Truman recommended:

1. Federal aid for hospital construction
2. Enlarged federal aid for public health and for maternal and child health services
3. Federal aid for medical education and research
4. A national health insurance plan as part of "our existing compulsory social insurance system"
5. Disability insurance

The president's message evoked support from liberal physicians and labor leaders. Within three months of the delivery of the speech, many of these individuals and other supporters of the president's plan organized a Committee for the Nation's Health to help bring the plan into effect. The principal financial support for the committee came from labor. The president's message on health aroused not only support, but also the AMA's stubborn opposition to any health insurance program (including Blue Cross) not under the control of state and county medical societies.

Hill-Burton

The AMA opposed the Hospital Survey and Construction (Hill–Burton) Act, which was enacted by Congress in 1946. The preliminary studies of the Commission on Hospital Care, the cooperation of the Public Health Service, the lobbying effort of George Bugbee as part of the AHA support of the bill, and the active participation of Senators Lister Hill, Harold Burton, and Robert Taft in making this great hospital construction program possible have all been described in chapter 3. With the passage of the Hill–Burton bill, one aspect of the national health program was complete: the "experiment in health planning" mentioned by Roosevelt in 1940 was accomplished.

About the time of the passage of Hill–Burton, the AMA decided to hire an outside agency to evaluate its attitudes and its public positions and statements. The AMA retained Raymond Rich Associates, a public relations firm, for the job. The agency's report was critical of the NPC, of the total medical control of Blue Shield, of the type of economic "research" carried on for AMA, and the lack of opportunity for minority views in the profession to be expressed.

In 1948, about two years after the Raymond Rich Associates evaluation, the AMA hired another public relations firm, Whittaker and Baxter, to actively work against "socialized medicine." (Whittaker and Baxter, working for the California Medical Association, had been active in defeating California Governor Earl Warren's plan for state legislation for health insurance in 1944.) The AMA's opposition to any efforts to institute compulsory hospital insurance continued until after the Medicare and Medicaid legislation was passed in 1965.

In connection with the AMA's opposition to compulsory health insurance, Dr. Morris Fishbein, a genius of vituperation, should not be passed over. As editor of the *Journal of the American Medical Association* (JAMA), he was a strident opponent of national health programs. His phrases characterizing the recommendations of the Committee on the Costs of Medical Care in 1933 as "Communism" and "inciting to revolution" are probably best remembered. Beginning in 1924 and for about 25 years thereafter, Fishbein's pen was an effective weapon in the AMA's war against change in the health care system.

One of the features in JAMA in the 1940s was a column Fishbein wrote and labeled his "Pepys' Diary," after the work of the 17th century English diarist. Unfortunately for Fishbein, he made a slip in one of his columns describing his activities during a trip to England, and Nelson Cruikshank brought it up in a radio debate with him. Cruikshank pointed out that while Fishbein was reportedly making a study of the British National Health Service (NHS), he in fact merely picked up a few papers on the subject from the NHS office. Instead of studying, Fishbein had been socializing. There was no misbehavior on Fishbein's part, but the incident destroyed his credibility and effectiveness. He was removed as editor in 1949.

Insurance

President Truman, during his last years in the White House, continued to speak for health insurance, particularly for the aged and indigent, however nothing tangible came of it.

A conference on aging was held in 1950. Although little of direct consequence can be pointed out, there was evident a rising concern about the problem of illness among the aged and indigent.

In 1952 (the presidential election year), voices were raised for compulsory health insurance as a part of Social Security. Oscar Ewing, the federal security administrator and a Democratic presidential hopeful, advocated it. The Social Security Administration recommended it in its 1951 annual report, as did the President's Commission on the Health Needs of the Nation. That same year the Murray-Humphrey-Dingell-Celler bill, calling for the same thing, was introduced in Congress. These various efforts were to no avail.

Eisenhower and Health Care

The election of Dwight David Eisenhower ushered in a quieter period in the drive for and against a national health program. The medical profession seemed to think the president was with them. Furthermore, the growth in voluntary health insurance through commercial insurance companies and Blue Cross–Blue Shield plans made many persons in government conclude that the need for the federal government's participation might pass.

The new president believed in a moderate approach to a health program.[14] He proposed a plan to:

1. Extend Social Security to 10 million more persons and to increase benefits

2. Continue the construction of public housing at the rate of 35,000 units a year for at least four years

3. Bring four million and more persons under unemployment insurance

4. Increase grants for the construction of hospitals and clinics

Another idea broached during the Eisenhower years was for the federal government to reinsure health insurance policies written by nongovernment agencies. The goal of this proposal was to ensure that the needy would have insurance protection. Although the idea was incorporated into legislative language, the bill never got out of committee.

There was nothing really new about Eisenhower's ideas; they were mainly just a conservative progression of existing programs.

Even though Eisenhower's plans for health were moderate, there was an obstructive force abroad, one based on vindictiveness. The Department of Health, Education, and Welfare was formed early in Eisenhower's first term. The president appointed Oveta Culp Hobby, a capable woman who had headed the Women's Army Corps during World War II, as HEW's first secretary. Hobby was a Democrat and a newspaper publisher from Houston. Unfortunately, she had also been active in Democratic party politics in Texas; thus she appeared to Sam Rayburn, the Democratic leader of the House and also a Texan, as a deserter. Anything she officially proposed was likely to be opposed by Rayburn, thus Hobby was at a disadvantage as a proponent.

One outstanding health program during the Eisenhower years was the development of the Salk polio vaccine and the administration of it to millions of children. Before this time, the nation worried about outbreaks of the disease every autumn, since there was little remedy and no prevention. The production of a large amount of vaccine and the administration of a nation-wide program of inoculation was plagued by delays and confusion, but the program was finally a success.

On the legislative front, the Forand bill, a labor-backed bill calling for health insurance for Social Security beneficiaries, was introduced in Congress in 1957. It proposed benefits of 60 days of hospital care as well as surgical and nursing home coverage. This bill aroused the opposition of the medical profession, so in 1959 Forand dropped the surgical and nursing home benefits. The bill was still unable to get a favorable vote in the Ways and Means Committee. Nelson Cruikshank describes this action in his oral history.[15]

Throughout the closing months of Eisenhower's second term, pressure was mounting for health insurance for the elderly and needy. One product of this pressure was the passage of the Kerr-Mills bill, which proved to be inadequate, as Cruikshank discusses in chapter 4.

The last days of the Eisenhower administration were capped by the White House Conference on Aging. The conference was planned by the Republicans, however it was covertly managed by the Democrats and labor. Cruikshank describes this in chapter 5.

Kennedy and Health Care

President John F. Kennedy sent a special message to Congress about a month after his inauguration advocating health insurance under Social Security. This was on February 10, 1961. Three days later, the King–Anderson bill, which was referred to as "Medicare," was introduced.

Arthur M. Schlesinger, Jr.,[16] who was close to the president, believed Kennedy did not expect Medicare to pass in 1961 or 1962 but felt that, since he had sent up a message to Congress and an administration bill had been introduced, there would be committee hearings and publicity. All of this he expected would lead to passage of the legislation later.

To add to the publicity and support for Medicare legislation, the presidential Task Force on Health and Social Security for the American People made a report early in 1961 that was favorable to Medicare.

Many of the health insurance events during the Kennedy years have been reported in the Medicare section of this book. Suffice it to say that, although Medicare legislation did not pass in that congressional session, the momentum that was generated helped carry it through under the guidance and energy of Lyndon B. Johnson.

Johnson and Health Care

Wilbur Mills, the chairman of the Ways and Means Committee, felt increasing pressure for a Medicare bill after Lyndon Johnson was elected president in 1964. Johnson was striving to pass the social legislation initiated by President Kennedy, and one of the most important pieces was Medicare. There was a great wave of sympathy and a wish to carry out the programs of the assassinated president, however one should not overlook the great power Johnson wielded in Congress. He turned some of that power on Wilbur Mills and demanded action on Medicare. Mills up to this point had faced a very close vote on Medicare in his own Ways and Means Committee. With the landslide election of Johnson and the Democrats, however, the makeup of the Ways and Means Committee changed and Mills could get a favorable vote. Mills was a skilled tactician, and he suddenly presented a plan that pleased Democrats and Republicans alike—the three-layer cake compromise described in the Medicare chapters of this book.

The final flourish was the signing of the bill by President Johnson in the presence of former President Truman in Independence, Missouri, on July 30, 1965.

Medicare and Medicaid changed the American health care world forever. The elderly and needy gained new access to care. Hospitals found themselves with a new but restricted source of revenues. Physicians were raised to new economic levels. The federal and state governments were faced with health care demands and costs beyond the imagination of the best of the actuaries. The history of the time from the mid-1960s to the mid-1980s has been one of trying to adjust to this and accompanying events, which revolutionized the practice and economics of health care.

The Pathways of the Future

In the early 1960s, before Medicare, Walter J. McNerney, then president of the Blue Cross Association, and Wilbur Cohen, later to be secretary of HEW, were on the University of Michigan campus on the same day. An impromptu meeting of the hospital administration faculty and these distinguished visitors was called. The conversation was focused on how American health care delivery and financing would develop in the future. Many pathways were discussed, ranging from a broad national health program to one with only the slightest federal participation. After some discussion, a consensus emerged. The American way was not likely to be monolithic, but pluralistic. Many ideas for health care delivery and financing would be tried, some of them simultaneously. Now, more than 20 years later, this statement is still valid.

Pluralism implies different approaches to problems, and in many cases opposing views. A few approaches likely in the future are suggested below, with no assessment of degree of magnitude or possibility of occurrence.

Hospital versus Health Center. It would seem that the movement toward the hospital's becoming more and more the center of diagnosis and treatment of disease will continue. Physicians, dentists, therapists, home care services, and community mental health services could be linked so that all diagnostic and therapeutic inpatient and outpatient services would be provided in the most efficient and convenient way.

Hospital versus Ambulatory Centers. The urgency of containing costs has encouraged the use of ambulatory care, walk-in clinics, one-day surgery, and other services in freestanding centers. Although investor-owned centers have sprung up, it would seem that alert hospitals would establish such centers, if they do not have them already, in order to compete with the freestanding units. Furthermore, patients may find ambulatory units more convenient to use and may thus choose them.

Solo versus Group Practice. Physicians have learned in the past few years that group practice has many advantages over solo practice. Specialties and subspecialties have multiplied to such a point that a cooperative group can offer much better care over a varied patient load than can a solo practitioner. Further, working hours, office routines, vacations, and leisure time can be arranged more conveniently in groups.

New Technology. Technology has changed so rapidly that, as one radiologist put it, a radiologist today can no longer finish his residency with competence and training that will last for some years; today a radiologist must realize he is destined to continue his education unremittingly for the rest of his professional life in order to try to keep up with the advances in his field. In fact, one radiologist has said that, with CAT, NMR, PET, and ultrasound, it is possible to diagnose conditions for which there is no known treatment—and that is only in radiology![17] Technology is going to challenge the best brains in all fields of medicine to keep abreast in therapeutics.

Voluntary versus Investor-Owned. Investor ownership of hospitals and other health facilities is a phenomenon that has become strikingly noticeable in the past ten or more years. The Hospital Corporation of America, for example, grew during that time from one doctor-owned hospital to about 400 hospitals, owned or managed, with a total of about 57,000 beds. Sheer size and purchasing power of corporations, ready access to capital needs, excellent managers, a wide range of computerized data for management analysis and research, self-insurance potential, and audiovisual facilities for training employees and medical staff are a few of the reasons voluntaries are finding it difficult to compete as individual institutions.

Voluntaries, however, have learned from investor-owned chains in many ways. They are moving toward hospital systems and networks of voluntary hospitals, and this would seem to be the pathway to the future for them.

Women versus Men. In the last 20 years, women have been entering professional schools (in addition to the traditional ones of nursing and education) in increasing numbers. Medical schools now have a high percentage of female students (as much as 50 percent in some schools). The same is true of programs in health administration, pharmacy, physical therapy, and related professions. Women in medicine may supply an element some people say is missing in the profession—an understanding of the social problems of patients and of how they affect health and health care.

Blue Cross versus Commercial Insurance. The insurance picture has become so complex that few individuals have a broad view of it. Gone are the days when Blue Cross just sold full-service benefits in hospitals and the commercial insurance companies paid specified dollars for certain services (indemnity insurance). Instead, insurance policies today are tailor-made to fit the needs of the group purchaser, even to the extent of designing partial self-insurance schemes. Furthermore, many insurance entities are offering optional plans, including HMOs. This trend seems likely to grow.

Providers. Federal money is paying a large percentage of health care costs in the United States. Because these costs have been rising faster than the national inflation rate, regulations are becoming more restrictive. The most recent plan, that of using prospective pricing (diagnosis-related groups) for determining payment to hospitals for care of Medicare patients, may set a pattern for other payers.

Political Voice. The AHA has traditionally been the national voice in Washington for hospitals, while the state association has been the voice for hospitals at the local level. In fact, action has not been as independent as that statement might imply, because national, state, metropolitan, regional, and sectarian hospital associations have found that they can cooperate and complement each other in the political arena. This rather complicated cooperation has to be carefully orchestrated for the full benefit of all concerned. The AHA, because of its national scope, should attempt to keep improving this working relationship, because the future seems to promise more legislation and more regulation in health care.

Unionization. Unions will be a more important factor in health care operations in the future. A distinct change is taking place in the organization of workers in health facilities: whereas the greatest number of union members may now be the service workers (housekeeping, dietary, laundry, mainte-nance), nurses are becoming organized and unions are increasingly looking to white-collor workers for future membership growth.

Research. With the growth of the voluntary and investor-owned chains of health care institutions—and with the information age upon us—masses of data covering whole regions of the country will give us a new profile of patients, diseases, treatments, accounting, personnel, and management. These data will be a gold mine for researchers. Our picture of health care in the United States should be more finely tuned in the coming years and so guide our efforts toward exellence in care.

The Elderly. As everyone knows, elderly persons are increasing in num-ber. With this increase will come both new and increased demands for health care services.

The American care of the elderly in nursing homes is not a shining example of success. More thought must be put into the problem. More nursing home beds must be built to keep up with the growing need. Better management and regulation are needed. Some persons recommend that the federal government go into nursing home operations, as some other national governments have done.

Not all elderly persons, nor even all old-old (over 85 years of age) persons are in nursing homes, although many of them need a specially de-signed residence. A few proprietary groups are experimenting with resi-dences for the ambulatory elderly. These elderly individuals need the company and companionship of others; they need activities they can enjoy; and they need regular, planned meals. Many of the elderly can afford these pleasant living conditions for a monthly fee. For those who cannot finance such care out of their own resources, another way must be found to meet the cost.

One of the basic beliefs since the founding of our nation has been that there would be continuous progress, that life would be better and better for each generation. Inventions, new technology, better social conditions, and new understanding of the problems facing our nation would lead to that progress and a better life. Along the way there have been some setbacks, depressions and wars. The dream of progress, however, seems inbred and carries over from generation to generation. The future therefore continues to be bright, simply because we believe we shall find answers to our problems.

Notes

(Transcripts of the oral histories cited here are housed in the library of the American Hospital Association, 840 North Lake Shore Drive, Chicago, Illinois 60611. The Oral History Collection is a joint project of the Hospital Research and Educational Trust and the AHA.)

1. Altmeyer was an assistant secretary of labor, director of the technical committee of the

Committee on Economic Security, a member of the Interdepartmental Committee to Co-ordinate Health and Welfare Activities, a member of the first Social Security Board, and Social Security commissioner when that entity became part of the new Federal Security Agency formed in 1939. Altmeyer also held administrative positions in several wartime agencies.

2. Witte of the University of Wisconsin headed the Committee on Economic Security. The data and information gathered by that committee were used in the writing of the Social Security bill.

3. See Profiles of Participants, in the center of this book, for biographical information.

4. Michael M. Davis, *Medical Care for Tomorrow* (New York: Harper 1955), p. 274.

5. Bacon was a Chicago hospital administrator and treasurer of the AHA.

6. For further information on the minority report, see Appendix C.

7. Slogan used by Huey Long.

8. Arthur J. Altmeyer, *The Formative Years of Social Security* (Madison: The University of Wisconsin Press, 1966), p. 3.

9. Ibid., pp. 93–96.

10. J. Joseph Huthmacher, *Senator Robert Wagner and the Rise of Urban Liberalism* (New York: Atheneum, 1968), pp. 263–67.

11. Ibid., p. 265.

12. Rosenman was an early political adviser and speech writer of Franklin D. Roosevelt—even before Roosevelt was elected governor of New York in 1928. Rosenman was a member of the Brain Trust, which worked for Roosevelt for president in 1932. Roosevelt appointed him to the New York Supreme Court in 1932, and Rosenman worked closely with Roosevelt outside government until 1943, when the president urged him to resign from the judiciary and become counsel to the president, which he did.

13. Davis, *Medical Care*, pp. 280–81.

14. Robert J. Donovan, *Eisenhower: The Inside Story* (New York: Harper, 1956), p. 228.

15. *Nelson Cruikshank, In the First Person: An Oral History.*

16. Arthur M. Schlesinger, Jr., *A Thousand Days: John F. Kennedy in the White House* (Boston: Houghton Mifflin, 1965), p. 710.

17. "Medical Milestone," *Wall Street Journal,* October 3, 1984, pp. 1, 22.

APPENDIX A

The Committee on the Costs of Medical Care

Ray Lyman Wilbur, the chairman of the Committee on the Costs of Medical Care, wrote the following words in the final report of the committee, which was published by the University of Chicago Press in 1933.

> Pain, sickness, and bereavement have shadowed mankind throughout the ages; today there is a vast amount of unnecessary sickness, and many thousands of unnecessary deaths. Each year, over a hundred thousand babies die during the first year of life, many of them needlessly. Of the many thousand victims of tuberculosis, over 88,000 died in 1930 alone. Pellagra and hookworm disease reduce the economic efficiency of a large proportion of the people of the South. Syphilis and gonorrhea destroy fertility, deform babies, and wreck homes. Over one-third of a million persons are mentally diseased. The death rates for cancer, diseases of the heart, and diabetes are rising. A large portion of the people, young and old, are handicapped by one or more defects—particularly by decayed teeth, enlarged or diseased tonsils, defective vision, partial deafness, and weak feet. For the hundreds suffering from specific diseases, thousands are rendered inefficient for their various occupations because of common colds, constipation, headaches, rheumatism, and other minor ailments.

In a more hopeful expression, the report enumerated the many advances in the previous half-century, much of it based on the work of Louis Pasteur, Robert Koch, and Joseph Lister. Scientific advances brought many communicable diseases under control and helped lengthen the average life span. The feared scourges such as yellow fever and bubonic plague had been virtually wiped out by the 1930s. In addition, typhoid fever and smallpox had been greatly diminished.

Considering the advances that had been made by then in the knowledge, technology, and equipment to improve the health of the public, Wilbur looked ahead 50 years (to our present time) with great anticipation. In spite of the advances, Wilbur stated, the knowledge, technology, equipment, and trained personnel that were available were not being used to full capacity. Those advances that he saw 50 years in the future could be attained, at least partially, fairly soon with the proper use of present resources. Two reasons were mentioned for the lack of use of those resources. One was the cost involved. The other was the poor distribution of services.

The cost of medical care was not only an important factor in keeping some patients from seeking health care, it also affected physicians' incomes, and the quality of the hospitals where they worked.

Wilbur heard the concerns of leaders in medicine, public health, and social science about the problems of delivering adequate health care. He invited many of them to a meeting in Washington, D.C., on April 1, 1926. The problems discussed at that meeting resulted in the appointment of a Committee of Five to investigate the possible need for a course of action. The committee questioned about 75 prominent citizens by mail. Their responses almost unanimously favored establishing an organization to carry out extensive research, particularly about the economic problems of the delivery of medical care.

As a result of the mail survey, a conference was called in Washington on May 17, 1927, to coincide with the annual meeting of the American Medical Association. About 60 persons, comprised of physicians, public health officers, social scientists, and representatives of the public, attended. The Committee on the Costs of Medical Care was created, and an executive committee was appointed. Subsequently a study director was named to develop a proposed course of studies. On February 13, 1928, a five-year program of research in 17 areas was adopted by the executive committee. (As the studies progressed, some changes were made.)

For most of the five-year period, the CCMC consisted of 50 members from private medical practice, medical institutions, the social sciences, and the general public. The committee met twice a year to study data developed in the research. During the final year there were three meetings to consider drafts of the committee's recommendations.

The executive committee met monthly, except during the summer. This committee examined all research reports before they were submitted to the general committee. Wilbur praised the executive committee for having "given freely of their time at a sacrifice of personal obligations. The total value of the work done by the General and Executive committees, if paid for in money, would have cost many thousands of dollars."

The research staff and supporting professional and technical personnel proved to be very efficient. Twenty-six reports of studies were produced during the allotted period. At the beginning of the research, the executive and general committees tended to take responsibility for the details of the reports. As the work progressed and the staff demonstrated their skills, the committees gave the staff members increasing freedom in their work decisions and reports.

The CCMC developed a public relations staff to keep the public up to date on the results of the committee's work. Although the 26 study reports were written for health professionals, the public relations staff circulated abstracts to various other interested persons.

The five-year program was made possible through the financial support of eight foundations: the Carnegie Corporation, the Josiah Macy, Jr., Foundation, the Milbank Memorial Fund, the New York Foundation, the Rockefeller Foundation, the Julius Rosenwald Fund, the Russell Sage Foundation, and the Twentieth Century Fund. Special studies were supported separately. The Social Science Research Council gave a grant for a special study, as did the Vermont Commission on Country Life for a research project on a subject of special interest to it.

The American Medical Association, the American Dental Association, the National Bureau of Economic Research, the Metropolitan Life Insurance Company, and the National Tuberculosis Association all did supplementary studies that assisted the CCMC greatly. The U.S. Public Health Service also helped, by tabulating the mass of data gathered by the CCMC in family surveys about the incidence and costs of sickness. Other groups aided in the field work of the CCMC research. These groups included state and local departments of health, visiting nurse associations, and others that collaborated in many studies without cost to the committee. The work contributed by these groups would have cost the committee thousands of dollars to complete.

The study of the CCMC was scheduled for completion by January 1, 1933. The final output was 27 volumes, consisting of 26 study reports and a summary volume containing the committee report and recommendations. There were also reports of two minority groups of the committee.

Working on the assumption that the physical and mental health of the people were the country's greatest asset, the CCMC recommended future action that it believed to be, according to Wilbur, "a scientific basis on which the people of every locality can attack the perplexing problem of providing adequate medical care for all persons at costs within their means."

The Committee on the Costs of Medical Care

OFFICERS
>Ray Lyman Wilbur, M.D., Chairman
>>U.S. Department of the Interior
>Charles-Edward A. Winslow, Vice Chairman
>>Yale University School of Medicine
>Winthrop W. Aldrich, Treasurer
>>Chase National Bank
>Harry H. Moore, Study Director
>>Washington, D.C.

EXECUTIVE COMMITTEE

C.-E. A. Winslow, Chairman
Walter P. Bowles, M.D.
Michael M. Davis
Mrs. William Kinnicutt Draper
Haven Emerson, M.D.
George E. Follansbee, M.D.
Walton H. Hamilton
Walter R. Steiner, M.D.

ADMINISTRATIVE STAFF

Harry H. Moore, Study Director
Alden B. Mills, Executive Secretary
Allen Peebles, Field Secretary

RESEARCH STAFF

I.S. Falk, Associate Study Director
Maurice Leven, Statistician
Martha D. Ring, Editor

Niles Carpenter
Hugh Carter
Robert P. Fischelis
Cameron St. C. Guild
Don M. Griswold
Lewis W. Jones
Margaret C. Klem
Louis S. Reed
C. Rufus Rorem
Nathan Sinai
Gertrude Sturges

APPENDIX B

Recommendations of the Committee on the Costs of Medical Care

Group Practice

The committee favored providing medical care through organized groups of physicians, nurses, dentists, pharmacists, and other health care personnel. It advocated groups organized around hospitals and capable of furnishing "complete home, office, and hospital care." It recommended that the organization maintain and preserve the high standards of the professions, and develop and preserve good personal relations between doctors and patients.

Public Health Service

The committee recommended the extension of all basic public health services, whether provided by government agencies or not, so that they would be available to all persons when needed. This action implied more financial support for health departments and more trained health officers and staff—with tenure dependent only on professional and administrative experience.

Group Payment

Group payment to defray the costs of medical care through an insurance plan, through taxation, or through a combination of those methods was recommended by the committee. Group payment could be optional and in addition to the existing plan of individuals' paying fees for services. Cash benefits from workmen's compensation should be considered "separate and distinct" from medical services.

Medical Service Appraisals

State and local medical service appraisals were recommended through agencies to be formed for studying and coordinating medical service. The committee said that coordination of rural and urban services should be given special attention.

Professional Education

Several suggestions were made about professional education.

1. The training of physicians should emphasize the teaching of health and preventive medicine, and more effort should be made to train health officers.

2. The social aspects of medical practice should be given proper attention.

3. The practice of specialties should be restricted to persons well qualified.

4. Dental students should be given a broader education.

5. The education of pharmacists should stress opportunities for public service.

6. Nursing education should be remolded to provide well-educated and well-qualified registered nurses.

7. Trained and competent nurse's aides and attendents should be provided.

8. Adequate training should be provided for nurse-midwives.

9. Opportunities should be provided for the systematic training of hospital and clinical administrators.

APPENDIX C

Principal Minority Report of the Committee on the Costs of Medical Care

The authors of the minority report were all physicians except A.M. Schwitalla, who was a priest and president of the Catholic Hospital Association. The eight physicians who signed the minority report were also a minority of the physicians on the CCMC.

The principal minority group made several recommendations.

Government Competition

Government competition in medicine should be discontinued and its activities restricted to: care of the indigent and patients with diseases that could only be cared for in government institutions; promotion of public health; support of the medical departments of the army, navy, coast guard, and geodetic service, which have patients who, because of their location, cannot be served by the general medical profession; and care of veterans suffering from service-connected disabilities and illnesses, except for tuberculosis and nervous and mental diseases.

Care of the Indigent

Government care of the indigent should be expanded, with the ultimate object of relieving the medical profession of the burden.

Medical Service Appraisals

The minority concurs with the majority in recommending that state and local agencies study, evaluate, and coordinate medical services and give special attention to the coordination of rural and urban services.

General Practitioner

A concerted effort should be made to restore the general practitioner to a central place in medical practice.

Corporate Medicine

The corporate practice of medicine, being financed through intermediary agencies, should be vigorously and persistently opposed as being economically wasteful, inimical to the continued and sustained high quality of medical care, and unfairly exploitative of the medical profession.

Careful Trial

New methods should be given a careful trial that can be fitted into present institutions and agencies without "interfering with the fundamentals of medical practice."

Planning by Medical Societies

State and county medical societies should develop plans for medical care.

A.C. Christie, M.D.	N.B. Van Etten, M.D.
George E. Follansbee, M.D.	A.M. Schwitalla
M.L. Harris, M.D.	Olin West, M.D.
Kirby S. Howlett, M.D.	Robert Wilson, M.D.
A.C. Morgan, M.D.	

APPENDIX D

*Introductory Statement of the Commission on Hospital Care**

The attention of the entire nation has been focused upon the need for adequate preventive and curative health services for all the people. At no other time has so much emphasis been placed upon the role of good physical and mental health in the welfare and development of the nation.

Education in matters of health is begun with infants and developed in organized courses of instruction throughout elementary school, high school, and college years. It is continued, for the adult, with discussions of health problems and explanations of new scientific discoveries in books, magazines, newspapers, and movies, and on the radio. Through education, a demand has been created for more and better services for the maintenance of health, the prevention of disease, and the cure of illness. The public is evidencing an ever-increasing awareness of the importance of good health and is voicing its desire that health services be made more generally available.

We have boasted of our fine institutions, of the number of hospital beds per unit of population, and of the high standards of hospital care that exist in the United States. Yet both physical facilities and the arrangements under which they operate leave much to be desired. Many of our hospitals are old and outmoded. Some are housed in makeshift adaptations of buildings designed for other purposes. In many urban communities, there is wasteful duplication of facilities created and continued by special interests, individual ambitions, and prejudices. There are many regions in the United States in which hospital care is quite inadequate. It is wholly lacking in some rural areas.

Emphasis has been placed on the care of certain special types of illness, but there is a partial, sometimes even a total, disregard for the needs of persons suffering from other diseases. Advances in medical science have made it possible to prevent many diseases and to increase materially the efficiency of diagnosis and treatment of many acute illnesses. However, there has been little increase in our knowledge concerning the prevention and treatment of chronic diseases and of mental illness. In general, there has been gross negligence in providing for the care of patients afflicted with these conditions.

The principle of public responsibility for hospital care of the indigent

---

*Used with the permission of the Commonwealth Fund.

has been generally accepted, but in many instances public funds have not been sufficient to meet the cost of such service. While progress toward solving the problem of financing hospital care for people of the middle income group has been made, much remains to be done.

We frequently refer to our splendid system of hospitals, whereas actually there is none. Governmental units, church bodies, philanthropists, industries, and individuals have participated in the construction of hospital facilities. The diversity of background and objectives of the sponsoring interests has resulted in widely disparate patterns of organization, administration, and control of hospitals. There is very little coordination. In some instances, there even may be competition. Because of the rapid development and the nature of hospital service and the independence of the sponsoring agencies, we find disorganized, unrelated, and oftentimes overlapping patterns of hospital care. Critics describe them as uneconomic and ineffective. Patrons admit there is room for improvement.

In most states, anyone can establish the most meager facility for the bed care of the sick and call it a hospital. There is little supervision of the establishment, the organization, or the quality of care in our hospitals. A few states have passed legislation designed to raise the quality of care. Professional organizations have established standards with which hospitals may voluntarily conform. These efforts at improving the quality of service have had a wholesome influence. But the supervision of hospitals has been very largely extralegal in that each institution has been permitted to rest its case with the public it serves. For the most part, the current program of supervision has not resulted in effective controls, particularly in the case of the many very small institutions, because public judgments usually are based upon incomplete information or misunderstanding of the elements which contribute to a high quality of hospital care.

Many of the deficiencies in our hospital program have resulted from our inability to keep pace with the rapid development of medical science. The progress of medicine has changed the concept of the hospital from that of a domiciliary type of institution providing bed and nursing care to that of a complex, scientific organization capable of providing all the adjunct services necessary to assist the physician in the diagnosis and treatment of illness.

The contingencies of world-wide economic depression and war during the past fifteen years have throttled the growth of hospitals. Hospitals are now on the threshold of a period of development which will mark the beginning of a new era in the advancement of human welfare. The base of their financial support must be broadened, their services strengthened, and their availability extended to all people so that a complete and systematic service will be the heritage of the new generation.

The haphazard development of hospital service of the past should not be extended to the future. The public must be made aware of and must assume its responsibility for the development and support of adequate hospital care on a community-wide basis. The expansion and development of individual institutions must be in accord with an over-all planned program for the community. There is some evidence of a future dispersal of the population prompted by the recent war experiences with area bombing. Planning bodies should anticipate this movement of people from large urban centers to rural and suburban communities in hospital construction programs. Direct benefit will accrue to both hospitals and public through organized effort in the intelligent planning of hospital care. If planning groups, consisting of the representatives of the hospitals, the professions, and the public, fail to take full advantage of their opportunity to realign hospital care to match the needs and demands of the public, they will contribute to the bankruptcy of voluntary effort in the hospital field. Intelligent planning now will provide hospitals with an opportunity for future growth—growth in effectiveness, service, and public appreciation.

The hospital situation never is static. Constant improvement in the methods of treatment of illness, together with the continuous development of new technical equipment and advances in medical science, dictates the need for alertness and vigilance in the hospital field. Ceaseless study is necessary to coordinate the development of an economic and effective hospital program with advances in medicine and public demand. Coordination of study among the various health service groups is prerequisite to a full understanding of the intricate problems involved.

APPENDIX E

*Foreword to the Report of the Commission on Hospital Care**

This report is presented to the American people as a guide to the future development of hospital care. It appears at a time when there is wide interest in the problem and great need for extending hospital facilities. The Commission has developed a plan for integrating and extending hospital service in a way which it believes is workable and desirable—one which will strengthen and improve the present method of organization and distribution of hospital care. It is hoped the report will prove useful in planning the expansion of hospital facilities throughout the country.

Neither funds nor time permitted a comprehensive study of all phases of hospital care and interrelated health services. Rather than spread its work thinly over the entire field of institutional care, attention was focused upon the function and scope of service of the general hospital. It is urged that other groups add to this report through studies of other types of hospital service.

The Commission recognized that hospital care is a personal service which must be organized and effected by the residents of the area who use the facilities. Therefore, major emphasis during the two years of the Commission's work was placed upon the establishment and guidance of study groups in the various states. In its pilot study in Michigan, the staff developed procedures and methods of study and outlined a basic plan for that state which would serve as a work pattern for other states. The Commission's proposed study procedure is being used in forty states where studies are under way, and it is expected it will be followed in other states when studies are launched.

The results of the work of state study groups will be far-reaching and will continue to be felt as long as they function effectively. The state study phase of the Commission's efforts can be reported now only in terms of number of projects begun and their present status. The history of the state study action program will record the long-time value and full extent of the work of the Commission on Hospital Care. Through this program, a means has been established whereby the planning phases of its activity will be given purpose and meaning.

In its study of the general hospital, the Commission inquired into the

---

*Used with the permission of the Commonwealth Fund.

manner in which service was organized and the ways in which it could be made more effective. It studied methods by which hospital care could be extended to greater numbers of people. It prepared formulas by means of which the need for hospital facilities can be determined. It assembled background material for use by students of hospital problems so that they might better understand the influences and forces which have combined to create the present pattern of hospital service.

These assembled data are offered as a source book of basic information and suggestions to individuals and groups who are responsible for or interested in the improvement of hospital care.

The Commission was fortunate in having the assistance of many national organizations, especially those in the hospital, medical, dental, and nursing fields. We are deeply indebted to these groups as well as to many other organizations and individuals who contributed much to this study.

I cannot let this opportunity pass to express to Doctor Bachmeyer and the staff who worked with him my personal appreciation for their untiring efforts throughout all stages of this study. Without their diligence, cooperation, and willingness to give unselfishly, not only of their services but of themselves as well, the successful completion of this project could not have been accomplished.

Thomas S. Gates
Chairman

APPENDIX F

Excerpts from the Testimony
of George Bugbee
before the Senate Committee
on Labor and Public Welfare,
March 19, 1954*

The American Hospital Association and the 5,500 member hospitals it represents are interested in the health of the American people. They have joined together to make the highest possible quality of care available to all the people. It became obvious to us many years ago that the kind of health care available to any segment of the population was directly related to the availability of hospital services.

The hospital is fundamental to the modern practice of medicine and is the means by which the advancements of medical science can be brought to the people. Further, the establishment of standards and controls by the medical profession which are essential to the welfare of the people are best attainable within hospitals. Thus, the existence of good hospitals makes for better medical care, and the absence of hospitals may result in very limited or no medical care. The lack of hospital facilities in many areas of the country is a serious deterrent to meeting the health needs of the people residing there.

It was with this background of thought that the American Hospital Association adopted the position that Federal funds were necessary to assist in providing hospital facilities in needy areas. A mechanism of providing Federal funds on a matching basis to the states was visualized. Therefore, the active support of the Hospital Survey and Construction Act by this Association was a natural consequence.

In general, we are highly pleased that past operations of the Hospital Survey and Construction program have so warranted public support through accomplishments under the Act that additional expansion is recommended. We believe the proposals embodied in S. 2758 are constructive in character. We are appearing before the Committee to raise certain questions which occur to us and to suggest technical changes which we think might more satisfactorily accomplish the objectives of the sponsors of S. 2758.

Representatives of the American Hospital Association have regularly

*Published by the American Hospital Association (Chicago: AHA, 1954). Used with permission.

had opportunity to appear before this Committee in regard to hospital construction grants, this being the thirteenth time we have been privileged to
present testimony on the subject before a Congressional Committee. We
would like to quote very briefly from testimony in March 1946 before the
House Interstate and Foreign Commerce Committee. What was said then is
equally true today.

Aware of the Need

"The American Hospital Association is concerned with this Act because
it will vitally affect our own field of humanitarian endeavor. We were one
of the first organizations to offer our support to this legislation, and we have
followed its legislative progress closely, because we are keenly aware of the
need for the additional hospital facilities that may be provided under it, while
on the other hand we are apprehensive of the dangers involved if this program
is not wisely and carefully carried out. . . .

"The Hospital Survey and Construction Act proposes Federal grants-
in-aid to assist the states to build hospitals and health centers in communities
and areas where they are most needed. The nationwide program is to be
under the general supervision of the Surgeon General of the United States
Public Health Service, who will consult with a Federal Hospital Council of
experienced hospital authorities in establishing over-all standards and regulations and in approving state construction programs. The administration of
the program in each state will be carried out by authorized state governmental
agencies.

"The program has two purposes: First, to inventory existing hospitals
and survey the need for additional hospitals and develop programs for the
construction of such public and other nonprofit hospitals as will, in conjunction with existing facilities, afford the necessary physical facilities for
furnishing adequate hospital, clinic and similar services to all of the people
and, second, to construct public and other nonprofit hospitals in accordance
with such programs.

"In other words, the design of this legislation is to develop an *integrated*
system of hospitals and health centers that will make these facilities more
readily available to an increased number of people, especially to serve rural
or needy areas. The program is thus directly related to the health and welfare
of the nation. . . ."

The success of this Federal program is a direct result of the care with
which the original legislation was drafted to insure that certain principles
were followed. Intimately concerned with the revision of the legislation in
the Senate Committee were Senator Lister Hill of Alabama, a sponsor of the
legislation, and the late Senator Robert A. Taft of Ohio.

Rights of the States

Senator Taft's particular contribution to this legislation, much of which he personally rewrote, related to the specific delineation in the Act of the intent of the legislation with a minimum granting of latitude to the Federal administrative agency for the interpretation of Congressional intent. Second, he was insistent that within the carefully spelled out purposes of the Act that the states be given maximum administrative authority.

Further, the requirements that the states were to comply with in order to be granted funds by the Federal Government were clearly stated and the Act unequivocally orders the Federal administrative agency to grant funds where the states comply with these requirements.

There are other broad philosophical concepts in the Act which are not there by chance. The Act requires local participation as an earnest of assumption of local responsibility for the successful operation of the facility. The Act requires that each state shall inventory all facilities and develop a state plan to delineate those hospital facilities which should be constructed to bring present facilities up to a proper level.

Further, the state plan must order proposed construction projects by priority before granting funds, which insures that local applications in each state will receive attention on the basis of priority of need rather than on the basis of political pressures.

The Act insures that the Federal administrator will not act in an arbitrary manner, as it requires regulations and other administrative actions be approved by the Federal Hospital Council. Backing of the Federal Council also permits the Federal Administrator to administer the Act in an objective manner.

Inventory Avoids Duplication

The requirement for surveys is one of the most important features of the Act. For the first time, the Act provided for an actual inventory of all of the hospital resources within a state. . . . These studies and the ideal plan for hospitals which each state must prepare provided a guide for all construction, whether Federally aided or not. The plan avoids duplication and insures adequate facilities for all of the people within a state.

Much more could be said of the consistent and thoughtful study given to the preparation of this legislation. The Association participated in this study and has contributed to the very best of its ability not only in the preparation of the initial legislation and later amendments, but in its administration. We believe this is a proper function of our Association. We are, of course, proud of the accomplishments under the Act in bettering hospital care for the people of this country.

We are sure this Committee knows that this Act has been described as a model of local, state, and Federal partnership in meeting an important national need. We have endeavored, not only at the Federal level, but in states and localities, to stimulate and insure continuing participation in the successful accomplishment of these important objectives. . . .

Shortly after the enactment of this legislation in the spring of 1948, the Association with the approval of the Public Health Service held working conferences country-wide with representatives from official state agencies and hospital administrators representing state and local hospital associations.

Annually, the American Hospital Association has cooperated with the association of directors of the state agencies administering this Act in providing opportunity for them to meet and discuss not only the day-to-day problems of operation under the Hospital Survey and Construction Act, but all aspects of hospital care which might affect administration of this program to insure adequate hospital facilities country-wide.

In the past two years, two members of the Association staff made visits to every newly operating hospital in four states which had received Federal aid under this Act to study the success with which these hospitals were providing community service. . . . A third member of the staff recently surveyed a number of health centers being constructed in the Southern states. . . .

It is not the purpose of this testimony to delineate all of the efforts of the Association to insure the success of the program under the Hospital Survey and Construction Act. We are, however, endeavoring to establish for the Committee the responsible position that the Association has taken in order that our comments on the amendments may be evaluated in proper perspective. . . .

Comments on S. 2758

The broad purposes, as stated in S. 2758, are substantially the purposes as stated in (the Hill-Burton Act) covering the survey and construction of hospitals. We presume that the amendments are suggested for two purposes:

—To provide for survey and construction of facilities not now covered under present legislation, or

—To provide a higher priority in the construction of certain types of facilities, even though they may be provided for under present provisions of the Act.

Our comments will be first directed to the examination of the four classifications of facilities outlined . . . and defined in the amendments proposed. . . .

In general, there has been difficulty in the field from the standpoint of classifying hospitals because hospitals generally were not constructed on the basis of any over-all planning. They grew up to meet local needs. Individual hospitals were developed to utilize the medical manpower available and to facilitate the type of practice being carried on in a community.

Generally, there is no clear-cut line of demarcation between the physical plants of different types of hospitals, whether they be the typical community general hospital or for the care of mental illness, tuberculosis, or other chronic illnesses. The type of patient to be treated, whether requiring long-term or short-term care, and, among other factors, the size community, have all affected the gathering together of facilities in the individual hospital.

We find some hospitals primarily classified for the care of chronic illness with laboratory, x-ray and all the facilities which would be present in the usual general hospital. On the other hand, we find some small general hospitals with no more in the way of diagnostic equipment than might be expected to be found in some units for the care of chronic illness or even a nursing home.

The American Hospital Association, concerned with the lack of standardization of definition of hospitals and related institutions in January of 1953, called together 29 individuals experienced in hospital operations, hospital statistics, prepayment for hospital care, and hospital licensure, in both this country and Canada, including representatives of the Public Health Service and of the Census Bureau of the Federal Government. These individuals were invited because of their experience with the problems created by lack of definition of a type of hospital. . . .

The significant findings of the Conferences were the following definitions:

> *Hospitals and Related Institutions:* A hospital or related institution is any establishment offering services, facilities, and beds for use beyond 24 hours by two or more non-related individuals requiring diagnosis, treatment, or care for illness, injury, deformity, infirmity, abnormality, or pregnancy.
>
> The above broad definition was subdivided into hospitals, nursing and convalescent homes, and domiciliary institutions. These were defined as follows:
>
> > *Hospitals:* A hospital is any establishment offering services, facilities, and beds for use beyond 24 hours by two or more non-related individuals requiring diagnosis, treatment, or care for illness, injury, deformity, infirmity, abnormality, or pregnancy, and regularly making available at least (1) clinical laboratory services, (2) diagnostic x-ray services and (3) treatment facilities for

(a) surgery or (b) obstetrical care or (c) other definitive medical treatment of similar extent.

Nursing and Convalescent Homes: A nursing or convalescent home is any establishment offering services, facilities, and beds for use beyond 24 hours by two or more non-related individuals requiring treatment or care for illness, injury, deformity, infirmity, or abnormality, including at least room and board, personal services, and nursing care.

Domiciliary Institution: A domiciliary institution is any establishment offering services, facilities, and beds for use beyond 24 hours by two or more non-related individuals requiring room and board and personal services which they cannot render for themselves because of a deformity, infirmity, or abnormality.

Careful examination of these definitions will indicate that, without any question, an institution providing care for chronically ill patients may often be classified as a hospital. On the other hand, there will be many institutions, some of which are now called hospitals, which, because of lack of laboratory, x-ray, and intensive day-to-day medical care, would better be classified as a nursing and convalescent home.

We do not believe that the definition of "hospital for chronically ill" and "nursing home" in Senate Bill 2758 clearly indicates the type or classification of facility that the Bill is intended to benefit. In fact, we question that it will accomplish its purpose on the basis of such a differentiation. The basic problem is to provide more beds for the patients in need of long-term care, a group presently inadequately cared for and one which, because of the aging of the population, is increasing greatly in number.

The chronically ill need care in facilities of different types, and the grouping of these types of facilities is affected by the size of the community and various other factors.

On Needs of the Chronically Ill

Some chronically ill patients are in need of surgery and other intensive care which requires all of the diagnostic and treatment facilities of the general hospital. A second group of chronically ill patients may need only some of the facilities available in a general hospital, but for an extended period. For example, they may need physical therapy, occupational therapy, as well as periodic medical and diagnostic services.

Where a sufficient number of this second group of patients can be gathered together, they may be cared for in a special unit of a general hospital or in a chronic hospital, which will be somewhat less expensive to construct.

Such patients may need less nursing care, and operating costs will be less than for care of the typical acutely ill patient receiving short-term care in a general hospital.

A certain number of the chronically ill may not require extensive medical care and concomitant facilities, for example, patients with inoperable cancer or with disabling forms of heart trouble, and those badly crippled with arthritis. Such patients primarily need kindly attention, adequate nursing care, and some recreational facilities. Depending on the degree of acuteness of their illness, such patients may be cared for in a nursing home.

It is sometimes possible, where there are large numbers of chronically ill, as in a metropolitan community, to have facilities specially constructed and staffed for patients who are classified by degree of medical and nursing care required. Where this is possible, if the average patient needs less treatment and nursing care than is available in the average general hospital, the cost of the facility and the cost of maintenance of the facility decrease.

An example of the complexity of caring for patients, separated by classification, was illustrated in the discussions in the Classification Conference to which we have referred. That group generally agreed that most homes for the aged were nursing homes, as the aged who need only domiciliary care at time of admission to the home, during their period of residence inevitably became ill and required nursing care.

It is undoubtedly true that some homes for the aged would not have such nursing care available even when needed, and, indeed, it is one of the dangers of establishing institutions with limited care that patients who require more nursing care or more intensive medical supervision may suffer because the specialized facility is not equipped to meet their need. The conferees concluded that homes for the aged inevitably became nursing homes.

Danger in Varied Facilities

A particular danger of multiple grades of facilities for the care of long-term patients is the tendency for patients to remain in a facility having a relatively low level of care when professional services and technical facilities available in a higher type of facility are required for good care and rapid rehabilitation.

It is generally agreed that many patients receiving long-term care in nursing homes and in chronic hospitals might be rehabilitated or made more nearly independent of care if they had opportunity for intensive medical care in a general hospital. From this standpoint alone, construction of different types of facilities often may be inadvisable.

In the small community of the size in which most hospitals have been built under the Hospital Survey and Construction Act, it would be likely that the one hospital is for not only the patient acutely ill and in need of general short-term hospital care, but, in addition, the acutely ill chronic patient who might be cared for in a chronic hospital or in a nursing home.

The degree to which these patients might be wisely segregated in separate facilities from the standpoint of adequate care rendered on an economical basis has never been fully delineated. Strong argument can be made that, in such a small community, all patients except those needing solely nursing care with only occasional medical care might best be treated in one unit.

This interweaving of type of hospital and type of patient is an important factor in the hospital field. Many times, facilities are interchangeable. While beds built for long-term patients *can* be less expensive than similar facilities for the care of patients staying for a short time, this is not always true. As a practical matter, we have repeatedly heard of an older but usable facility which has given many years of service for the short-term patient being replaced by new physical facilities, with the older quarters being then used for patients needing less technical care for chronic illness.

Definition Questioned

We might, incidentally, call to your attention, the wording . . . "not acutely ill" as a part of the definition of patients to be admitted and cared for in a "nursing home." We believe this would not accomplish the intended purpose of the amendment. The patients generally cared for in nursing homes are not necessarily "not acutely ill." As a practical matter, many of them are acutely ill but are not in need of and cannot benefit from intensive medical care. For example, terminal cancer patients may be very acutely ill and require intensive nursing care even though the need of day-to-day medical care may be very limited.

We believe that without question the definition of a hospital in the Hospital Survey and Construction Act was intended to include the type of patient facility this Committee wishes to provide for in hospitals for the chronically ill and probably in nursing homes. In support of that, we call to the attention of the Committee the definition which is embodied in the present (Hill-Burton) Act:

> (e) the term 'hospital' (except as used in section 622 (a) and (b)) includes public health centers and general, tuberculosis, mental, chronic disease, and other types of hospitals, and related facilities, such as laboratories, out-patient departments, nurses' home and training facilities, and central service facilities operated in connection with hospitals, but does not include any hospital furnishing primarily domiciliary care;

Referring to the definition of hospitals and related institutions, which this Association's special conference committee developed, it will be seen that domiciliary institutions are defined and that they include the only types of facilities which were not intended under the original Act and do not appear to be contemplated under S. 2758. On the other hand, hospitals for chronic disease are clearly envisoned under the present Act.

The testimony of this Association on the Hospital Survey and Construction Act presented in 1946 to your Committee pointed out that facilities alone do not provide a complete health service for the American people. The Association, at that time, recommended that the Federal Government, in an act structured like the Hill-Burton program, stimulate the assumption at local and state level of the responsibility for adequate financing for the care of non-wage and low-income groups.

More Resources Needed

To a great extent, those persons suffering chronic illness will be found in the non-wage and low-income groups. Without more resources than have been made available to date through private charity and local welfare funds there can be no broad increase in the number of beds for chronic patients. We particularly call to your attention the exhaustive studies of the Commission on Financing of Hospital Care, an organization sponsored by the American Hospital Association, which, following an expenditure of $550,000, has so clearly delineated this difficulty.

We would suggest that this Committee request the Public Health Service to determine whether applications for beds for the care of chronic disease have been refused by state agencies for lack of adequate priority within each state.

Our experience . . . leads us to believe that this Committee will find that there have been almost no such refusals, that, on the contrary, most of the state agencies have done everything within their power to stimulate applications from government and nonprofit agencies to provide beds for the treatment of chronic illness, which they fully understand is an area of high priority of unmet need.

The main deterrent to the construction of chronic disease beds, in the opinion of this Association, will not be affected greatly by the provisions of S. 2758. Correction will only come if local, state, and Federal Government provide added funds for payment of care for those with chronic illness in order that there may be funds available to operate the type of facilities we are discussing.

Diagnostic or Treatment Centers

The over-all purpose of Title VI of the Public Health Service (Hill-Burton) Act is to provide facilities for the diagnosis and treatment of patients.

The Act (Public Law 725) clearly specifies that it includes "clinic" and "out-patient." There is not agreement in the hospital field or in the medical profession on the meaning of the terms "clinic" or "out-patient diagnostic facilities." These terms are used synonymously to mean various types of facilities for the care of ambulatory patients. At the present time, ambulatory patients are cared for, for the most part, in the offices of private physicians.

These physicians may be working solo or in group practice. There is a growing tendency to locate offices in connection with hospital facilities. Groups of doctors practicing medicine together often call these facilities "clinics." The term clinic is also used to indicate the out-patient facility operated by a hospital and also facilities operated by other agencies for the care of indigent and medically indigent patients. In fairly recent years a number of so-called "clinics" have been set up by hospitals for out-patient facilities for private patients.

All of the major studies in the hospital field in recent years and most recently, the studies of the Commission on the Financing of Hospital Care, point out the importance of utilizing out-patient services, whenever possible. This will often make in-patient admissions unnecessary. This would include diagnostic and treatment services in doctors' offices, which would avoid the heavy expense of in-patient admission.

One of the major criticisms of much prepayment of hospital and medical care is that it does not provide for out-patient services for diagnosis and treatment, with the result that great pressure is stimulated for in-patient admissions. Both the prepayment plans and the hospitals are fully aware of this situation and some experimentation is going on.

However, there is a great difference of opinion as to the advisability of providing out-patient services through health insurance because of the difficulties of controlling over-use and resulting heavy demand on the funds of the prepayment plan. Without careful study and planning, the whole prepayment movement could be damaged seriously.

Services and Facilities

From the first discussions of the Hospital Survey and Construction Act in 1945, there has been confusion in understanding the difference between providing services which the community may want and need as contrasted with solely the construction of facilities. Neither the Hospital Survey and Construction Act nor S. 2758 will do more than provide facilities. No funds are provided for maintenance, and the funds for facilities are granted only on application by the local community or the state.

New facilities are most significant and have certainly greatly improved the distribution of medical and hospital service, but the construction of facilities alone cannot force new concepts of medical care.

There is no question of the need for more adequate diagnostic services country-wide. Careful and accurate diagnosis is one of the most difficult and challenging day-to-day responsibilities of physicians. Physicians can be assisted in performing this service by having adequate x-ray and laboratory facilities and other diagnostic tools available.

However, facilities in themselves do not lead to the pooling of the knowledge of a group of specialists, and facilities for diagnosis should not be constructed to serve ambulatory patients unless there is assurance that they will be used by the medical profession in a community to provide services and are so badly needed as to justify Federal funds.

S. 2758 proposes the construction of diagnostic or treatment centers. However, such centers are not clearly defined. It would be difficult to know what facilities are to be inventoried within a state using the definitions in S. 2758, or to establish necessary standards without a clearer definition.

Medical Cooperation Vital

All doctors' offices are diagnostic and treatment centers as defined in S. 2758. Hospitals are diagnostic and treatment centers, and, in that sense, the present Hospital Survey and Construction Act is providing such centers.

It is not clear in this bill just what out-patient facilities are to be given the priority of a separate classification with an appropriation of $20,000,000 per year. If private-pay out-patient facilities, as part of a hospital, are to be built to care for patients who now go to doctors' private offices or to the offices of private groups of doctors, then there will need to be developed a new type of plan of medical practice in many communities. This will need the cooperation of the medical profession or it cannot succeed. The bill provides that such facilities must be sponsored by nonprofit or governmental agencies and not a clinic owned and operated by physicians.

Some consideration has been given to the advisability of constructing facilities in outlying communities which might be used by one or two physicians practicing in such a community. Such a facility would provide, at a minimum, x-ray and laboratory equipment and technical personnel for the tests needed by these physicians. In most instances, it would be presumed that physicians in such communities could provide the minimum type of equipment and facilities needed from their own resources. However, in sparsely settled communities, the provision of such facilities by the town or county might encourage a physician to practice in such a setting and give him the assistance of diagnostic or treatment facilities needed for good medical care.

The Kellogg Foundation, in some of the western counties in the lower peninsula of Michigan, has experimented with the construction of such facilities. It is our information that these facilities, once provided, have not been easy to operate. In such a small community, it is difficult and expensive to obtain and retain the x-ray and laboratory technicians needed for good quality of care. Physicians who are specialists in radiology and pathology are needed to supervise the work of the technicians and interpret the diagnostic tests for the physicians. Such professional services are very difficult to secure in an outlying community.

Expensive to Operate

Under the present Hospital Survey and Construction Act, a number of states have constructed "community clinics" which were equipped with minimal x-ray and laboratory equipment and a few beds for patients needing emergency care who could not be transported to a larger hospital. However, very few states have constructed such facilities as they are expensive to operate, particularly so if adequate quality of service is to be maintained.

If the "community clinic," with a few beds, or with no beds but only simple diagnostic facilities, is contemplated for construction as a "diagnostic or treatment center," we would raise questions as to whether such facilities should be given the encouragement implicit in the special appropriation of $20 million and the priority provided by S. 2758.

We suggest that the development of diagnostic and treatment facilities in areas where there are hospitals, which are not to be in any way associated with these hospitals, should be studied very carefully. It would appear to be contrary to the whole progressive development of health services in this country and not in keeping with the economies which must be practiced in behalf of the public.

S. 2758 recommends that each state, with funds provided for surveys, inventory all "diagnostic or treatment centers" and provide a plan under regulations to be promulgated by the Surgeon General for a sufficient number of such units to serve the entire population. We believe that all of the comments we have listed above raise particular questions as to the practicality of an inventory and state plan required by S. 2758 for this type of facility.

Rehabilitation Facilities

We are in complete agreement that not enough is being done to rehabilitate the sick and injured. Nevertheless, that is the primary function of all physicians and all hospitals and they are most conscious of that responsibility. The question is, what new type of facility emphasis is needed?

There are rehabilitation centers connected with hospitals in this country which are doing an outstanding job. In many respects, the difficulty is not a lack of facilities or funds for facilities but rather a lack of trained physicians and other personnel interested in the special medical and psychological problems needed to carry rehabilitation to levels not reached at present. Success has been very much a matter of the dynamic leadership of a few specially trained physicians.

We recognize the difficulties involved in making a state plan for the type of rehabilitation facility defined in S. 2758. In many areas of the country the proposal to build such facilities separate from rather than in relationship to general hospitals will be seriously questioned.

Survey and State Plan

S. 2758 provides for a survey of the four categories: diagnostic or treatment centers, hospitals for the chronically ill, rehabilitation facilities, and nursing homes. The original Act required that all states survey all facilities defined as hospitals, including many of the facilities here contemplated. It would seem that a new state plan solely for four classifications of facilities is very cumbersome, and that, with a new Federal appropriation for inventorying and making a plan, it would be necessary to inventory all hospital facilities as well as these four separate categories which are so unclearly defined.

The basic Act requires that the state shall periodically revise its state plan. In many instances, it has been some time since the states have had sufficient resources to carefully re-inventory all hospitals. It would appear that it would be wise, in appropriating funds, to require a re-inventory of all hospitals, including the four categories suggested in S. 2758.

A new plan of all hospitals facilities would be helpful in every state and would insure a re-evaluation of all priorities for all the different classifications of hospitals which may be aided in construction under Public Law 725.

The proposals in S. 2758 that states match survey funds with 50 per cent state matching money and that each state be granted a minimum of $25,000 of Federal matching money seem wise.

General Comments

Earlier, it was suggested that the purposes of S. 2758 must be either one or both of the following:

—To provide for survey and construction of facilities not now covered under present legislation, or

—To provide a higher priority in the construction of certain types of facilities, even though they may be under present provisions of the Act.

Considering S. 2758 in relationship to these purposes, the following comments are offered:

1. Chronic hospitals are clearly eligible for a construction grant under Public Law 725.
2. Nursing homes may be eligible under the Act and could be brought under it by regulation, even though that has not been true up to the present time.
3. All hospitals often care for patients who are chronically ill, and certainly all facilities for the long-term care of patients should be planned in an integrated system as all classifications very much interweave and are inter-related and may wisely all be provided for in some communities in one unit.
4. The categorization of appropriations for chronic hospitals and nursing homes, while admittedly giving a priority, may lead to separate construction or may prevent the construction of other facilities which will generally contribute to the care of chronic patients.
5. No type of diagnostic or treatment facility for ambulatory patients seems to warrant a priority or need for Federal construction money which would justify a separate definition of facility and the priority given by a separate appropriation.
6. Categorization of facilities in five types which are but variations of hospitals will tend toward the construction of separate types of facilities where one facility might much better serve multiple purposes.
7. Separate appropriations for each of the types of facilities authorized . . . will result in a very small allocation of money to each state and may well not be applied for in every state by any eligible applicant during the period for which it is available.
8. Two separate state plans for facilities which can often not be wisely separated seems cumbersome and would better be handled on one survey.

As we have tried to visualize the problems involved in carrying out the intent of S. 2758, we are concerned with the difficulties involved in establishing priority for the various facilities to be constructed. The funds as stipulated must be maintained separately, and it will not be possible to shift funds from one category to another in the event it seems desirable to do so.

If it is found through experience that there is little or no demand for funds in a state for one or more types of facilities suggested in the proposed amendments, it would be well to allow the expenditure of these funds for other needed facilities. This would avoid the accumulation of especially allocated funds and major criticism of the over-all program. All of the facilities envisoned under the present Act and S. 2758 are believed to contribute to better health care in each state.

With all the reservations as to the wisdom of the technical approach to accomplish the stated objectives in S. 2758, and with a definite impression that without correction wise administration will be difficult, it is suggested that, at a minimum, the following amendment would be helpful in correcting certain of the difficulties, though it is realized that such an amendment would reduce the planned priority:

> "Sums allotted to a state for a fiscal year and remaining unobligated at the end of such year shall remain available to such state for the purpose for the first six months of the next fiscal year (and for such six months only) in addition to the sums allotted to such state for such next fiscal year, and thereafter shall be available to such state for obligation during the next six months for construction of any projects eligible under part C of this title."

We believe that a more effective accomplishment of the objectives might be attained by the following amendments to Public Law 725, the Hospital Survey and Construction Act:

1. Define and include nursing homes.
2. Define and include rehabilitation facilities.
3. Assign priority to all facilities for the care of long-term patients with the exception of those for the care of mental illness or tuberculosis.
4. Require a re-inventory and re-survey providing additional funds for Federal matching on a 50 per cent basis with a minimum allotment to each state of $25,000.

President Eisenhower, in his health message to Congress, recognized the need for additional facilities and the major problem of the care of the chronically ill, and the ever-growing number of aged in the population. He has suggested that the Hill-Burton grants-in-aid program be utilized as a basis for working out solutions to these problems.

The American Hospital Association is fully in accord with the President, both as to the seriousness of the problems and the need for a solution as well as the wisdom of considering the Hill-Burton Act as a means of assisting in finding the answers. We are, however, greatly concerned that no amendment weaken a highly successful and workable program or fail to achieve the successful results which S. 2758 is planned to accomplish.

The Hospital Survey and Construction Act was a non-partisan proposal. The American Hospital Association is a non-partisan organization. We believe that the health goals for the American people enunciated by President Eisenhower and by the sponsors of S. 2758 are universally acceptable, but that their successful achievement is more likely through modification by changes which we are prepared to submit to the Committee. . . .

We wish to reiterate our strong desire to cooperate with this Committee and with the Administration in the development of legislation to further meet the health needs of the American people along sound lines.

Excerpts from Interrogation of Mr. Bugbee by Members of the Senate Subcommittee

Senator Lister Hill (interrupting Mr. Bugbee's description of AHA support of the Hospital Survey and Construction Act). You speak of your support of that act. I think you are very modest. You and I know the inspiration which you gave, the thought you gave, to bringing that act into being and, of course, you recall how you sat in day after day and week after week with Senator Taft and myself and other members of the subcommittee as we wrote that legislation. You, along with the representatives of the Public Health Service, sat right in our executive session when we were trying to write that act, and get the best act we could.

Mr. Bugbee. I appreciate, Senator Hill, that recognition of the fact that we have followed it very closely, and it gives me an opportunity to express our appreciation of the time and effort that you have given to the act, too, through the years to make it an effective program.

Senator Hill. One of the most important things was writing into this act the fact it was to be administered and operated at the state level and not from Washington.

Mr. Bugbee. Yes, sir.

Senator Hill. Isn't that true?

Mr. Bugbee. It is true, and it was fundamental to the Association's support of the legislation.

Senator Hill. The Association insisted on that and met with a ready response from both Senator Taft and myself; isn't that true?

Mr. Bugbee. That is correct, sir.

*   *   *

Senator Hill. In other words, you not only sat in and helped all you could in writing this act, but you and your Association through the years have kept in touch with its operation and have kept what we might call a continuing study; is that right?

Mr. Bugbee. We have tried to do so.

Senator Hill. Of the act and its operations and results and effects?

Mr. Bugbee. That is correct.

Senator Hill. Is that correct, sir?

Mr. Bugbee. That is correct, and it is very complicated legislation aimed at meeting an important need; and, to the degree we could, we have tried to be helpful.

*   *   *

Senator Hill. We have a declaration in the budget as to the $62 million which would be authorized under this bill, but, of course, that is not a budget estimate as yet, and it couldn't be a budget estimate until the legislation was passed, but we have a budget estimate for the next fiscal year of only $50 million. Now, isn't this true: that most of the things this bill would provide in the way of construction can be done under the original act?

Mr. Bugbee. Yes.

Senator Hill. Is that correct?

Mr. Bugbee. I would think most of the types of facilities could be, Senator, though I believe there may be merit to making very clear that they are included.

Senator Hill. I understand, but most of them could. For instance, a chronic hospital—

Senator Hill. Yes.

Mr. Bugbee. There is no question—

Senator Hill. Chronic hospital is written out, and even the word "clinic" appears here, and out-patient departments for ambulatory patients, and those sorts of things.

Now, what I am thinking of is, if we are only able to use $50 million, have only $50 million for next year, or most of next year, what will that do to the program we have been carrying on now since about 1947, or thereabouts?

Mr. Bugbee. Well, I think the 50 million alone would be less than could be spent wisely—it is, of course, the smallest appropriation that has been made under the basic act. On the other hand, as we have suggested in our testimony, we are hoping that the suggested supplemental appropriation will be made for the broad purposes of the act, with whatever additional priority need be given the types of facilities described in 2758.

Senator Hill. You would hope, then, that more than $50 million would be available this coming fiscal year?

Mr. Bugbee. Our Association would certainly hope so on the basis of the need for the construction of facilities.

Senator Hill. Did your surveys, the conferences you had here a year ago and other surveys that you made, show there is still a very great need for general hospitals, mental hospitals, and tuberculosis hospitals, as well as chronic hospitals?

Mr. Bugbee. The Public Health Service, of course, has the summary of the figures developed by the state plans, as to the degree of need for beds, but the four conferences held country-wide approached that same problem and there was much discussion as to the backlog of applications which could not be met out of the appropriations up to that period, and without exception the states reported that they had multiple applications for hospitals in areas where they were needed.

Senator Hill. According to the testimony we had yesterday from the Public Health Service, there is a need if we continue through the Hospital Survey and Construction Act to meet those needs, the needs we have since the act was passed, or certainly since about '47, for almost 600,000 additional general, mental and tubercular beds and some 240,000 chronic disease beds.

Mr. Bugbee. Senator, it is a very substantial number. I would not be prepared to confirm those figures as necessarily exactly right, but we are far enough away from having the needed beds so that it has not been a question of worrying about national over-construction.

Senator Hill. I sit as a member of the Appropriations Committee and I have heard a good deal of testimony. I know surely there is a crying need not only for general hospital beds, but for beds for mental patients; isn't that true?

Mr. Bugbee. That is correct, sir.

Senator Hill. Isn't it true that so many of our mental hospitals and institutions for the mentally ill are terribly crowded and inadequate today?

Mr. Bugbee. Certainly the figures would prove that, and from what knowledge I have that is certainly true.

Senator Hill. Mr. Chairman, I have here a letter which just came this morning . . . written by Mr. Clay H. Dean, director of the Hospital Planning Division of the Department of Public Health, Montgomery, Alabama. He is the man immediately in charge of the hospital construction under the Hospital Survey and Construction Act and, among other things, I note—as I say, I haven't had time to read the letter in full, but I notice—this:

> We also feel the requirement for matching survey funds would work a definite hardship on Alabama and other states whose legislatures do not meet until 1955.

> Since the Legislature does not meet until the summer of 1955, it would be impossible to get any state funds for matching purposes.

That is for the survey.

I just bring this out because it poses the problem I had sought to pose in the earlier questions. It takes time to get this job done, just as it took several years, as I recall, before the last state finally met the conditions of the survey and of the state plan and having that plan approved in order to come in and start construction. Wasn't that true?

Mr. Bugbee. That is my memory of it, Senator; yes.

Senator Hill. Mr. Bugbee, you stated:

> We believe that the health goals for the American people enunciated by President Eisenhower and by the sponsors of S. 2758 are universally acceptable, but that their successful achievement is more likely through modification by changes which we are prepared to submit to the committee.

Mr. Chairman, I would like to ask, if it is agreeable with the Chairman, if Mr. Bugbee may, not at this time, but in the next day or two, submit those changes to the committee.

Senator Purtell. We would be very happy to receive them, Senator.

Mr. Bugbee. I shall do so.

* * *

Senator Hill. On the record now.

I do want to commend Mr. Bugbee for his very excellent, fine, analytical, helpful statement here this morning.

Mr. Bugbee. Thank you very much.

Senator Purtell. I want to thank you, too, Mr. Bugbee . . . and it may be—I know you are most anxious to cooperate, as you always have been—the staff of this committee may wish to consult with you at a later time, and I know you will extend whatever you can in the way of help.

APPENDIX G

Foreword to the Report of the Commission on Financing of Hospital Care*

This volume presents the report of the Commission on Financing of Hospital Care on *Factors Affecting the Costs of Hospital Care*. This is one of the three volumes being published by the Commission and contains the detailed study report on factors which affect the cost of hospital care and the recommendations of the Commission as formulated and adopted at meetings held in October, November, and December 1953.

Out of concern for better understanding of the current problems involved in financing modern hospital care at the lowest possible cost to the public, the American Hospital Association sponsored the organization of the Commission on Financing of Hospital Care. The Commission, an independent non-governmental agency, was established in late November 1951 to function for a two-year period.

Funds for the Commission's study program were made available by grants from the Blue Cross Commission of the American Hospital Association, Health Information Foundation, John Hancock Mutual Life Insurance Company, W. K. Kellogg Foundation, Michigan Medical Service, Milbank Memorial Fund, National Foundation for Infantile Paralysis, and Rockefeller Foundation. A total of $556,000 was contributed by these organizations to the American Hospital Association to finance the work of the Commission.

The task undertaken by the thirty-four persons constituting the Commission was two-fold: "to study the costs of providing adequate hospital services and to determine the best systems of payment for such services."

In fulfillment of the objective "to study the costs of providing adequate hospital services," this report of the Commission on *Factors Affecting the Costs of Hospital Care* is being published. In this volume the Commission has been concerned with the rise in hospital expenditures that has accompanied the increase in the quantity and quality of hospital services received by the people of the United States. The Commission has addressed itself to such questions as the following:

How much of the increased cost of hospitalization is due to expanded service?

---

*Taken from *Financing Hospital Care in the United States,* vol. 1, *Factors Affecting the Costs of Hospital Care* (New York: Blakiston, 1954), pp. ix–xii. Used with permission of McGraw-Hill Co., successors of Blakiston Company, Inc., the original publishers.

How much is due to higher costs of labor and materials?

By what means may costs of care to the public be held to a minimum without impairing quality of services?

In fulfillment of the objective "to determine the best systems of payment for such services," two volumes are being published: *Prepayment and the Community* and *Financing Hospital Care for Non-wage and Low-income Groups.*

In its evaluation of voluntary prepayment the Commission has been concerned with the amount of protection available today and the actual amount purchased by the public and with the extension of prepayment coverage to groups now without protection. Special attention has been given in the report on *Prepayment and the Community* to the problem of economical use of funds paid by the public to prepayment agencies.

In the report on *Financing Hospital Care for Non-wage and Low-income Groups* the Commission recognized that there are many persons who, for reason of inability to work or for reason of marginal income, are unable to pay for hospital care at the time of illness or to budget for care through prepayment. Adequate financing of hospital care for these persons is a problem of major significance to many communities as well as to many hospitals.

The Commission's task has been a difficult one, for there were no easy solutions to the problems studied by the Commission. Each community and each hospital has its particular problems. The Commission members, individually and as members of study committees, have devoted many hours to the assigned task. The Commission's recommendations are the subject of this summary report. It is our hope that the Commission's reports will make a constructive contribution to the thinking of the people of the United States.

What may prove to be one of the most important effects of the Commissions' many meetings and extensive discussions is not fully reflected in the reports to the public. During the two years of our deliberations persons representing various points of view and fields of interest have spent many hours together discussing the questions about which policy decisions needed to be made. The broad base of agreement reached by the Commission has required an understanding and appreciation of many different points of view. Thinking through the problems confronting the Commission has helped to bring closer together divergent points of view. The virtual unanimity* of thinking as expressed in the Commission's recommendations is not only

---

*Commission member E. J. Faulkner dissented with respect to one recommendation and Commission members Stanley H. Ruttenberg and Boris Shishkin filed general statements taking issue with the scope of the report and with several of the positions taken.

Lewis L. Strauss has requested that, although familiar with the study reports, his concurrence should be considered of general character since he has been unable, because of the pressure of his national security responsibilities, to participate in committee and Commission meetings in recent months.

gratifying but has undoubtedly established a sounder foundation on which to build in the future.

The study reports, in their detail, cover areas in which all points of view could not be entirely reconciled and, for that reason, reflect a consensus. Also, it has not been possible for the study reports to receive the same concentrated attention of all the Commission members which was devoted to the recommendations.

Inherent in the Commission's recommendations to the public is the need for further study and examination of the problems discussed. In every community and in every state, representatives of the public, of hospitals, of physicians, and of prepayment and other health and welfare agencies will need to test the Commission's recommendations in the light of their own particular problems. The lasting effectiveness of the Commission's work is dependent on such community action. We believe that our recommendations provide a basis for organized community action.

I wish to express, on behalf of the entire Commission, appreciation for the cooperation given us by the panel of consultants who met with the committees and who, in other ways, gave us assistance. Also, special acknowledgement should be given to the various organizations and groups, and the several thousand hospital administrators, who supplied us with information and generously gave us help in countless other ways. Particularly, I wish to express appreciation for the indispensable assistance given us by the American Hospital Association, the American Medical Association, the Blue Cross Commission of the American Hospital Association, organizations representing the insurance industry, and the Social Security Administration and the Public Health Service of the Department of Health, Education and Welfare.

My comments on the Commission's work would be incomplete unless I made special reference to the contributions of the staff to the successful conclusion of the study. Staff members often worked under trying and difficult circumstances. Their task was not made easier by the fact that circumstances presented the Commission with three different directors in the course of the project.

Graham Davis was the first director of the Commission's work. During the year he served in this capacity, the Commission was organized, key staff members were recruited, a general pattern of its work program was outlined, and work on the project was formally inaugurated. When Mr. Davis resigned because of ill health, Dr. Arthur C. Bachmeyer was enthusiastically selected as the choice of the Commission for his successor.

Special reference should be made to Dr. Bachmeyer's contributions to the Commission study. Long before the Commission was actually established, he worked on plans for the study. At the first meeting of the Commission, of which he was a member, he was of great assistance in setting up the necessary procedures for activating the study program. As a member of the Executive Committee and during the five months he served as Director of Study until his death on May 22, 1953, which occurred immediately following a meeting of the Commission, his firm and experienced judgment was a major factor in many decisions which were made. I feel that the energy and time he devoted to the Commission's program were an added burden that he should not have assumed, but it was something that he wanted to do and he gave to it, as he did to all things, his best efforts. Our studies reflected his wisdom and his concern that the people of the United States have the highest standards of hospital care at the lowest possible cost.

John Hayes was drafted at approximately the time of his retirement from the superintendency of Lenox Hill Hospital in New York to fill the gap created by Dr. Bachmeyer's untimely death. Mr. Hayes' unusual understanding of hospital problems, reflecting his long experience as a successful hospital administrator, was of material assistance to the Commission during the latter months of the Commission's work when recommendations were being formulated and the final report was being compiled. Largely through his efforts, the Commission's timetable was maintained, in spite of the two interruptions in continuity of the directorship of the program. He contributed greatly as a counselor to both Commission and staff members.

From the beginning and throughout the entire period of the Commission's efforts, Harry Becker served as Associate Director of Study. He developed basic survey procedures, undertook responsibility for major sections of the report and provided continuity to the work program. His energy and stimulating guidance were reflected in the dedication and unremitting efforts of the entire staff.

On behalf of the Commission, I wish to express appreciation and gratitude for the professional assistance which the entire staff provided to the Commission in its analysis of voluminous data presented in an objective manner.

In this report the Commission presents for the consideration of the American people its studies and its recommendations based on such studies. It is our hope that the material contained in this volume will be of help to the people of the United States in better understanding the various factors that affect the cost of hospital care.

Gordon Gray
Chairman
Chapel Hill, NC

APPENDIX H

Preface to the Report of the
Commission on Financing of Hospital Care*

The establishment of the Commission on Financing of Hospital Care in November 1951 as an independent, non-governmental agency was a natural sequel to the work of the Commission on Hospital Care, which made its report to the public in 1947 after a two-year study. The twenty-two members of the Commission on Hospital Care, representing a cross-section of public interest, were responsible for the nation's first comprehensive study of the general hospital. That study was primarily concerned with an evaluation of the general hospital's function as a community institution and its role in the care of all types of illness.

In its 181 principles and recommendations the Commission on Hospital Care established a guide for the provision of more effective hospital care. The soundness of these recommendations is evidenced by their widespread application today in hospital administration and community planning for hospital services.

Thus that Commission, sponsored by the American Hospital Association, gave the leadership which, in large measure, resulted in the planned and orderly manner in which communities and states have approached their post-war hospital improvement and expansion programs. The Commission, however, recognized in its report and recommendations that a subsequent study program would be needed to analyze the various problems associated with financing the care which hospitals are dedicated to provide. Lack of facilities and time did not then permit the Commission on Hospital Care to conduct the companion study on the financing of hospital services.

Within a year after the report of the Commission on Hospital Care was made public, the American Hospital Association organized its Council on Prepayment Plans and Hospital Reimbursement. At its first meeting, with Dr. E. Dwight Barnett as chairman and Maurice Norby, who was Associate Director of the Commission on Hospital Care, as secretary, the Council stated that it was unrealistic to expand hospital facilities without considering methods for financing the wider scope and higher quality of services being

*Taken from *Financing Hospital Care in the United States,* vol. 1, *Factors Affecting the Costs of Hospital Care* (New York: Blakiston, 1954), pp. xiii–xv. Used with permission of McGraw-Hill Co., successors of Blakiston Company, Inc., the original publishers.

made available. This recognition of the concern of both the public and the hospital with the problem of financing hospital care was the first of a series of steps which culminated in the formation of the Commission on Financing of Hospital Care.

In 1950 the Board of Trustees of the American Hospital Association directed that a planning committee be established to outline a specific study program on the broad problem of financing hospital care. This planning committee recommended the creation of an independent agency *"to study the costs of providing adequate hospital services and to determine the best systems of payment for such services."* The planning committee's recommendations were adopted by the Board of Trustees, and the Association's president at that time, Dr. Charles F. Wilinsky, and its executive director, George P. Bugbee, were authorized to proceed with the details of fund raising and organization of this independent group. Gordon Gray, President of the University of North Carolina, was asked to serve as chairman of the new study group, which was named by the Commission on Financing of Hospital Care. On November 28, 1951, the Commission held its first meeting in Washington, D.C., and accepted its assigned task of preparing a report to the public on financing hospital care.

Graham Davis was designated director of the program. On his resignation in December 1952, for reasons of ill health, Dr. Arthur C. Bachmeyer assumed responsibility for direction of the Commission's program. Dr. Bachmeyer, who had been director of the earlier Commission on Hospital Care, was a member of the Commission's Executive Committee from its inception and had actively assisted the staff in setting up the study program. Immediately following a meeting of the Commission on May 22, 1953, at which the results of Dr. Bachmeyer's five months of intensive work with the staff in planning the study reports were reviewed and acted upon by the Commission, he died suddenly at the Washington National Airport. John H. Hayes, who for twenty-seven years was administrator of Lenox Hill Hospital, New York City, and a past president of the American Hospital Association, interrupted his retirement plans in July 1953, to complete the task undertaken, with particular responsibility for the studies concerned with the costs of hospital care.

Harry Becker was appointed the Commission's Associate Director in December 1951 and has served throughout the entire period of the study.

From the beginning it has been the Commission's desire to direct its attention primarily to those areas of immediate concern to:

1. The public;
2. Hospital administrators and hospital boards;
3. Prepayment agencies;

4. Other interested groups.

During the early months of the study a series of five regional conferences was held throughout the nation to formulate the Commission's major areas of study in consultation with persons who, from day to day, were directly concerned with the provision of community hospital services. Around the conference tables sat physicians, hospital administrators, nurses, workers in health, welfare, and community services, and representatives of industry, labor, and the general public.

The conference participants posed questions which they thought, from their own local community experience, should receive Commission attention.

More than 400 questions were presented to the Commission at the regional conferences. These questions were classified and reviewed by the staff, by a special technical advisory committee appointed by the Commission, and by the Commission itself to determine as objectively as possible the definitive areas in which intensive study by the Commission would be most helpful to states and communities. The areas of greatest interest, as established by analysis of the conference questions, were adopted by the Commission in April 1952. They were:

1. *Voluntary prepayment*—an evaluation of its effectiveness for the public, for the hospital, and for the community, and proposed steps for strengthening prepayment in the public interest.

2. *Improved methods of financing hospital care for groups unable to afford prepayment or in other ways to pay for care*—a determination of means for assuring hospitals and communities of an adequate and orderly provision for meeting the costs of hospital care for persons unable to pay for care.

3. *Why does hospital care cost what it does?*—an appraisal of the elements of hospital cost and an evaluation of various methods for control of hospital costs.

Chairman Gordon Gray, with the approval of the full Commission, appointed the Commission membership to three working committees, with each Committee assigned one of the three study areas. A member of the Executive Committee served as chairman of each working committee and a staff member was assigned as committee secretary. In the spring and summer of 1952 the committees outlined their study program in consultation with the assigned staff personnel and with a panel of consultants appointed to work with each of the committees. Each committee developed its study program in the manner that seemed most appropriate for the particular study area.

During the fall of 1953 the committees met to review their study reports and to formulate proposed principles, considerations, and recommendations for submission to the Commission. The full Commission devoted two days to each committee's report. It used the reports as background for the formulation of principles and the adoption of recommendations.

APPENDIX I

Excerpts from C. Rufus Rorem's Report on Group Hospitalization to the American Hospital Association's 1933 Annual Convention*

As long as hospital bills are unpredictable as to amount, people will complain about them. It is important to silence a popular, present-day criticism of hospitals by explaining that hospitals are efficiently managed or that hospital bills are reasonable. . . .

The function of group hospitalization is not to make easier the problems of the individual and of the public who own the hospitals. . . .

Group hospitalization, by definition, is a device by which people pool their resources by fixed and equal periodic payments, the total being used for the payment of hospital services to members who require such care. Group hospitalization plans are not primarily for the benefits of the hospitals . . . but for the benefits of people.

The experience of the last several years . . . has demonstrated that the people can and will budget their hospital bills if given an opportunity. . . .

The council on community relations and administrative practice (following the action of the trustees endorsing the principle of group hospitalization) has specified certain characteristics (or criteria, or essentials, or points) which would characterize successful and ethical group hospitalization plans. Let us examine them now and test their validity, both by logic and by experience.

The first principle was that a group hospitalization plan should place primary emphasis upon public benefit and secondary emphasis upon hospital finance. . . . Group hospitalization is a method by which people pay their bills, not a product to be sold by a hospital executive, although the public will require the active cooperation of hospital directors in outlining the administering of their plans. . . .

The second essential was that group hospitalization shall be limited to hospital services. The term "hospital service" was purposely not defined, but it means merely that the plan should include only those services which the hospital regularly provides. . . .

As one man said to me in Boston: "What is the objection to including

---

*Rorem presented this report in his capacity as consultant to the AHA's council on community relations and administrative practice.

the physician's bill?" I merely replied, "I have no objection, and the public has no objection. Whenever physicians want medical bills included, some arrangement can be made."

The third criterion was that it should involve participation by all hospitals of standing in the community. This policy avoids competition among individual hospitals.

The fourth point was that plans should be economically sound. The rates should be sufficient to cover the costs of services and payments to the hospitals, and payments to the hospitals should be sufficient to remunerate them for the care rendered on behalf of sponsorship.

The fifth point was that group hospitalization should have community sponsorship. A group hospitalization plan should be established for the people and by the people. The initiative may come from hospital superintendents, professional groups, industrialists, social workers, unions, or people in the various trades.

The sixth and last characteristic is that it should be promoted on a noncommercial basis. No intermediary group should be allowed to take the position of promoter or sponsor with the idea of a net profit or a net loss made from the success of this plan.

[These criteria were ultimately developed into the standards which served as the basis for formal approval of Blue Cross plans by the AHA.]

APPENDIX J

Excerpts from C. Rufus Rorem's Report on Group Hospitalization to the American Hospital Association's 1934 Annual Convention*

Group hospitalization is a way of putting hospital care in the family budget. It is not primarily a way of putting money into the hospital budget. The public has no particular interest in problems of hospital finance, but the ordinary citizen has a lively interest in the problem of his personal finance. Group hospitalization is a way by which people pay hospital bills and not a way by which the hospital pays its own bills. . . .

Group hospitalization applies the principle of insurance, of removing the uncertainty of a large hospital bill and replacing it with the certainty of a small hospital bill. . . . No one can tell when he is going to be sick or what his sickness will cost him. If he could tell, there would be no discussion of group hospitalization. . . .

The average cost of medical care is not high; the average cost of hospital care is not high. . . . But if a bill of $65 or $165 is presented to a patient, it is no comfort to the patient to know that hospitals are well managed. He is interested only in some plan by which he can pay the hospital bill. . . .

It is sometimes said that if people would be as careful about budgeting their hospital bills as they are about keeping up their installments on the radio and automobile, we would not have all this talk about the cost of hospital care. This is true. But the individual's sickness is unpredictable. On the other hand, the sickness of a group of individuals can be predicted with reasonable accuracy. . . . It is possible for a group of people to do what is impossible for an individual, namely, to place hospital care in the family budget. . . .

Group hospitalization, as officially endorsed by the American Hospital Association, applies to hospital bills only. The question of the inclusion of the physician's fee is often raised by members of the general public as well

---

*Rorem presented this report in his capacity as consultant to the AHA's Council on Administrative Practice and Community Relations. It is reprinted from Rorem's *A Quest for Certainty: Essays on Health Care Economics, 1930–1970* (Ann Arbor: Health Administration Press, 1982), pp. 83–85.

as by physicians. The question may be answered this way: "Whenever physicians want their fees included it will be done."

One-third of the population requiring hospital care for acute illnesses receives it at government expense or through philanthropy. In 1929 not more than five percent of the people were receiving relief for food, clothes, and shelter, yet a third of the people were receiving relief in the form of hospitalization. The standards of ability to pay for hospitalization are different from those for ability to buy economic commodities which can be budgeted. . . .

How far down in the economic scale must you go before you find a person who cannot pay a hospital bill? One-third of the population is now receiving free hospital care. Who cannot afford to subscribe to a group hospitalization plan at five, six, seven, or eight dollars a year? Only the unemployed. . . .

An acquaintance of mine who is on "relief" explains that he now rolls his own cigarettes. In this way he makes a 5-cent package last two days. Five cents every two days, two and a half cents a day, is about $9.15 a year—more than the rate for a group hospitalization plan providing semi-private accommodations. . . .

I do not say that people should give up tobacco for hospitalization. I merely say that hospital care could be budgeted (and should be budgeted) along with sweets, chewing gum, and tobacco, without the aid of governments or philanthropy. . . .

The following characteristics of a group hospitalization plan are set forth as desirable features from the points of view of public welfare and hospital support:

1. Nonprofit sponsorship and control.

2. Provision of initial working capital and reserves . . . from contributions or loans, rather than from accumulation of subscriptions.

3. Lowest possible annual subscription rates. A low annual rate is desirable even if it requires limiting the subscribers' benefits to the use of the lower-priced hospital accommodations.

4. Widest possible coverage as to types of subscribers. Plans should ultimately be developed for membership by employees and families: large groups, small groups, individuals, women, children, unemployed dependents.

5. Greatest possible coverage as to special diagnostic and treatment services.

6. Minimum of exclusions as to cases accepted for hospitalization. Exclusions should be dictated by facts as to other coverage, such

as workmen's compensation or governmental provision for mental, tuberculosis, or communicable diseases cases. Subscription rates may well include services for maternity cases, without extra charge, or at discounts from regular rates.

7. Free choice of hospital service should be available in all hospitals of standing in the community, and to some degree in other communities.

8. Adequate payments to group-hospitalization employees, on a basis which will not jeopardize quality of service.

9. A uniform schedule for remunerating hospitals for the same types and classes of service. This may be accomplished by an all-inclusive day rate, or a schedule for each type of service, such as board and room, operating room, laboratory, X-ray, etc. The maximum liability of the association . . . should be stated in the agreement.

10. Admission for hospital care only upon recommendation of a medical practitioner and for treatment only while under his care.

11. Definite statement as to liability of participating hospitals or the hospital service association when "specific performance" of service is impossible.

12. Compliance with existing state legislation covering hospital service associations and insurance companies.

Interest in the periodic payment plan for the purchase of hospital care continues to grow. The widespread discussion among hospital executives which began two years ago, and which resulted in the official endorsement of group hospitalization by the American Hospital Association, has now spread to the medical profession and the general public.

Hardly a meeting of medical men occurs but the subject of the principle of insurance becomes one of the topics for presentation or debate. The offices of the American Hospital Association receive inquiries almost daily for the information on the development of group hospitalization throughout the United States, and I have been called upon frequently to explain or describe many of the problems of organization.

Examples of the types of organizations before which I have appeared are local, state, and county medical societies, state hospital associations, boards of trustees of individual hospitals, organizations such as the Chicago Conference of Personnel Managers, Kiwanis International, Illinois Parent-Teachers' Association, General Federation of Women's Clubs, and many others.

All of the city-wide group hospitalization plans which were in existence a year ago have continued to expand their membership. . . . In general, the single-hospital plans in cities with more than one hospital have met with stubborn resistance in the enrollment of subscribers, even where there was no criticism of the financial stability of these hospitals or the quality of professional work. In several cities where competing hospital plans are in effect, the number of subscribers has been much smaller than might have been achieved if the institutions had worked together.

During the past year, city-wide plans have been introduced in a number of places, including St. Paul, New Orleans, Washington, D.C., and Durham, N.C. . . . An interesting development of the past year is the formation of the Elkin Mutual Aid Association in Elkin, N.C., a community of approximately 2,500 urban inhabitants and 2,500 farmers. . . . In Kingston, Ontario, a special type of plan reimburses the subscriber for the payment of hospital bills rather than make payment directly to the hospital for this service.

As a result of advice and suggestions from the offices of the American Hospital Association, the Youngstown Sheet and Tube Company has established a group hospitalization plan for its own employees, modeled to a great extent on that of the Goodyear Tire and Rubber Company.

Within the last year announcement has been made of group life insurance plans with the benefits for hospital care, issued by the Prudential Insurance Company and the Equitable Life Assurance Society of New York. The former has completed a contract with the 12,000 employees of the Firestone Tire and Rubber Company and the latter with the General Tire and Rubber Company.

There is a definite trend in all voluntary nonprofit group hospitalization plans toward the inclusion of service to dependents and the liberalization of the policy to cover more types of disease and more types of care. . . .

The question whether group hospitalization is "insurance" has been replaced by the question whether it is good for the public and for the participating institutions. Legislation has been revealed in the Ohio statutes which makes it unnecessary for nonprofit hospital service corporations to be organized under the laws of insurance companies.

During the past year, enabling legislation has been enacted in New York providing for special regulation of nonprofit hospital service corporations. In the public interest, it is necessary that group hospitalization plans receive the type of regulation which will protect the interests of both subscribers and hospitals. The regulations originally established for the control of life insurance companies are not necessarily those most appropriate for the control of nonprofit hospital service corporations.

Group hospitalization in some forms will probably continue to hold the imagination and interest of the public and will ultimately develop under some type of auspices. Whether or not the hospital will retain control of this development and keep it on a private, nonprofit basis will depend upon courage and prompt action. There is, to be sure, some financial risk in inaugurating group hospitalization plans. But this risk is small compared to the costs daily incurred for rendering services to part-pay cases and giving free care to people who would be able to and eligible to participate in group hospitalization plans.

There is need for development in the United States of contributory schemes, based on the English principle, by which the subscription rates are intended only to cover a part of the cost, the balance to be paid through taxation or philanthropy. Such plans, which might be sold at rates from two to four dollars a year, would enable subscribers to pay from half to two-thirds of the cost of services which they are now receiving free, at the expense of philanthropists and taxpayers.

It is significant that in England at the present time (1934) the hospital contributory schemes have enrolled more beneficiaries than are entitled to the services of general practitioners under the National Health Insurance Act.

In the United States, where hospital care has been regarded as a commodity rather than as a charity, the movement toward group hospitalization cannot be regarded as complete until it reaches from 15 to 20 million wage earners. If this is not developed under the auspices of nonprofit corporations, it will ultimately be developed by private insurance companies or by a system of taxation which will rest directly upon the potential beneficiaries.

Some plans have been sponsored directly by the subscribers. The function of the hospital is merely to "take the money." The fund pays the bills, according to the agreement with the subscribers. The hospital renders the service and is paid from the fund. Such a plan, of course, makes possible free choice, because the fund pays bills in any approved hospital, and not merely in those hospitals which sign a contract. . . .

It is the moral obligation of the executives and trustees of nonprofit hospitals to investigate carefully the economic and financial significance of group hospitalization plans from the standpoint of both hospital revenue and ultimate public benefits. If people of limited means are to utilize the voluntary hospital, they must develop some plan by which hospital care can be placed in the family budget. If this is not developed, encouraged, and experimented with by executives or representatives of hospitals, it will be developed by other bodies which may not be sympathetic to the problems of hospitals and may influence hospital policies in such a way as to interfere—for the time being, at least—with the quality of professional service.

APPENDIX K

Excerpts from the Testimony of C. Rufus Rorem before the Senate Committee on Education and Labor, 1946*

We are here to present the facts about the 21,400,000 members of Blue Cross plans for hospital care, a program which has enrolled more participants in less time than any voluntary movement in the history of the world. We are directly concerned with the administration of voluntary health services, and its management and achievements. We are anxious to expand its virtues and remove its defects and thus increase its services to our nation. We believe it should not disappear from the American scene as a noble experiment.

We participated 17 years ago in establishing many of the estimates which have been submitted as evidence that no one can tell either when he will be sick or what his sickness will cost him. It is now generally recognized that the costs of severe illness weigh heavily upon a small number of people, whereas the larger proportion are faced with only small annual expenditures for necessary health services. The burden of sickness costs thus can be most effectively carried by application of the law of averages to the payment of hospital bills. The basic question before your committee is the method and degree of such application at the present time.

What Is Blue Cross?

A Blue Cross plan for hospital services is a nonprofit corporation, a community organization which accepts regular and equal payments from groups of members, the combined funds being used to pay hospital bills for those members requiring care. The hospital protection may be supplemented by a medically sponsored plan for medical and surgical care. The cost for hospital plan membership is approximately seventy-five cents a month per person or two dollars per family. Subscription rates for doctors' services in hospitalized cases are about the same.

The governing body of a Blue Cross plan is a board of directors (which

---

*From Rorem's *A Quest for Certainty: Essays on Health Care Economics, 1930–1970* (Ann Arbor: Health Administration Press, 1982), pp. 99–113. At the time of this testimony, a national health insurance program (S. 160) had been presented to Congress and had been referred to this committee. Rorem spoke as the director of the Blue Cross Commission.

includes leaders from industry, medicine, labor, welfare, hospitals, agriculture, government) who serve without pay, just as do the trustees of a church, social agency, or educational institution. These persons have no financial interest in the success of the Blue Cross plans, yet they devote many hours to professional and administrative policies. Their only reward is participation in a program of community service.

Benefits are available as hospital service rather than cash allowances. The services to subscribers are guaranteed by contracts with more than 3,500 community hospitals throughout the United States. Benefits are usually provided in semi-private accommodations and include the special services necessary for diagnosis and treatment. Benefits are available for each family member, usually for three to four weeks of "full coverage," with extended periods at discounts from regular hospital charges.

Blue Cross plans are supervised through an approval program conducted by the trustees of the American Hospital Association, and in the various states are regulated and supervised by the insurance department or other appropriate body. The American Hospital Association's requirements for approval include nonprofit organization, free choice of hospital and physician, hospital guarantee of service benefits, and representation of subscriber interests in control. The standards also provide for the establishment and maintenance of contingency financial reserves to protect the interests of subscribers and member hospitals.

It is not accidental that protection for hospital bills has expanded so rapidly throughout the nation. The hospitals of America belong to the people, and hospital service is generally recognized as a community responsibility. Hospitals have assumed a moral, and sometimes legal, obligation to accept emergency cases, regardless of their ability to pay. Instances where a patient is refused emergency care are so unusual as to make headlines or be the subject of editorial comment.

Blue Cross Enrollment Growth Rapid

Enrollment in Blue Cross has accelerated during the past few years, and particularly the last few months. Growth during the war years was not entirely due to increased employment and high wages. The three-month period ending March 31, 1946, witnessed the largest total net increase in the history of the movement; nearly 1,400,000 persons joined during that period. This growth occurred in spite of conversion from war to peacetime industry, and in spite of many strikes in certain industries where Blue Cross protection had been especially well accepted.

The percentage of population enrolled under Blue Cross has been highest in the eastern and northern states, where large portions of the population are engaged in industry. Yet, of the twelve states which show a total of more than 20 percent of their population now protected under Blue Cross, four may definitely be said to be rural in character.

Recent Developments in Blue Cross

We now turn to a set of affirmative statements which are presented to explain the progress and prospectives of voluntary health programs. Frankly, we are doing much better than many of us had ever expected. Eight years ago, we were congratulated for having reached 1,000,000 subscribers. Now we are criticized for merely exceeding 21,000,000 participants. Friends and critics alike are emphasizing the unfinished task rather than the work already done.

Most of the American population is now eligible for participation in a nonprofit prepayment plan for hospital care. Nonprofit Blue Cross plans now serve 43 states and the District of Columbia, and it is expected that the number will reach 47 by the end of the year. Residents of small towns are being protected through community enrollment; farm groups are being served through the activities of the farm bureaus, granges, and unions and the establishment of special organized county health improvement associations. Rural producers and consumers co-operatives also have served as enrollment and collection agencies. In many urban areas, enrollment privileges for self-employed persons are being introduced, and Blue Cross is giving increased attention to those groups.

Over half of the 80 U.S. Blue Cross plans offer complete protection for catastrophic illness through co-ordination with plans for medical or surgical protection. This coverage does not meet the full need of the American people, but it removes most of the economic burden of sickness from the shoulders of the individual.

The Blue Cross program has proved adequate for the mobile population of recent years. Blue Cross plans permit convenient transfers of memberships from one Blue Cross plan to another, and they allow continuance of membership when a subscriber leaves his place of original enrollment. Liberal out-of-town benefits are provided. These privileges have been achieved through formal agreements among the various Blue Cross plans.

Blue Cross plans are representative of the entire community: employers, employees, agriculture, hospitals, the medical profession, welfare groups, and others. The social significance of this voluntary sponsorship and guidance cannot be overemphasized. It is consistent with human values derived from permitting individuals to act voluntarily in removing the uncertainty of their sickness costs. The economic and social foundation of a community hospital is as broad as the population itself. And the combined resources and support of a group of hospitals in a community of a state may be said to represent the combined resources and support of the entire public.

Hospital administrators and trustees regard themselves as administrators and trustees of public funds. The primary purpose of both Blue Cross plans and hospitals is to maximize service for the people who have built the hospitals, who use them, and who support them. Critics of Blue Cross plans have sometimes described them as "producer co-operatives," implying that their trustees were concerned only with maintaining the status quo of hospital operations and finance. The analogy is something less than complete. For, although the hospitals sponsor and guarantee the Blue Cross plans which enroll potential patients, the net savings are distributable only to the subscribers as increased benefits or reduced subscription rates.

The proof of the pudding is not in the recipe. Blue Cross plan trustees have typically been able to strike a balance between the interests of subscribers, who provide the money, and the hospitals, which provide the service. They have used the subscribers' funds economically, having regard for the necessity of maintaining professional standards through adequate payments.

Wage agreements between labor unions and management are often written to provide partial or full payment of prepaid health benefits by the employer. Blue Cross has been specially popular in such agreements because of their non-profit service-benefit features and the policy of permitting continuance of membership when employment is interrupted by strike, layoff, or change to another firm. The advantage of protection has been demonstrated by a number of organizations during recent strikes. Some of the larger corporations in the country have permitted employees to authorize advances during a strike or temporary layoff. Conversely, Blue Cross plans have often permitted protection to continue, with the idea that payments would be made upon return to work.

The largest employer in the United States (the federal government) does not yet permit the privilege of voluntary payroll deduction. The Blue Cross Commission office receives letters daily from units of the United States government asking for the privilege of protection. Yet there are only 300,000 federal employees and their dependents participating in voluntary plans because of the difficulties involved in handling organization and payment details through voluntary group leaders who are employees of the federal government. Mutually satisfactory arrangements are not possible without the privileges of payroll deduction. Undoubtedly the existing makeshift enrollment and collection procedures have in many instances proved to be inefficient for the government departments involved as well as for the plan.

Overhead costs have been remarkably low, considering the rapid rate of growth.

The average operating expense for the entire country, for all Blue Cross plans, was approximately 12 percent of the total income during the year 1945. In some of the larger organizations with established memberships, the operating expenses are less than 10 percent of the total subscribers' payments. On the average, about three cents of the subscriber's dollar has been used for consumer education and enrollment activities. About nine cents has been required for accounting and billing procedures and the payment of benefits. The expenses for general administration are being reduced. Plans are now using streamlined methods for maintenance of enrollment records, authorization of hospital admissions, and other administrative economies consistent with good business practice and efficient public service.

Many of the Blue Cross plans have increased their benefits during their period of operation without corresponding increase in subscription rates to the beneficiary. The increased benefits have been made possible through better "selection" among subscribers and [the] decision to apply reserves to provision of immediate benefits. Blue Cross plans are, of course, concerned with providing protection for all costs of hospitalized illness. In some cases, increased costs for labor and supplies in hospitals have necessitated increased rates to the subscribers. Usually, however, this has also been accompanied by increased benefits. But the problem of inflation and its effects upon increased costs of hospital care still face Blue Cross and any program of health service, voluntary or governmental, if the quality of availability of care is to be increased and assured.

Voluntary plans have been accepted by many veterans as a genuine opportunity for family protection. Even though veterans are entitled to care under existing GI legislation, they recognize that at least three-fourths of the care in their families is received by wife and children. Moreover, Blue Cross benefits permit free choice of hospital and doctor, which are not available at the present time for nonservice-connected disabilities. Blue Cross plans have exempted returning veterans from the group requirements imposed upon members of the general public, and thousands are being added daily to the Blue Cross rolls.

Suggested Readings

Abdellah, Faye G., and Levine, Eugene. *Better Patient Care Through Nursing Research*. New York: Macmillan, 1965.

Abernethy, David S., and Pearson, David A. *Regulating Hospital Costs: The Development of Public Policy*. Washington, D.C.: AUPHA Press, 1979.

Aday, Lu Ann, and Andersen, Ronald. *Access to Medical Care*. Ann Arbor: Health Administration Press, 1975.

Altmeyer, Arthur J. *The Formative Years of Social Security*. Madison: The University of Wisconsin Press, 1968.

Ambrose, Stephen E. *Eisenhower, the President*. New York: Simon & Schuster, 1984.

Anderson, Odin W. *Blue Cross Since 1929*. Cambridge, Mass.: Ballinger, 1975.

_____. *The American Health Services: A Growth Enterprise Since 1875*. Ann Arbor: Health Administration Press, 1985.

Anderson, Odin W., and May, J. Joel. *The Federal Employees' Health Benefits Program, 1961–1968: A Model for National Health Insurance?* Chicago: Center for Health Administration Studies, Graduate School of Business, University of Chicago, 1971.

Austin, Charles J. *The Politics of National Health Insurance*. San Antonio: Trinity University Press, 1975.

Ball, Robert M. *Social Security Today and Tomorrow*. New York: Columbia University Press, 1978.

Bellin, Lowell Eliezer, and Weeks, Lewis E., eds. *The Challenge of Administering Health Services: Career Pathways*. Washington, D.C.: AUPHA Press, 1981.

Blue Cross Association–American Hospital Association. *Financing Health Care of the Aged*. 2 vols. Chicago: The Associations, 1962.

Campion, Frank D. *The AMA and U.S. Health Policy Since 1940*. Chicago: Chicago Review Press, 1984.

Cohen, Wilbur J., Gill, David G.; Schorr, Alvin I.; Merriam, Ida C.; Wolkstein, Irwin; Haber,

William. *Social Security: The First Thirty-Five Years*. Ann Arbor: Institute of Gerontology, University of Michigan–Wayne State University, 1970.

Commission on Education for Health Administration. *Education for Health Administration*. 3 vols. Vol. 3, *A Future Agenda*. Ann Arbor: Health Administration Press, 1975, 1977.

Commission on Financing of Hospital Care. *Financing Hospital Care in the United States*. 3 vols. New York: Blakiston, 1954–1955.

Commission on Professional and Hospital Activities. *The International Classification of Diseases, 9th Revision, Clinical Modification*. 3 vols. Ann Arbor: The Commission, 1978.

Corning, Peter A. *The Evolution of Medicare*. Washington, D.C.: Office of Research and Statistics, Social Security Administration, 1969.

Creel, George. *Rebel at Large*. New York: Putnam's, 1947.

Davis, Michael M. *Medical Care for Tomorrow*. New York: Harper, 1955.

Donabedian, Avedis. *Aspects of Medical Care Administration*. Cambridge, Mass: Harvard University Press, 1973.

Donabedian, Avedis; Axelrod, Solomon J.; and Wyszewianski, Leon. *Medical Care Chartbook*. 7th ed. Washington, D.C.: AUPHA Press, 1980.

Donovan, Robert J. *Eisenhower, The Inside Story*. New York: Harper, 1956.

———. *Conflict and Crisis: The Presidency of Harry S. Truman*. New York: Norton, 1977.

Douglas, Paul. *In the Fullness of Time*. New York: Harcourt Brace Jovanovich, 1972.

Falk, Isidore S.; Rorem, C. Rufus; Ring, Martha D. *The Costs of Medical Care: A Summary of Investigations on the Economic Aspects of the Prevention and Care of Illness*. Chicago: University of Chicago Press, 1933.

Feder, Judith; Holahan, John; and Marmor, Theodore. *National Health Insurance: Conflicting Goals and Policy Choices*. Washington, D.C.: Urban Institute, 1980.

Ferrell, Robert H. ed. *Harry S. Truman*. New York: Harper & Row, 1980.

Filerman, Gary L., with Shattuck, Frances. *The Senate Rejects Health Insurance for the Aged*. Ann Arbor: University Microfilms, 1967.

Fine, Sidney. *Frank Murphy: The New Deal Years*. Chicago: University of Chicago Press, 1979.

Flexner, Abraham. *Medical Education in the United States and Canada: A Report to the Carnegie Foundation for the Advancement of Teaching*. New York: Carnegie Foundation, 1910.

Flexner, James Thomas. *An American Saga: The Story of Helen Thomas and Simon Flexner*. Boston: Little, Brown, 1984.

Flook, E. Evelyn, and Sanazaro, Paul J., eds. *Health Services Research and R&D*. Ann Arbor: Health Administration Press, 1973.

Furnas, J.C. *Great Times*. New York: Putman's, 1974.

Ginzberg, Eli. *The Limits of Health Reform*. New York: Basic Books, 1977.

Goldman, Eric F. *The Tragedy of Lyndon Johnson*. New York: Knopf, 1969.

Griffith, John R. *Quantitative Techniques for Hospital Planning and Control*. Lexington, Mass.: Heath, 1972.

Griffith, John R.; Hancock, Walton M.; and Munson, Fred C., eds. *Cost Control in Hospitals*. Ann Arbor: Health Administration Press, 1976.

Harris, Richard. *A Sacred Trust*. New York: New American Library, 1966.

Huthmacher, J. Joseph. *Senator Robert F. Wagner and the Rise of Urban Liberalism*. New York: Atheneum, 1968.

Katcher, Leo. *Earl Warren: A Political Biography*. New York: McGraw-Hill, 1967.

Kipnis, Ira A. *A Venture Forward: A History of the American College of Hospital Administrators.* Chicago: The College, 1955.

Kovner, Anthony R. *Really Trying: A Career Guide for the Health Services Manager.* Washington, D.C.: AUPHA Press, 1984.

Lave, Judith R., and Lave, Lester B. *The Hospital Construction Act: An Evaluation of the Hill-Burton Program, 1948–1973.* Washington, D.C.: American Enterprise Institute for Public Policy Research, 1974.

MacColl, William A. *Group Practice and Prepayment of Medical Care.* Washington, D.C.: Public Affairs Press, 1966.

McNerney, Walter J.; Barlow, Robin; Diokno, Antonio; Fitzpatrick, Thomas B.; Foyle, William R.; Gottlieb, Symond R.; Griffith, John R.; Morgan, James N.; Payne, Beverly C.; Riedel, Donald C.; Skinner, Charles G.; Spaulding, P. Whitney; Wirick, Grover C., Jr. *Hospital and Medical Economics.* 2 vols. Chicago: Hospital Research and Educational Trust, 1962.

McNerney, Walter J., and Riedel, Donald C. *Regionalization and Rural Health Care.* Ann Arbor: Bureau of Hospital Administration, The University of Michigan, 1962.

Manney, James D., Jr. *Aging in American Society.* Ann Arbor: Institute of Gerontology, The University of Michigan–Wayne State University, 1975.

Martin, George. *Madame Secretary, Frances Perkins.* Boston: Houghton Mifflin, 1976.

Miller, Nathan. *FDR: An Intimate History.* Garden City, N.Y.: Doubleday, 1983.

Neely, James R. *Hospital Associations in Change.* Chicago: American Hospital Association, 1981.

Neuhauser, Duncan. *Coming of Age: A 50-Year History of the American College of Hospital Administrators and the Profession It Serves.* Chicago: Pluribus Press, 1983.

Numbers, Ronald L. *Prophetess of Health: A Study of Ellen G. White.* New York: Harper & Row, 1976.

Patterson, James T. *Mr. Republican: A Biography of Robert A. Taft.* Boston: Houghton Mifflin, 1972.

Perkins, Frances. *The Roosevelt I Knew.* New York: Viking Press, 1946.

The President's Commission of the Health Needs of the Nation. *Building America's Health.* 5 vols. Washington, D.C.: Government Printing Office, 1952.

Pringle, Henry F. *Theodore Roosevelt.* New York: Harcourt, Brace, 1956.

Rorem, C. Rufus. *Private Group Clinics.* Chicago: University of Chicago Press, 1931.

————. *A Quest for Certainty: Essays on Health Care Economics, 1930–1970.* Ann Arbor: Health Administration Press, 1982.

Rucker, T. Donald, ed. *Pharmacy: Career Planning and Professional Opportunities.* Washington, D.C.: AUPHA Press, 1981.

Russell, Louise B. *Technology in Hospitals: Medical Advances and Their Diffusion.* Washington, D.C.: Brookings Institution, 1979.

Schlesinger, Arthur M., Jr. *A Thousand Days: John F. Kennedy in the White House.* Boston: Houghton Mifflin, 1965.

Schwarz, Richard W. *John Harvey Kellogg, M.D.* Nashville: Southern Publishing Association, 1970.

Somers, Herman Miles, and Somers, Anne Ramsey. *Doctors, Patients, and Health Insurance.* Garden City, N.Y.: Doubleday, 1962.

————. *Medicare and the Hospitals: Issues and Prospects.* Washington, D.C.: Brookings Institution, 1967.

Sorensen, Theodore C. *Kennedy.* New York: Harper & Row, 1965.

Southwick, Arthur. *The Law of Hospital and Health Care Administration*. Ann Arbor: Health Administration Press, 1978.

Starr, Paul. *The Social Transformation of American Medicine*. New York: Basic Books, 1982.

Stevens, Robert, and Stevens, Rosemary. *Welfare Medicine in America: A Case Study of Medicaid*. New York: Free Press, 1974.

U.S. Congress. House Committee on Ways and Means. Subcommittee on Health. *Proceedings of the Conference on the Future of Medicare*. 98th Cong., 2d sess., 1984.

Weeks, Lewis E., and Berman, Howard J. *Economics in Health Care*. Germantown, Md.: Aspen Systems, 1977.

Williams, Greer. *Kaiser-Permanente: Why It Works*. Oakand, Calif.: Henry J. Kaiser Foundation, 1971.

Witte, Edwin E. *The Development of the Social Security Act*. Madison: The University of Wisconsin Press, 1963.

Zuckerman, Howard, and Weeks, Lewis E. *Multi-Institutional Hospital Systems*. Chicago: Hospital Research and Educational Trust, 1974.

Index

About the Authors

The authors have been collaborators for 15 years, beginning when both were at the Program and Bureau of Hospital Administration of the University of Michigan. Their joint publications include *The Financial Management of Hospitals* (five editions have been published, and a sixth is in preparation); *The Economics of Health Care* (coeditors); and *Financing Health Care* (coeditors with Gerald E. Bisbee, Jr.).

LEWIS E. WEEKS was editor of *Inquiry* from 1976 to 1984 and is now conducting oral history interviews of leaders in the health care field for the Lewis E. Weeks Series of the Hospital Administration Oral History Collection housed in the Library of the American Hospital Association, Asa S. Bacon Memorial, in Chicago. Weeks received his master's degree in history from the University of Michigan and his doctorate in communication arts from Michigan State University.

HOWARD J. BERMAN became president of Blue Cross and Blue Shield of Rochester, New York, on July 1, 1985. Before that he was Group Vice President of the American Hospital Association and President of the Hospital Research and Education Trust. He is on the advisory board of the Cooperative Information Center for Health Care Studies at the University of Michigan and is a member of the editorial boards of *Inquiry* and *Topics in Health Care Financing*. He is also executive editor of *Health Services Research*. He is a graduate of the University of Illinois in finance and holds a master's degree in hospital administration from the University of Michigan.